AF478555

Modeling
of
Cancer Genesis
and
Prevention

Authors

Nicolae Voiculetz
Head, Chemical Carcinogenesis and
Molecular Genetics Department
Institute of Oncology
Bucharest, Romania

Alexandru T. Balaban
Polytechnical Institute — TCH
Department of Organic Chemistry
Bucharest, Romania

Ion Niculescu-Duvăz
Institute of Oncology
Chemical Carcinogenesis and Molecular Genetics Department
Bucharest, Romania

Zeno Simon
Biophysics Department
University of Medical Sciences
Timişoara, Romania

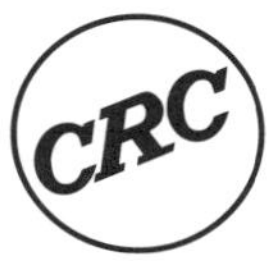

CRC Press
Boca Raton   Ann Arbor   Boston

Library of Congress Cataloging-in-Publication Data

Modeling of cancer genesis and prevention/authors, Nicolae Voiculetz
   ...[et al.].
       p. cm.
     Includes bibliographical references.
     Includes index.
     ISBN 0-8493-6379-9
     1. Carcinogenesis—Computer simulation. 2. Cancer—Prevention-
-Computer simulation. 3. Carcinogens—Structure-activity
relationships. I. Voiculetz, Nicolae.
     [DNLM: 1. Antineoplastic Agents—analysis. 2. Carcinogens-
-analysis. 3. Models, Chemical. 4. Neoplasms—chemically induced.
5. Neoplasms—prevention & control.   QD 480 M689]
RC268.5.M58   1990
616.99'4071'0113—dc20
DNLM/DLC
for Library of Congress   90-2505
                                                                          CIP

PREFACE

The cancer phenomenon was well documented to be multifactorial in its etiology and multistep in its development. The main environmental factors inducing cancer are chemicals. If they could be identified and eliminated, a major fraction of human cancers would be avoided. Therefore, the first problem is to detect the chemicals with carcinogenic properties. The second is to remove them from the environment. Because their removal in a rapidly developing technological society is a difficult, if not impossible, task, other strategies must be adopted.

In contemporary oncology a large amount of studies are devoted to carcinogenesis, mechanisms of action of carcinogenic substances and more recently to pharmacological agents exhibiting cancer prevention properties. The elaboration of predictive screening for both cancer-inducing and cancer-preventing compounds is a goal of obvious importance for cancer prevention. A useful predictive capacity is the privilege of quantitative models. However, the complexity of the carcinogenesis and anticarcinogenesis mechanisms raises many difficulties in the accomplishment of this task.

Nevertheless, the growing capabilities of the computers furnished a powerful impetus to the development of modeling methodology. The quantitative modeling of kinetic processes, of structure-activity relationships (QSAR), the introduction of new topological and geometric indices expressing the molecular shape and size, the use of molecular graphics and molecular mechanics, as well as a more sophisticated mathematical apparatus, obviously contribute to enhance the predictive capabilities of such models.

ACKNOWLEDGMENTS

The authors are grateful to their collaborators Floria Lupu, Mariana Arnăutu, Monica Hoffman, Adriana Colovai, Adriana Stoica, Gerald Stoica and Ioana Marinescu for assistance in the preparation of this book.

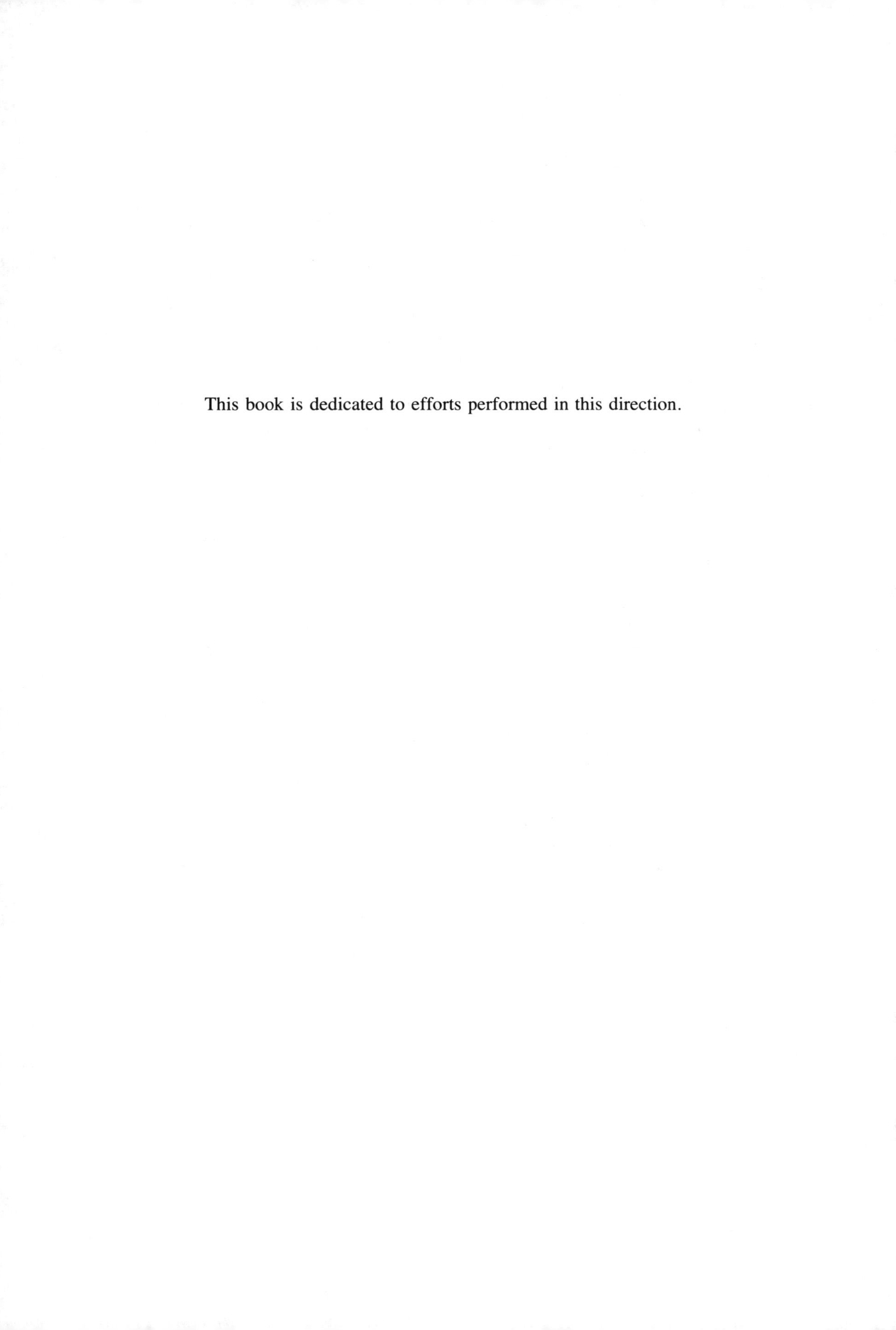

This book is dedicated to efforts performed in this direction.

THE AUTHORS

Nicolae Voiculetz, Ph.D., D.Sc., born in 1929, is the head of the Chemical Carcinogenesis and Molecular Genetics Department and Scientific Director of the Institute of Oncology, Bucharest, Romania. He was IAEA fellow in Belgium (1965) and an Eleanor Roosevelt fellow at Stanford University Medical School, California (1970 to 1971). His current research efforts are focused on the study of carcinogenesis and anticarcinogenesis processes. Dr. Voiculetz is the author of 4 books, 13 chapters in monographs, and more than 150 papers. He is a member of the Council of Romanian Oncology Society, European Association for Cancer Research and member of other scientific societies. Dr. Voiculetz's biographical data is available in the International Book of Honor, Who's Who in Atoms, Who's Who in the World and Men of Achievement.

Ion Niculescu-Duvăz, Ph.D., is senior research scientist at the Chemical Carcinogenesis and Molecular Genetics Department in the Institute of Oncology, Bucharest, Romania. He was AIEA fellow at Istituto per lo Studio dei Tumori — Milan, Italy. He is author of more than 100 papers, a book, 6 chapters in monographs and more than 25 patents.

Born in 1937, he has been interested in anticancer drugs (design and synthesis), chemical carcinogenesis inhibitors and QSAR approaches.

He was appointed as expert of IAEA/UNDP Agency (1971), and was invited to give lectures at NCI Institute, Chester Beatty Research Institute, Jules Bordet Institute, Mario Negri Institute, etc.

He is assistant treasurer of EACR for Romania and member of other scientific societies.

Alexandru T. Balaban, Ph.D., was born in 1931, graduated in Bucharest as dipl.-chemical engineer, attended a post-graduate training in radiochemistry, and obtained a Ph.D. in organic chemistry in 1959 in Bucharest. He has taught organic chemistry and related topics since 1953 at the Bucharest Polytechnic.

Between 1956 and 1974 he was head of the Laboratory of Isotopically Labeled Compounds at the Institute of Atomic Physics in Bucharest; between 1966 and 1970, he served as senior research officer at the International Atomic Energy Agency in Vienna.

He became corresponding member of the Roumanian Academy in 1963, and in 1990 he was elected as academician. He is a fellow of the New York Academy of Sciences and of the World Academy of Theoretical Organic Chemists.

He is a member of editorial boards of 11 international journals, has published 8 books and edited 4; he has published over 30 book chapters and 400 papers. Research interests are heterocyclic chemistry, chemical applications of mathematics and particularly graph theory, stable free radicals and aromaticity.

His biographical data may be found in Who's Who in Science in Europe and Men of Achievement.

Zeno Simon, Professor of Biophysics, School of Medicine, Timişoara. He graduated from the University of Bucharest in 1957 with a Ph.D. in Chemistry. He is author of more than 100 scientific papers. He is interested in quantum biochemistry and the application of topology and topological computational procedures to molecular biology, in trigger theory and in QSAR. He is the author of three books; the last one was published by Wiley and is about the MTD (Minimal Topological Differences) method.

CONTRIBUTORS

Alexandru T. Balaban, Ph.D.
Professor
Polytechnical Institute — TCH
Department of Organic Chemistry
Bucharest, Romania

Dan A. Ciubotariu
Associate Professor
Polytechnical Institute
Department of Organic Chemistry
Timişoara, Romania

Ion Niculescu-Duvăz, Ph.D.
Senior Research Scientist
Chemical Carcinogenesis and
Molecular Genetics Department
Institute of Oncology
Bucharest, Romania

Zeno Simon
Professor
Department of Biophysics
University of Medical Sciences
Timişoara, Romania

Nicolae Voiculetz, Ph.D.
Head, Chemical Carcinogenesis and
Molecular Genetics Department
Institute of Oncology
Bucharest, Romania

TABLE OF CONTENTS

Chapter 1

GENERAL MECHANISMS OF CARCINOGENESIS AND ANTICARCINOGENESIS

Nicolae Voiculetz

TABLE OF CONTENTS

I. INTRODUCTION

We decided to write this monograph keeping in mind the idea to select and clear up primarily the quantitative aspects regarding both carcinogenesis and cancer prevention (anticarcinogenesis). The chosen topics are less familiar to the molecular biologist and cancerologist, and also to many other specialists involved in this area, because some specific knowledge of organic chemistry, physical organic chemistry, quantum chemistry and even mathematics is needed. For these reasons, we tried to comprehensively discuss those models which allow a quantitative prediction of both carcinogenic and anticarcinogenic properties of chemicals, insisting sometimes on the experimental methodology used to obtain satisfactory data.

Cancer may be considered as an alteration of the control mechanisms involved in cell division and differentiation. This leads to a permanent and anarchic multiplication of transformed cells according to a kinetic law which is quantitatively different from that of the normal cells from which they originate. This hereditary transmittable modification (from the neoplastic cell to its daughter cells) represents the final stage of a series of biochemical, genetical, morphological and biological events, originating in an event at the molecular level, whose nature is not yet fully elucidated.

The carcinogenesis process actually consists of a series of discontinuous steps, triggered by a rare molecular event, and separated by selection periods, the sequence of many irreversible (or reversible) alterations leading to the preneoplastic, neoplastic, premalignant and finally malignant cells.[1] This complex development has a conspicuously stochastic aspect, and may be characterized by three major features: (1) the sequentiality of modifications which involves the successive replacement of a type of molecular or cellular lesion by another; (2) the apparition of characteristic cellular subpopulations for every step of the carcinogenesis process and (3) the stochastic character, specific to the selection process, which also depends on the frequency of the first events.

The fundamental problem of carcinogenesis lies in the elucidation of the malignant transformation and the mechanisms which underlie this process. Important progress was made during the last years in the knowledge of these mechanisms, and a powerful argument supporting this assumption is that now a satisfactory prediction of the carcinogenic potency of many chemicals may be achieved on the basis of their chemical structure.

Anticarcinogenesis was created in experimental oncology, and is conceptually based on the possibility of modeling the carcinogenesis — by means of chemicals or biological agents with inhibitory properties — aiming finally at the prevention of malignant transformation.

Because of their close connection, we shall briefly present the basic knowledge and strategy of both carcinogenesis and anticarcinogenesis, in order to subsequently discuss the pharmacological agents employed in the chemoprevention (anti-initiators and antipromoters) of several types of cancer as well as the Quantitative Structure — Activity Relationship (QSAR) methods for the selection and design of more efficient agents.

II. CARCINOGENESIS

The carcinogenesis process is triggered by a number of rare molecular and cellular events, caused by several chemical, physical or biological agents. These events are separated by multiple periods of selection. Thus, carcinogenesis is considered to be a multifactorial process in its etiology and a multistep process in its evolution.

At least three steps can be theoretically distinguished:[2] (1) carcinogenic initiation; (2) promotion steps, which underlie the triggering of cellular transformation and apparition of the first neoplastic cells and (3) the progression step, involving the survival and proliferation of this cancer cell and involving the entire process of maintenance and evolution of malignancy (Scheme 1). In the present report, we shall not deal with this last step.

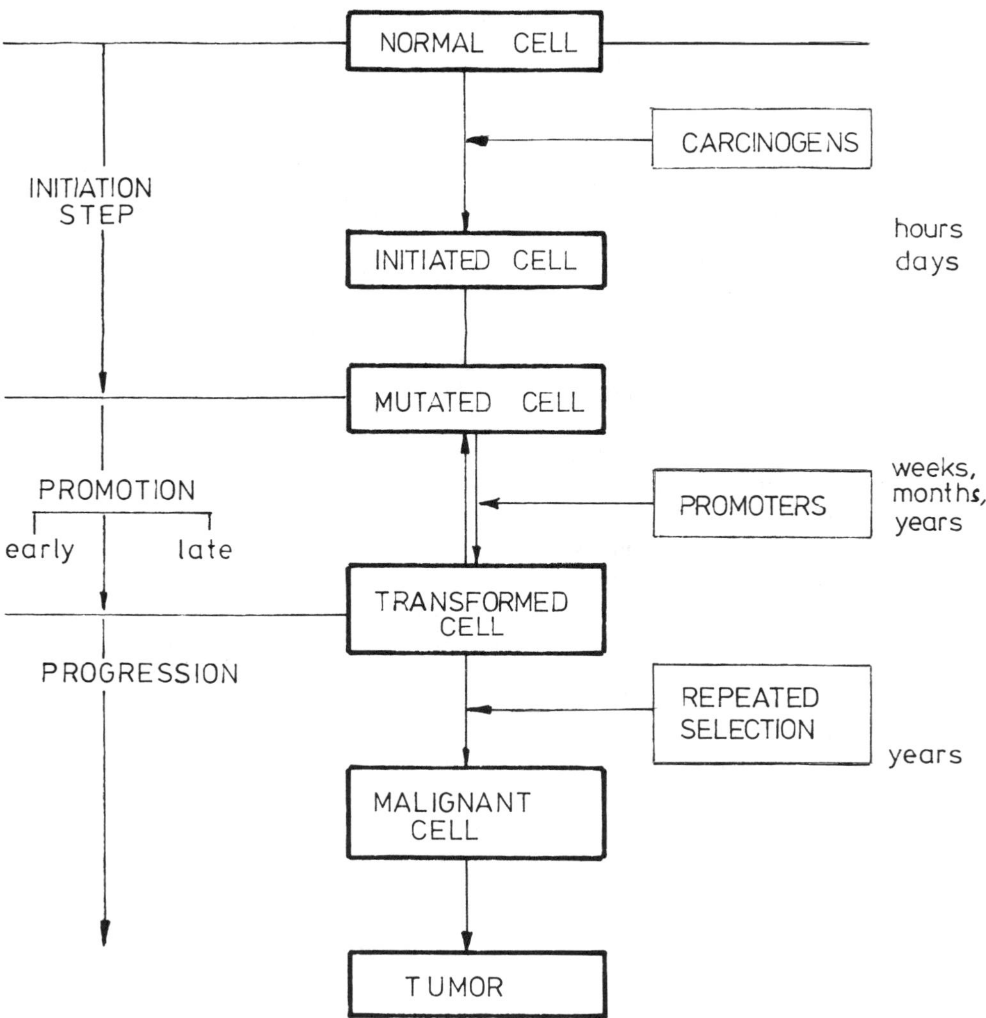

SCHEME 1. Schematic representation of carcinogenesis process.

A. THE INITIATION STEP

Initiation was studied *in vivo* in a large number of tissues and organs (mouse skin,[3] urinary bladder,[4] colon,[5] pancreas,[6] mammary gland[7] and respiratory tract[8]), as well as *in vitro*. Biologically, in a cell, it is associated with the induction of a structural modification which might become a permanent character after a round of cell replication.[9] Biochemically, initiation consists in the direct or indirect damage of cellular DNA by a carcinogenic agent, which causes a permanent and transmittable alteration at the level of this informational macromolecule. Initiation occurs rapidly (minutes or hours), and consists of the damaging of genetic information by chemical modification of DNA. This alteration may occur directly (i.e., chemical and physical carcinogens interacting with DNA) or indirectly (i.e., physical carcinogens, hormones, peroxisomes proliferators, etc.). Also, biological agents may directly or indirectly affect the informational machinery located at DNA level. However, without promotion, the initiated cell can remain in this state indefinitely, without producing adverse effects and without being recognized by the immunological system of the organism because it does not manifest itself phenotypically. Mention should also be made so that some of the carcinogenic alterations of DNA can be repaired during this delay. However, not every chemical modification at the DNA level is a carcinogenic lesion triggering the transformation process, but only a small fraction of specific modifications leads to carcinogenesis. For instance, promutagenic lesions, able to induce mutations by miscoding are carcinogenic. Insertion of an active viral promoter before a proto-oncogene is another such process. It is not our intention to develop this aspect. After initiating the first molecular event, which triggers the malignant transformation, the carcinogenic agent may disappear.

The number of cells initially damaged by the carcinogenic agent is enormous with respect to the number of morphological lesions which are identified in the subsequent phases. The number of transformed cells considerably decreases (in time) until one or several cells reach the final stage of malignant cells.

Concerning the initiation, the DNA damage has been axiomatically claimed as the key-step of carcinogenesis. The most suggestive picture of the carcinogenesis process is furnished by the large amount of studies on benzo(a)pyrene, an ubiquitous carcinogen.[10,11] This compound is inactive per se, but its activation (by the cytochrome P-450 dependent monooxygenasic system and other peroxidases) leads to highly reactive metabolites (ultimate carcinogens) that covalently bind to DNA.[12,13] During this complex process multiple modifications are produced in DNA structure and/or function. They are reflected by important changes in the expression of a number of genes,[14,15] some of them yet unknown, which contribute to the cellular growth and division.[16] The initiation step is explicitly linked to the carcinogenic potency of chemicals. This aspect was developed in Chapter 3, where the quantitative models allowing a satisfactory prediction of this biological property were discussed. One of the most interesting ways to design quantitative models with predictive capabilities is obviously the QSAR analysis. The methodology of this approach will be discussed in Chapter 5 and many examples were given for the chemical carcinogenesis area. Finally, a special emphasis was placed on the role of topological indices to increase the accuracy of such predictive models, this topic is developed in Chapter 4.

B. TYPES OF GENES INVOLVED IN INITIATION

It is nowadays unanimously accepted that the molecular substrate of malignancy lies in the genome of every normal human or animal cell.[17] During the last years, the discovery of proto-oncogenes gave a powerful impetus to carcinogenesis research. When oncogenes isolated from human or animal tumor DNA (induced chemically or by irradiation) are transfected to NIH 3T3 cells, the latter acquire several features of malignant cells. It was clearly demonstrated that oncogenes are the modified versions of normal genes called *proto-oncogenes*.[17-19]

According to experimental data, cellular proto-oncogenes represent direct targets for chemical and physical carcinogenic agents and also for some viruses.[20] The modifications thus produced can underlie the mechanisms of initiation of the carcinogenesis process (Table 1).

Several mechanisms are known to activate proto-oncogenes, namely:

1.   Point mutations at specific codons which result in the transcription of a structurally and probably functionally altered protein (protein kinases); among the proto-oncogenes activated by a single mutation are the genes of the *ras* family[21] from which codon 12, 13 and 61 modifications trigger cellular transformation (Table 2).

    The same point mutations were found in the transduced viral genes radiations, as well as in cell lines derived from various human tumors (Table 3). The hypothesis that proto-oncogenes underlie the initiation mechanism is supported by the mutagenic ability of most carcinogenic agents;[22] DNA-sequence specificity was demonstrated for some of them. Another argument is the presence of *H-ras* oncogenes in most papillomas appeared in skin tissue subsequent to classical induction with 7,12-dimethyl-benz(a)anthracene (DMBA) (followed by promotion). The involvement of the *ras*

TABLE 1
Oncogenes Identified in Chemically Induced Tumors in Rats

Chemical agent	Induced tumor	Oncogene	Oncogene containing tumors (%)
NMU	Mammary gland carcinoma	H-*ras*-1	86
DMBA	Mammary gland carcinoma	H-*ras*-1	23
DMN	Renal carcinoma	K-*ras*-2	40
ENU	Neuroblastoma	neu	100
NMU	Schwannoma	neu	70
MMS	Nasal carcinoma	—	100

TABLE 2
Point Mutations Leading to *ras* Oncogenes Activation in Cell Lines Derived from Human Tumors

Oncogene and cell line	Tumor of origin	Altered codon	Modified base	Modified amino acid
H-*ras* T-24	Bladder carcinoma	12	G → T	GLY → VAL
K-*ras* Hs-242	Lung carcinoma	61	A → T	GLY → LEU
K-*ras* CALU-1	Lung carcinoma	12	G → T	GLY → CYS
H-*ras* SW-80	Colon carcinoma	12	G → T	GLY → VAL
N-*ras* SK-N-SH	Neuroblastoma	61	C → A	GLU → LYS
K-*ras* SW-1271	Lung carcinoma	61	A → G	GLU → ARG

TABLE 3
Oncogenes Identified in Chemically or Radiation Induced Tumors in Mice

Inducing agent	Induced tumor	Oncogene	Oncogene containing tumors (%)
DMBA	Skin carcinoma	H-*ras*-1	90
X-rays	Lymphoma	K-*ras*-2	57
NMU	Lymphoma	N-*ras*-1	85
3-MC	Fibrosarcoma	K-*ras*-2	50
Hepatic carcinogens	Hepatoma	H-*ras*-1	100

oncogene in initiation does not preclude its activation in other stages of tumor development, as well as by other mechanisms. Actually, in some experimental systems, cellular transformation appears much more reduced as compared to the cell number having undergone point mutations.[23]

2. Activation by overproduction; this mechanism consists of the derepression of the systems controlling the activity of proto-oncogenes, thus leading to a structurally unmodified but exacerbated expression of the protein. Deregulation could result from the following processes: (1) chromosomal translocation; (2) genic amplification; (3) insertion of a viral promoter; (4) intragenomic transposition of DNA sequences and (5) other intragenomic rearrangements,[14,16] possibly also by defects in transcriptional regulation. In some tumors, the *ras* oncogene appears amplified, thus demonstrating the lack of specificity of the activation mechanisms for this proto-oncogene. Activation by chromosomal translocation or by retroviral insertion was noticed as an early event in the development of numerous animal and human tumors. It involves, however, another type of proto-oncogenes (*myc, myb, abl,* etc.), as well as other types of genes.[21,24]

Approximately 100 proto-oncogenes have been discovered up until now, and no more than 300 are expected to exist. Surprisingly, they were found in only 15 to 20% of all human tumors. This might be due either to the insufficient sensitivity of the detection methods or, much more probably, to the involvement in carcinogenesis of other genes or DNA segments operating on entirely different principles.

The control system of the normal cell growth must be altered in at least 2 to 3 points before the anarchic cell division may occur.[25] Therefore, safety mechanisms intrinsic to this system were assumed to exist and also mechanisms able to annihilate the activity of individual oncogenes.

During the last years, these safety mechanisms were identified with the growth suppression genes (antioncogenes) blocking the signal for cell division.[26] The existence of genes limiting cell growth has been presumed for a long time, since it had been noticed that cells somehow "feel" the situation when they should stop multiplying.[27] Typical in this respect is the contact inhibition. This contact produces, probably by second messengers, a signal which reaches the nucleus and activates several genes which, in turn, stop the cell growth and division. Thus, the presence of such genes is required in the cell in order to counteract the activity of proto-oncogenes (or oncogenes).

A first clue of this behavior resulted from the investigations undertaken on retinoblastoma. It was shown that either the loss of both *Rb* alleles on chromosome 13, or the alteration of their function leads to malignancy.[28]

A gene such as *Rb,* when it is intact, counteracts an oncogene. It was recently demonstrated that the deletion of the *apc* gene located on the long arm of chromosome 5 is responsible for the Gardner syndrome and for at least a part of the sporadic colon cancers. This gene is actually also an antioncogene.[29,30]

C. THE PROMOTION STEP

Promotion may be defined as the sequence of events following the repeated action of a promoter on an initiated cell, resulting in the transformation of the latter into preneoplastic or neoplastic cells and histologically detected as benign tumors.

This phenomenon requires a longer period (weeks, months, even years) and may be followed over two stages: (1) early promotion — in which alterations of gene expression appear, leading to an accelerated proliferating activity which is transmittable to offspring cells and (2) late promotion — in which a clonal expansion of cells (i.e., papilloma) is achieved.[31]

Promotion consists in events interfering with the genetic program of proliferation and especially differentiation.[32] The promoted cell does not recognize the differentiation signals removing it from the replicative population. The balance between the expression of programs for growth and differentiation is under stringent control in normal cells, whereas in promoted cells imperfections emerge, resulting possibly in: deficient control of cellular growth and differentiation; autocrine production of growth factors and lowered sensitivity of growth inhibitors and increased sensitivity to growth factors secreted by other cells.

These phenomena and possibly others could lead to a selection advantage in the clonal expansion for the preneoplastic and neoplastic cells.

The best studied promoter is 12-*O*-tetradecanoyl-phorbol-13-acetate (TPA). In the first stage it inhibits proliferation and differentiation; afterwards, it induces a pleiotropic proliferative answer at epidermal level, stimulating cell growth.[33] In contrast with initiators, promoters do not bind DNA, their main target being the cell membrane. Their behavior is consistent with epigenetic mechanisms of action. For instance, the effect of TPA is mediated by protein kinase C, considered as the potential receptor of this promoter. Following this interaction, protein kinase C is activated and induces, by a cascade of second messengers, a number of phenotypic effects which may be divided in three categories: (1) mimicking the transforming phenotypes; (2) inhibition or induction (modulation) of differentiation and (3) membrane effects regarding the control of transport, cell-cell communication, etc.[34]

In the second messenger system, protein kinase C activates by phosphorylation other protein kinases; these in turn phosphorylate cytoplasmatic and nuclear proteins which are involved in cell proliferation and differentiation. Thus, the type of phosphorylation of several proteins involved in transduction signals to the nucleus is altered. This results in the modulation of specific gene expression, for instance of genes involved in the synthesis of ornithine and histidine decarboxylase, as well as in the synthesis of plasminogen activator, prostaglandins, and, possibly, γ-interferon, calcitonin, prolactin and glycoforine. Several proto-oncogenes (c-*fos*, c-*myc*, c-*myb*) transcribing nuclear proteins involved in cell proliferation also represent potential targets for protein kinase C. Similarly to lymphocyte activation, protein kinase C could induce the expression of other genes involved in growth factor activation, thus promoting a long-term cell proliferation.[35]

Recent data demonstrated the existence of gene determining, or contributing to events specific to tumor promotion. In neoplastic mouse epidermal cell lines (JB6) two genes were identified, separated, cloned and sequenced. They were named *pro 1* and *pro 2*, due to their ability to confer tumor promotion responsiveness (tumors are induced in the absence of exposure to carcinogenic agents, but only after TPA application) by transfection of these genes in P⁻ cells (lacking *pro 1* and *pro 2* genes); malignant transformation also occurs in these cells subsequent to TPA treatment.[36] Thus, sensitive (JB6P⁺) or resistant (JB6P⁻) cells are known according to the presence or absence of the *pro* genes.

These genes were also found in the genome of human and murine cells being preserved (similar to proto-oncogenes) during evolution. Moreover, the presence of both genes was also observed in a DNA isolated from cell lines derived from a human nasopharyngeal carcinoma. Transfection of the DNA-P⁻ mouse cells conferred their susceptibility to promotion, suggesting the involvement of *pro* genes in human carcinogenesis.[37]

Despite the fact that no structural homology was found between *pro* genes and other oncogenes, their involvement in cell transformation raises the question whether these genes are a new class of oncogenes.

Under these conditions, the level of the necessary sequence (initiation-promotion) in carcinogenesis (promotion being exerted only on initiated cells) must be reformulated. The data reported above demonstrate that a gene for promotion susceptibility may be transmitted by heredity. This is supported also by the fact that the promoter may remain effective, even when administered 6 weeks before initiation.[38]

A final argument supporting the mechanism of *noncompulsory sequences* is the involvement of the herpes virus as initiator, and of papilloma viruses as promoters of cervical cancer. Frequently, papilloma genes are expressed before transcription of herpes virus genes,[39] suggesting that a constitutive promotion stage could be achieved independently of initiation, and the sequence of events would be noncompulsory.

An analysis of the above data leads to the following conclusions:

1. At least two classes of genes (proto-oncogenes and antioncogenes) represent critical targets for carcinogenic agents; although the mechanisms by which gene alterations lead to malignancy could be different, both these sets of genes certainly contribute to the appearance of neoplastic phenomena. Oncogenes are dominant and induce malignant transformation by their presence, whereas antioncogenes lead to the same effect either by their absence, or by recessive mutated variants.
2. The large variety of structural or regulatory alterations leading to proto-oncogene activation suggests a direct correlation between the activated gene and the cellular phenotype, regardless of the activation mechanism (mutation, translocation, retroviral insertion or amplification).

3. Repeated involvement of the same proto-oncogenes in the development of numerous types of tumors emphasizes the biological unity of cancer. A good example is the *v-myc* gene which is able to transform a large variety of cellular targets. It can induce hematopoietic, mesenchymal and epithelial neoplasia in a susceptible target; *c-myc* can contribute to development or progression of tumors in all the above mentioned tissues in birds and humans.

4. Appearance of an oncogene is necessary but not sufficient for tumor induction.[40] The evolution from a normal to a tumoral cellular phenotype depends mainly on the accumulation of events that alter several types of genes (proto-oncogenes, antioncogenes, etc.) The altered genes function in cooperation in order to produce, maintain and direct the evolution of the malignant state. For instance, the alteration of two oncogenes and/ or one antioncogene precede the transformation of normal lung cells to tumoral ones.

III. ANTICARCINOGENESIS

The term anticarcinogenesis is of more recent extraction than carcinogenesis. However, this antonym seems to be as real as carcinogenesis. In fact the strategy of anticarcinogenesis is actually based on the possibility of controlling and modulating carcinogenesis at the biochemical level. Several arguments support this assumption.

First, a number of true anticarcinogenesis elements are contained by the cellular genome itself: the antioncogenes exist as a cue to proto-oncogenes. It was demonstrated that a cell continues to behave normally in the presence of antioncogene transcription products, even after a proto-oncogene is activated. Second, epidemiological data confirm the presence in the environment of chemicals with carcinogenesis inhibitory properties (anti-initiators and antipromoters) even in our food.[11,31,41,42] Third, there are a series of synthetic products (with widely different chemical structures, e.g., phenolic antioxidants such as 2(3)'-tert-butyl-4-hydroxyanisole (BHA), selenium derivatives, disulfiram, etc.) able to decrease the incidence of chemically induced tumors in animals.[42] As a matter of fact, anticarcinogenesis, as an area with a well defined research topic, resulted as a deeper insight in the understanding of the mechanisms governing this very complex process of carcinogenesis. In the last years a number of concepts regarding cancer prevention (e.g., chemoprophylaxis) and its strategy were formulated, based mainly on the possibility of modulating the effect of the environmental carcinogens (especially chemicals) using pharmacological agents able to activate, inhibit, or reverse their carcinogenic activity.[41,43]

Theoretically, nowadays the strategy of anticarcinogenesis involves the following concepts:

1. Destruction of the precarcinogen which could be formed *in vivo* subsequent to a reaction between two or more reagents. A typical example concerns vitamin C which prevents — in the stomach — the formation of carcinogenic *N*-nitroso-derivatives as reaction products following amines and nitrites interaction at acidic pH.

2. Prevent the interaction of the ultimate carcinogen with the critical molecular targets in the cell (especially DNA), by scavenging the ultimate carcinogens by nucleophilic compounds. The most efficient agents acting by such a mechanism are SH-compounds, ellagic and tannic acid.[11,44]

3. Inhibition of the nuclear translocation of the receptor-carcinogen complex[45] by competition with or destruction of the receptor.

4. Direct inhibition of the enzymatic systems involved in precarcinogen activation; this direct interaction between the inhibitor and the enzymatic system (e.g., cytochrome P-450 monooxygenases) lead either to the (enzymatic) inhibition of the activation process, or to the modification of the regio- and stereoselectivity of the same enzymes.

5.   Modulation at the genetic level (e.g., Ah locus, etc.) of the enzymatic systems involved both in activation and detoxification of carcinogens; stimulation of this latter process could be of special interest.

6.   Stimulating the protection mechanisms of the cell and organism in order to block the cellular transformation or to destroy and eliminate the transformed cells. This research field will be the main matter of future investigations, the strategy of such an approach depends on the progress in molecular biology. Investigations in this field will aim at maintaining intact active antioncogenes, blocking activation of proto-oncogenes or favoring error free repair of the lesions at DNA level induced by carcinogens. This means a better understanding of the role of growth factors and transformation inhibiting factors, and also a better knowledge of local and general immune surveillance.[46]

7.   Inhibit promotion and reversion of its early stages. This goal may be achieved by using the so-called ''suppression agents'' or antipromoters. From the several types of exhibiting such properties the retinoids are the most carefully studied.[47]

Clinical trials supporting the reality of the anticarcinogenesis could also be cited, although this type of action is very difficult to evaluate. Two of these trials stressed the general cancer prevention, whereas 21 other trials were focused on five major localizations: cervix, uterus, colon, esophagus, lung and skin.[48] In several programs, supplementation of daily diet with β-carotens, retinoids, vitamins B_6, B_{12}, C, E, folic acid, selenium and corn bran (wheat fiber) was demonstrated to reduce the incidence of some types of cancer. Only retinol can be regarded as a synthetic derivative, although it is present in small amounts in several natural products.[49]

Etretinate administered p.o. induces regression in 80% of patients with keratosis. Other clinical tests of retinoids (e.g., basocellular carcinoma) led to complete remission in 18% of the patients, and to partial remissions in 65% of the cases. Retinoids were also used in treatment of preneoplastic lesions of the oral cavity. Their application led to a regression of leukoplasia in 62% of patients, with a several month persistence. In cervical dysplasia, a complete regression was obtained in 55% of patients treated with all-transretinoic acid.[50] However, mention should be made that the data available covers too short a period of time, thus not even preliminary conclusions could be drawn. Nevertheless, epidemiological and experimental additional data suggest that retinoids could be effective in a large number of cancer types. Calcium was suggested to be of potential value in the prevention of colon cancer, especially to patients with multiple polyposis.

The use of antioxidants in human cancer prevention was also reported. This is, however, the first generation of such pharmacological agents, so that probably more effective carcinogenesis inhibitors will be designed in the future. New concepts completing this strategy suggest the modulation of antioncogene expression and the activation of error free repair systems at DNA level by specific factors of biological origin.

In Chapter 2 we briefly review and discuss some mathematical models of biological triggers able to explain some specific behaviors of initiated, promoted or transformed cells.

A part of these problems, as well as some quantitative models, used in cancer chemoprevention will be developed in Chapter 6. A QSAR-analysis of two series of carcinogenesis inhibitors (e.g., phenolic antioxidants and retinoids) was proposed, useful in the design of more efficient pharmacological agents.

We like to believe that the material presented here will give a comprehensive insight on some less known quantitative aspects of chemical carcinogenesis and chemoprevention. Maybe it will suggest new approaches to this fascinating domain.

REFERENCES

1. **Farber, E.,** Reversible and irreversible lesions in processes of cancer development, in *Molecular and Cellular Aspects of Carcinogen Screening Tests,* Montesano, R., Bartsch, H., Tomatis, L., Eds., IARC Publishing, Lyon, 1980, 143.
2. **Berenblum, I.,** Sequential aspects of chemical carcinogenesis skin, in *Cancer: A Comprehensive Treatise,* Vol. 1, edition 2, Becker, F. F., Ed., Plenum Publishing, New York, 1982.
3. **Slaga, T. J., Ed.,** *Mechanisms of Tumor Promotion,* Vol. 2, CRC Press, Boca Raton, FL, 1984.
4. **Cohen, S. M., Murasaki, G., Ellwein, L. B., and Greenfield, R. E.,** Tumor promotion in bladder carcinogenesis, in *Mechanisms of Tumor Promotion,* Vol. 1, Slaga, T. J., Ed., CRC Press, Boca Raton, FL, 1984, 131.
5. **Morson, B. C., Ed.,** *The Pathogenesis of Colorectal Cancer,* W. B. Saunders, Philadelphia, 1978.
6. **Denda, S., Inui, S., Saragawa, W., Takahashi, S., and Konichi, Y.,** Enhancing effect of partial pancreatectomy and ethionine — induced pancreatic regeneration on tumorogenesis of azaserine in rats, *Gann,* 69, 633, 1978.
7. **Cardiff, R. D.,** Protoneoplasia: the molecular biology of murine mammary hyperplasia, *Adv. Gann Res.,* 42, 167, 1984.
8. **Steele, V. E. and Nettesheim, P.,** Tumor promotion in respiratory tract carcinogenesis, in *Mechanisms of Tumor Promotion,* Vol. 1, Slaga, T. J., Ed., CRC Press, Boca Raton, FL, 1984, 92.
9. **Solt, D. B., Cayama, E., Sarma, D. S. R., and Farber, F.,** Persistance of resistant putative preneoplastic hepatocytes induced by N-nitroso-diethylamine or N-methyl-N-nitrosourea, *Cancer Res.,* 40, 1112, 1980.
10. **Niculescu-Duvăz, I., Safirman, C., and Voiculetz, N.,** Interacţiunea dintre ADN şi cancerigenii chimici. II., *Oncologia,* 4, 241, 1986.
11. **Voiculetz, N., Niculescu-Duvăz, I., Muresan, Z., Safirman, C., and Stoica, G.,** Some molecular aspects of chemoprevention of cancer, *Oncologia,* 2, 81, 1986.
12. **Nistoroiu, M., Stafidor, N., and Voiculetz, N.,** Importanţa sistemului monoxigenozic citocrom P-450 dependent pentru procesul de cancerizare chimica, *Oncologia,* 4, 267, 1986.
13. **Jeffery, A. M.,** DNA modification by chemical carcinogenes, in *Mechanism of Cellular Transformation by Carcinogen Agents,* Brungerger, D. and Goff, S., Eds., Pergamon Press, Elmsford, New York, 33, 1987.
14. **Weinberg, R. A.,** The action of oncogenes in the cytoplasm and nucleus, *Science,* 230, 770, 1985.
15. **Weinberg, R. A.,** Finding the anti-oncogene, *Sci. Am.,* 258(9), 34, 1988.
16. **Klein, G.,** *Cellular Oncogene Activation,* Marcel Dekker, New York, 1988, 302.
17. **Varmus, H. E.,** The molecular genetics of cellular oncogenes, *Am. Rev. Genet.,* 18, 553, 1984.
18. **Bishop, J. M.,** Cellular oncogenes and retroviruses, *Ann. Rev. Biochem.,* 52, 301, 1983.
19. **Bishop, J. M.,** The molecular genetics of cancer, *Science,* 235, 305, 1987.
20. **Voiculetz, N. and Niculescu-Duvăz, I.,** Mecanismele moleculare ale cancerogenezei chimice, Ed., Enciclopedică şi Stiinţifică, Bucureşti, in press.
21. **Nurse, R. and Berns, A.,** Cellular oncogene activation by insertion of retrovisal DNA; genes identified by provirus tagging, in *Cellular Oncogene Activation,* Klein, G., Ed., Marcel Dekker, New York, 1988, 302.
22. **Ames, B. N., McCann, J., and Yamasaki, E.,** Methods for detecting carcinogens and mutagens with the Salmonella/mammalian microsome mutagenicity test, *Mutation Res.,* 31, 347, 1975.
23. **Barbacid, M.,** *ras* oncogenes in human and carcinogen-induced animal tumors, in *Cellular Oncogene Activation,* Klein, G., Ed., Marcel Dekker, New York, 1988, 302.
24. **Weinstein, B.,** The origins of human cancer: molecular mechanisms of carcinogenesis and their implications for cancer prevention and treatment, *Cancer Res.,* 48, 4135, 1988.
25. **Land, H., Parada, L. F., and Weinberg, R. A.,** Tumorigenic conversion of primary embryo fibroblasts requires at least two cooperating oncogenes, *Nature (London),* 304, 596, 1983.
26. **Klein, G.,** The approaching era of the tumor suppressor genes, *Science,* 238, 1539, 1987.
27. **Pelech, S.,** How anticancer genes turn of tumors, *Sciences, (New York),* 29(1), 39, 1989.
28. **Knudson, A. G. J.,** Hereditary cancer, oncogens and antioncogens, *Cancer Res.,* 45, 1437, 1985.
29. **Bodmer, N. F., Bailey, C. J., Bodmer, J., et al.,** Localisation of the gene for familial polyposis coli in chromosome 5, *Nature,* 328, 614, 1988.
30. **Vogelstein, B., Fearon, E. R., and Hamilton, S. R.,** Genetic alteration during colorectal tumor development, *N. Engl. J. Med.,* 319, 525, 1988.
31. **Stoica, G., Lupu, F., Niculescu-Duvăz, I., and Voiculetz, N.,** Agenţi antipromotori, *Oncologia,* 4, 257, 1989.
32. **Carter, T. H.,** Regulation of gene expression by tumor promoters, in *Mechanisms of Environmental Carcinogenesis,* Barrett, J. C., Ed., CRC Press, Boca Raton, FL, 1987, 47.

33. **Fusing, N. E. and Samsel, W.,** Growth-promoting activity of phorbol ester TPA on cultured mouse keratinocytes fibroblasts and carcinoma cells, in *Carcinogenesis, Vol. II, Mechanisms of Tumor Promotion and Carcinogenesis,* Slaga, T. J., Sivak, A., and Bontwell, R. K., Eds., Raven Press, New York, 1978, 203.

34. **Dimond, L.,** Tumor promoters and cell transformation, in *Mechanisms of Cellular Transformation by Carcinogenic Agents,* Grunberger, G. and Goff, S., Eds., Pergamon Press, Elmsford, New York, 1987, 73.

35. **Nishizuka, Y.,** Perspectives on the role of protein kinase C in stimulus-response coupling, *J. Natl. Cancer Inst.,* 76, 159, 1987.

36. **Colburn, N. H.,** The genetics of tumor promotion, in *Mechanisms of Environmental Carcinogenesis,* Barrett, J. C., Ed., CRC Press, Boca Raton, FL, 1987, 81.

37. **Lerman, M. I., Hegamayer, G. A., and Colburn, N. H.,** Cloning and characterization of putative genes that specify sensitivity to induction of neoplastic transformation by tumor promoters, *Int. J. Cancer,* 37, 293, 1986.

38. **Furstenberger, G., Schweizer, J., and Marks, F.,** Development of phorbol ester responsiveness in neonatal mouse epidermis: correlation between hyperplastic response and sensitivity to first-stage tumor promotion, *Carcinogenesis,* 6, 289, 1985.

39. **Logue, T. and Frommer, D.,** The influence of oral vitamin C supplements on experimental colorectal tumor induction, *Aust. N.Z. J. Med.,* 10, 588, 1980.

40. **Duesberg, P. H.,** Activated proto-oncogenes sufficient or necessary for cancer?, *Science,* 228, 669, 1985.

41. **Waltenberg, L. W.,** Inhibition of neoplasia by minor dietary constituents, *Cancer Res.,* 43, 2448, 1985.

42. **Stoica, G., Safirman, C., Arnăutu, M., Voiculetz, N., Niculescu-Duvăz, I.,** Mechanisms of carcinogenesis inhibition, *Rev. Roum. Biochim.,* 24(3), 245, 1987.

43. **Hocman, G.,** Chemoprevention of cancer: phenolic antioxidants (BHT, BHA), *Int. J. Biochem.,* 20, 639, 1988.

44. **Galdean, D., Alangiu, P., Vray, Z., and Voiculetz, N.,** Efectul protector al Thiolei asupra genotoxicității benzo(a)pirenului la nivelul măduvei osoase la şoarece, *Oncologia,* 1, 223, 1983.

45. **Stoica, A. and Voiculetz, N.,** Rolul unor receptori in procesul de cancerizare, *Oncologia,* 3, 161, 1986.

46. **Oldham, R. K.,** *Principles of Cancer Biotherapy,* Raven Press, New York, 1987, 502.

47. **Niculescu-Duvăz, I., Voiculetz, N., and Simon, Z.,** The carcinogenesis inhibitory properties of retinoids: a QSAR-MTD study, in *Chemistry and Biology of Synthetic Retinoids,* Dawson, M. I. and Okamura, T., Eds., CRC Press, Boca Raton, FL, 1990, 575.

48. **Bertram, J. S., Kolonel, L. N., and Meysens, F. L., Jr.,** Rational and strategies for chemoprevention of cancer in humans, *Cancer Res.,* 47, 3012, 1987.

49. **DeCosse, J. J., Miller, H. H., and Lesser, M. L.,** Effect of wheat fiber and vitamins C and E on rectal polyps in patients with familial adenomatous polyposis, *J. Natl. Cancer Inst.,* 81(17), 1290, 1989.

50. **Browman, G. P., Arnold, A., Booker, L., Johnstone, B., Skingley, P., and Levine, M. N.,** Etretinate blood levels in monitoring of compliance and contamination in a chemoprevention trial, *J. Natl. Cancer Inst.,* 81(10), 795, 1989.

Chapter 2

TRIGGER MODELS FOR GENE ACTIVITY REGULATION IN CARCINOGENESIS

Zeno Simon and Nicolae Voiculetz

TABLE OF CONTENTS

I. INTRODUCTION

In the past few years, rapid progress has been made in a number of research areas which have considerably increased our knowledge of the biological processes occurring in cells under both "normal" and "pathological" conditions. Important advances have been achieved by molecular biology and biochemistry allowing a better understanding of the regulatory mechanisms involved in gene expression.[1-3]

Cells, as simple unicellular organisms, must proliferate at the highest possible rate in given environmental conditions, with a single alternative-sporulation, i.e., when these conditions become severe. In contrast to this behavior, in higher organisms several new regulatory mechanisms appear, allowing the integration of the eukaryotic cells into the whole organism. Cell growth, proliferation and differentiation are strictly controlled. Disruptions or defects in these control mechanisms can induce transformation into the neoplastic phenotype. The mechanisms leading to the initiation and proliferation of malignant cells are still poorly understood.

According to the "central dogma of molecular biology" as a basis for cell regulation, DNA-transcription, mRNA-translation, and enzymatic reactions can be considered as three consecutive amplification cascades. Regulation of gene activity at the transcription level would be the most efficient one. Genes involved in the transduction of signals required for normal cell proliferation commonly appear to be subverted in the carcinogenesis process too.

Recent discoveries have pointed out that some tumors may arise due to various genetic and epigenetic mechanisms[4] producing alterations in cellular gene regulation. Proto-oncogenes are a subset of cellular genes, some of them have been directly implied in the control of cellular proliferation. They are also able to induce cell transformation and tumor growth after insertion into retroviruses, or upon specific alteration in structure or regulation within the cell. The products of viral or cellular oncogenes are related to various kinases, growth factors and growth factor receptors which are modified or overexpressed. All these might contribute to a new picture of the general mechanisms for the induction of cellular proliferation. We shall discuss the peculiarities of gene regulation in eukaryotes, the alteration of the normal cellular machinery at various points which can determine the transformation of a normal cell into a malignant one. We consider that progress in understanding gene activity provides a better fundamental insight into molecular mechanisms of the cell, thus leading to a better knowledge of the runaway mechanisms in cancer diseases.

We shall present here a model involving a trigger with positive control as a hypothesis for gene activity regulation in eukaryotes (Ptashne's autoregulation of genes[5]) especially for the switches between inactive and active states in gene transcription. We shall demonstrate, by computer simulations, the adequacy of this model and discuss its involvement in growth control and carcinogenesis. Some earlier models for gene regulation will also be discussed insofar as they are involved in growth control, cell transformation and evolution of malignancy.

For this purpose, a short critical review of the main factors and mechanisms involved in cell regulation will be presented; we shall emphasize the data which are in accordance or in contrast with the mathematical model proposed here.

II. CELL REGULATION AND CARCINOGENESIS

A. THE REGULATION OF PROTEIN SYNTHESIS IN EUKARYOTES

Several textbooks[1-3] are a key source of references for gene regulation in eukaryotes. About 10% of the eukaryotic DNA represents the structural genes (SG) and only a small fraction of them is actually transcribed in the cells of a given tissue. While histones produce an unspecific blockage of transcription, the transcriptional control is mainly positive: it is exerted by nonhistonic proteins (NHP), which bind specifically to DNA control sequences (promoters, enhancers) and activate the nearby genes.

Whereas in prokaryote synthesis (structural) genes are under control of a few elements — the operon model of Monod and Jacob[6] — in eukaryotes each gene is regulated by many control elements, both positive and negative ones. Most of these control elements appear to be highly dependent on tissue specificity, i.e., to be selectively bound and inactivated in some cells. The large diversity of proteins probably accounts for the highly complex combinatorial system as a requirement for the control of gene expression in pluricellular organisms. The actual rate of protein synthesis is also influenced by various types of post-transcriptional, translational and post-translational controls. As the eukaryotic cells are embedded into the relatively constant internal medium of the organisms, no rapid adaptation to the changing environment is required, but the activation degrees of the cell genes must be stable, certain on and off switches occurring only during differentiation processes.

As an example of regulating translation in somatic mammalian cells, the modulation of intracellular pH and ionic strength (especially via Ca^{2+} ions) can be considered; this occurs when quiescent cells are stimulated by growth factors or serum. Numerous initiator factors, such as eIF-2 or eIF-4e were recently demonstrated in sea urchin eggs. In somatic mammalian cells the initiator factors equivalent to those found in sea urchin eggs undergo covalent modifications under conditions that modulate translation.[7]

The protein kinases also play a key role in cell regulation, especially for rapid responses in differentiated cells or during cell proliferation. About 1%, i.e., a substantial fraction, of the genes from the mammalian genome (approximately 1000 genes) probably code for protein kinases.[8] Of the human PKC (protein kinase C) isoenzyme family, the cdc2 protein kinase, for example, has a constant abundance throughout the cell cycle but its activity oscillates dramatically, reaching a maximum of the G2/M-boundary. This kinase is regulated by phosphorylation of a tyrosine site, which, in turn, is regulated by another protein.[9] Transfer of cell membrane bound, inactive PKCs to the cytoplasm or nucleus also has a main role in activation and is produced by Ca^{2+} ions, diacylglycerols and tumoral promotors such as phorbol esters. PKCs modulate the activity of several membrane receptors (the epidermal growth factor receptor, by phosphorylation, for example) enzymes, nuclear proteins and induce transcription of certain genes, DNA synthesis, etc. Increased PKC activity is found in human tumors or premalignant states (breast cancer, for example).

One may ask the reason why the negative control (repression), characteristic for bacteria, was often substituted by a positive control (induction) in higher organisms. On and off switches also occur in the Monod-Jacob model. An example could be the trigger of cross and feedback interrelated operons,[6] each operon synthesizes the repressor for the other. One reason might be that most of the eukaryotic genome is silent due to the unspecific histone blockage. Another possible reason may be the diploidy in higher organisms which increases the degree of reliability of cell function; mutations in both alleles being required to inactivate one enzyme. For positive control, dominant constitutive mutations can be avoided, as will be further proved (see Section V.E). In the operonic Monod-Jacob control, a single mutation in the operator gene may produce an uncontrolled, constitutive synthesis of the proteins coded by the operon genes.

B. GENE ACTIVITY AND GROWTH CONTROL

The mechanisms regulating gene activity in eukaryotes have not been completely elucidated until now. Among the processes involved one may cite: specific DNA-base methylation, histone-phosphorylation, gene loss, amplification and rearrangements.[10]

Positive control triggers based upon gene autoactivation by their own transcription or translation product were first considered for viruses and used to explain the lambda-phage cycle in lysogenic bacteria (SOS induction).[11,12] The most general model for gene regulation is the hierarchical model of Davidson and Britten.[13] A group of "integrator" genes or "master" genes are interrelated by the interaction between their synthesis products and their sensor DNA-sequences which control the activity of the other genes, the so called "slave" genes. Because it was easier to conceive the specific recognition of a sensor DNA-sequence occurring through a polynucleotide than through a protein, Britten and Davidson considered some nuclear RNAs as the interrelating gene products. However, recent data attribute this role to the NHP.

A theory for the control of cell and tissue growth was given by Bullough.[14,15] It is worth mentioning here, at least for its elegance and simplicity. According to Bullough there are three types of genes: mitotic genes involved in cell proliferation, "house-keeping" genes coding for the essential metabolic enzymes and histospecific genes whose expression is required by specific tissue functions. Each cell type synthesizes a histospecific growth inhibitor, the chalone, which acts only upon cell receptors of the same tissue. It decreases the activity of mitotic genes and increases the activity of histospecific genes, thus favoring differentiation toward mature, functionally active and nonproliferative cells. The increase in tissue mass results in an elevated chalone production and concentration, decreasing the cell proliferation rate. Tissue lesions result in chalone loss, and the decreased chalone concentration leads to an increase in cell proliferation. A simple mechanism for tissue homeostasis is given hereby. Chalones are diffusible, relatively small glycoproteins[16] which act upon cell surface receptors and produce secondary messengers. The cyclic AMP and cyclic GMP systems are probably involved in chalone control.

Several histospecific growth inhibitory factors were isolated together with less specific growth-inhibiting and various growth-enhancing factors.[17] The term chalone for specific growth-inhibiting substances has not been generally accepted, although several of the protein molecules involved in the control of tissue development (for example, those involved in the molecular control of blood cell development)[18] present several of the characteristics attributed by Bullough to the chalones.

Bullough developed an entire theory of carcinogenesis based upon his chalone concept, but no mention is made of features like cell adhesion and contact inhibition which are fundamental both for normal tissue formation and for the invasivity of tumors. Cell adhesion is based upon specific interaction between the so called RGD proteins, containing the Arg-Gly-Asp tripeptide sequence in different spatial conformations. Receptors for this tripeptide sequence are part of a supergene family of cell surface proteins, termed integrins. They are heterodimeric proteins made up of two subunits (mol wt 140,000 to 200,000 Da and 95,000 to 120,000 Da), present in a noncovalent complex at the cell surface.[19] The cell surface recognition molecules, such as the neural cell adhesion molecule (N-CAM), have an immunoglobulin-like structure.[20] Another fundamental phenomenon for normal tissue formation is the intercellular communication system through gap junctions, which allow a direct electric and metabolic contact between the cytoplasm of neighboring cells. In mammalian cells these allow the passage of ions and small molecules (up to mol wt 1200 Da) such as secondary messengers and possibly morphogens. Gap junctional communication is considered to play a role in the control of cell growth and in maintaining a harmonious tissue function. Besides the role played in cell-to-cell communication, gap junctions have been shown to affect the regulation of cell proliferation and specific gene expression, and their reduction could be involved in the early stages of carcinogenesis. In transformed fibroblasts[21] and in preneoplastic focal lesions or primary tumors induced by N-methyl-N-nitrosourea in rat liver,[22] the expression of the gap junction proteins was reduced or abolished (as detected by monoclonal antibody techniques). Generally, in cancer cells these gap junctions appear to be closed.[23-24] Junctional permeability is elevated by c-AMP and retinoic acid derivatives, and reduced by Ca^{2+} and the decrease of intracellular pH. A small group of genes regulating intercellular communication was recently identified, namely the *lin-12* gene and *glp-1* gene in *C. elegans* and the *notch* gene in *Drosophila*.[25]

Correct cell adhesion and normal tissue formation could be based upon an antigen-antibody type recognition between cell surface receptors and/or upon a regular and histospecific geometric pattern of these surface receptors and gap junctions, allowing strong contacts and intercellular communications only between cells of the same type.

From this brief outline of cell regulation one may expect several types of defects to lead to the loss of growth control and different degrees of malignancy, related to the nature of defects or to the number of defects accumulated within a cell.

C. DEFECTS IN CELL REGULATION AND CARCINOGENESIS

Human cancer appears as a consequence of various genetic and epigenetic mechanisms,[4] including inherited defects in certain genes.[26-29] The first suggestions came from epidemiological studies indicating a relationship between cancer incidence and exposure to environmental carcinogenic factors which are known for their mutagenic properties.

Carcinogenesis in various systems and even in man is considered to be a multiphasic process, comprising at least three distinct steps: initiation, promotion and progression.[30,31] Mutations and viruses have been lately considered as primary causes of cancer. The initial defect could diminish growth control, thus leading to an increased rate of cell division, followed by the accumulation of precancerous mutations. Cells with mutations which further reduce growth control will be selected out of this initial populations as the cells with low malignancy. The increased glycolysis in several tumors as compared to the original tissue (Warburg's theory),[32] may represent just a metabolic advantage acquired by such a selection process.

Bullough's theory assumes that carcinogenesis is produced by a defect of the chalonic system. Several types of cancer cells (epidermal carcinoma, chloroleukemia, etc.) were found to produce the chalone of the original tissue, but at the same time to have a reduced sensitivity towards chalones; much higher chalone concentrations are required to stop the proliferation of these cells.[33]

More recently, the so-called oncogenes have been considered to be the primary cause of cancer.[34] The silent forms (proto-oncogenes) are normal, highly conserved cell genes, expressed at a certain development stage or during normal proliferation; they might correspond to the so called ''mitotic genes'' of Bullough. Proto-oncogenes control the growth and they effect the differentiation of eukaryotic cells. Scientists recently reported evidence that, for instance, proto-oncogene *c-mos* influences meiosis in oocytes. This is the first direct evidence that a proto-oncogene has a specific function during germ cell maturation. The activation of oncogenes in mammalian cells can occur by two mechanisms: by a point mutation in the cellular proto-oncogene that results in a functionally altered protein, or by deregulation resulting in overexpression of the normal product. The deregulation can appear following: (1) chromosomal translocation; (2) insertion of a strong promoter, e.g., a viral one; (3) transposed active DNA sequence or (4) gene amplification.[34]

Although the complete implication of oncogenes in all human tumors has not been yet demonstrated, there is compelling evidence to support the conclusion that oncogenes do play a role in certain steps of neoplastic evolution.[35] The activation of proto-oncogenes by carcinogens (mutagens) provides direct evidence for mutational events in carcinogenesis processes. The proto-oncogenes of the *ras* family are activated and acquire transformation ability following the treatment of fibroblasts with known carcinogenic compounds such as: 3-methyl-cholanthrene, dimethylbenz(a) anthracene, nitroso-methyl-urea.[36] Studies concerning molecular alterations of the *ras* oncogene family demonstrate the existence of a single point mutation in codon 12, 13 or 61.

Gene amplification provides another mechanism by which oncogene expression may be increased. The amplification of oncogenes occurs in many tumor cell lines where double minute chromosomes (DMC) and homogeneously staining chromosomal regions (HSR) were observed, suggesting the role of this type of genetic alteration in the transformation and progression of malignancies.

In some cases, the amplified region contains a known oncogene (proto-oncogene) or a gene related to such oncogenes. In other cases, the use of DNA probes, complementary to oncogenes, shows that a particular oncogene is amplified, although the amplification is not necessarily detectable. The level of amplification is quite variable (5 to 1000 times) and it is not known whether the oncogene is of the wild type or has been mutated in addition to its amplification. The somatic amplification of specific genes appears as an adaptive cellular response to environmental stress. It is possible that gene amplification gives an advantage to the growth of the established tumor, rather than being an event involved in its initiation.

Cytogenetic analysis of animal or human tumors revealed many chromosomal disorders (translocation, deletion, inversion, addition and numerical variation).[28] Particular attention has been given to leukemias, Burkitt lymphomas and tumors associated with rare congenital chromosome changes.[36] In human chronic myeloid leukemia (CML) the cytogenetic hallmark is the Philadelphia (PH) chromosome, the result of the translocation between chromosome 9 and 22, t(9, 22) (q34, q11).[37] Molecular rearrangements result in the translocation of the proto-oncogene *abl* from the long arm of chromosome 9 to the long arm of the chromosome 22 juxtaposed with a specific region termed *Bcr* (breakpoint cluster region). This rearrangement leads to an mRNA which is structurally different from that observed in normal cells. This translocation generates a chimeric gene which produces a new mRNA and a new protein with a kinase activity specific for thyrosine residues. The production of the *Bcr/abl* chimeric gene appears to be essential to the few demonstrated ones, in which a gene translocated on another chromosome produces a new, composite mRNA, and a fusion protein of 210,000 Da, containing a fragment (about 140,000 Da) of the usual (145,000 Da) c-abl protein and a fragment (of about 70,000 Da) of the Bcr protein. Another example belongs to the B- and T-cell malignancies, particularly Burkitt lymphoma in which translocations involve chromosome 8(q24) and chromosome 14(q32), 2(q13), or 22(q11). In these translocation the *c-myc* oncogene is involved. This gene is located on chromosome 8 and by translocation it gets closer to the promoter of the immunoglobulin genes located on chromosome 14 (locus for heavy chain), chromosome 2 (locus for kappa light chain) or chromosome 22 (locus for lambda light chain). As the effect of these translocations, a constitutive overexpression of the oncogene *myc* occurs. The myc protein appears to be involved in DNA replication and, when it is overexpressed, it might lead to uncontrolled cell proliferation.

In solid tumors, especially in those associated with rare congenital chromosome alteration such as retinoblastoma and Wilms' tumor, the malignancy is supposed to be in connection with a recessive or "antioncogene" mechanism.[38,39] The loss of a gene containing the information for a negative regulatory protein could allow the uncontrolled synthesis of other gene products. Under these circumstances, if the new proteins are involved in cell proliferation, then uncontrolled growth and cell division could result. The inheritance of certain growth suppressing genes in a mutated form reveals susceptibility to cancer. The first such antioncogene to be isolated is the retinoblastoma gene (Rb-gene)-related to a predisposition to an eye tumor.[40] Its product, the Rb protein binds to the E1A-adenovirus protein and to the large T antigen of SV40. Possibly it has a general suppressor role for proteins implied in cellular growth.[41,42]

In several types of tumors, carcinogenesis can be connected to some gross modification of chromosome structure. The conversion from adenoma to carcinoma in the development of human colorectal tumors,[43] for instance, was found to be synchronous with the loss of a part of chromosome 17 and, in certain retinoblastomas and Wilms' tumors, with a constitutional deletion of both copies of chromosome 13(q14) or 11(q13), respectively. Thus, for various types of deletion, including monosomy, when present as primary changes in specific tumors, it has been suggested that a recessive mechanism is involved in the transformation process. These results support the idea that tumor suppressor genes exist in normal cells and control the expression of tumorigenicity when multiple oncogenes are activated in a cell. Nevertheless, in many cases the affected genes remain unknown and therefore we need to understand intragenomic rearrangements and phenotypic changes induced by oncogenic agents.

The proteins coded by known oncogenes were found to be protein kinases, GTP-ases, guanine nucleotide binding proteins (G-protein) and DNA-binding proteins, nuclear phosphoproteins, growth factors, growth factor receptors, factors regulating transcription (*jun* oncoprotein), factors involved in cell proliferation, DNA synthesis and probably in the initiation and evolution of malignancy.[44]

The protein of the *ras* proto-oncogene is similar to the G-protein bound to the inner side of the cellular membranes. When binding GTP, these proteins acquire an adenylate-cyclase activity, which soon disappears, due to the GTP-asic activity of these proteins, by loss of the bound GTP-molecule. A point mutation producing an amino acid substitution at position 12 of the *ras* protein decreases the GTP-asic activity and this mutated *ras* protein acquires an uncontrolled ATP-cyclasic activity.[45,46]

A nuclear protein directly involved in DNA synthesis, termed proliferating cell nuclear antigen (PCNA or cyclin), a cofactor of DNA polymerase, was recently identified.[47] An alteration of receptors for cell adhesion molecules (fibronectin receptors) was observed in leukemia cells.[48]

Finally, the disputed (or at least very rare) phenomenon of cancer reversion has given rise to the hypothesis of reversible switches in gene activity as a cause of spontaneous involution of certain malignancies.[49]

D. HOW MANY EVENTS ARE REQUIRED FOR CARCINOGENESIS?

The number of events required to produce cancer could be, theoretically, deduced from the dependence of tumor formation upon the dose of carcinogen, time, etc., but some very stringent conditions — such as absence of previous, accidental carcinogenic effects — would be required.

Interpretations of epidemiological studies in the context of the multistep model for carcinogenesis suggest that we are at, or beyond, the limits of observational precision to detect effects which would allow calculation of the number of steps implied in carcinogenesis.[50] At least two key steps, escape from cell senescence, and neoplastic transformation are required, but these two steps cannot alone explain all the results even for carcinogenesis in cell culture models.[51] Earlier results indicate that the probability of cancer in human beings roughly increases with the square of their age.[52] Direct evidence which supports the supposition of a two-mutation step carcinogenesis is based on the clinical observation concerning retinoblastoma or other familial cancers.[40,53] In retinoblastoma, persons who carry the gene for this disease have a 95% probability of developing retinoblastoma bilaterally. In noncarrier persons the probability is only 0.05% and the disease often appears unilaterally. The explanation of this clinical observation is based on a two-hit model,[54] in which two steps (mutations) are required to convert a normal cell into a malignant one. In individuals who carry one gene for the retinoblastoma, the first step is an inherited germ-line mutation and the second step (probably a second mutation) takes place in the somatic cells. In individuals who are noncarriers of this gene, both events must appear in the somatic cell. Recent molecular studies on retinoblastoma support the two-hit model in which two mutations are required for the inactivation of the gene of retinoblastoma (Rb-gene), a recessive human cancer gene which has a suppressive or regulatory function.[39]

An interesting fact related to this matter was offered by recent developments in the oncogene area. The evidence that two distinct genetic lesions might combine to produce a malignant transformation has been obtained from studies on cell cultures. The long latency period required in most carcinogenic systems could also be explained by the participation of more than one oncogene in the multistep development (initiation, promotion and progression) of a malignant cell population.[54] In order to produce a tumor cell, it is supposed that two or more distinct oncogenes might cooperate or complement each other. This was demonstrated using *c-myc* and *c-H-ras* oncogenes to transform embryo fibroblasts in transfection experiments.

It seems thus likely that at least two defects (mutations) are required as the first step in carcinogenesis. During the lifespan of a human organism, about 10^{16} cell divisions occur; the rate of spontaneous mutations being of about 10^{-6} per gene and cell division, each gene, including the silent proto-oncogenes, would undergo about 10^{10} mutations during a human life time. Why then is cancer so relatively rare?[52] Most mutations will produce a defective protein, without an increased activity. If two mutational events are required for both alleles, such an event will have a probability of only about 10^{-12} per gene and division, and only about 10^4 cancer cells would result during a human's lifetime. Our environment contains a multitude of mutagenic and carcinogenic factors which exert a continuous pressure on all living organisms, thus increasing the frequency of DNA damage. For survival and resistance to carcinogenic pressure, the cells use a variety of enzymatic mechanisms for repairing or tolerating the DNA lesions.[55] In this case, an error free (or, more exactly, with very low error frequency) repair process could play a very efficient role in cancer prevention. On the contrary, an error prone DNA-replicative process might play a direct role in the initiation of malignancy after chemical carcinogen exposure. In addition, due to the rapid cell proliferation in epithelial tissues (such as epidermis or duodenal lineage), most of the neoplastic cells will be carried with the flow of cells toward the surface, where they are shed. And, last but not least, the immune surveillance may destroy such cells, if they present a sufficiently modified pattern of surface antigens.

III. GENE CONTROL IN EUKARYOTES

A. STRUCTURE OF EUKARYOTIC CHROMATIN

In the nucleus of eukaryotic cells the DNA exists in the form of chromatin which is organized into higher order structures.[56] Eukaryotic chromatin consists of nucleosomes.[57,58] A nucleosomal core consists of 146 to 166 base pairs (bp) of DNA, wrapped around the octameric histone complex containing two molecules of each histone: H2A, H2B, H3, H4. The nucleosomal cores are connected by DNA linker regions of 20 to 100 bp which are particularly sensitive to staphylococcal nuclease. The histone H1 is associated both with the nucleosomal core and with the linker regions of DNA, thus stabilizing the nucleosomes. This "pearl string" structure is bound into a more compact superstructure, a spiralized superfiber with a diameter of 250 to 300 Å, the so-called "thick fiber", with about 45,000 bp of DNA. Physicochemical studies suggest that this fiber consists of a continuous coiling of core and linker regions of DNA which form a "solenoid". Each solenoidal turn has a helix with 6 to 9 nucleosomes which include about 1200 bp of DNA. In interphase nuclei and metaphase chromosomes the "thick fiber" appears to be additionally folded into structures termed loops or domains, comprising 35 to 90 kbp of DNA. This type of chromatin structure is considered to be anchored in a supporting structure in the nucleus, the so called matrix or scaffold.[59]

The effect of this structure is to enable sequence elements, separated by important distances along the genome, to come close to each other in chromatin and to render regions of DNA accessible or inaccessible to large proteins or environmental factors.

Vertebrate genes display a wide range of lengths up to 200 kbp, most often in the 50 kbp domain. Exon lengths are often correlated to functional domains of the encoded protein, the same exon being used in different genes. Variations in splicing of the transcribed DNA (precursor RNA) can produce more than one protein per gene.[2]

Active genes in transcription are found in euchromatin, while those inactive in transcription are located in heterochromatin. Active genes contain DNA sequences of 50 to 400 bp, usually — but not always — situated before the transcription initiation point, with up to 10 times increased sensitivity to DN-ase I digestion. There also exists hypersensitive domains with up to 100 times increased sensitivity. This sensitivity and hypersensitivity to DN-ase I digestion seems to be correlated with gene activation, i.e., with low and, respectively, high transcription rate of the nearby genes.[60]

Eukaryotic chromatin also contains tissue-specific nonhistonic proteins. As demonstrated with reconstituted chromatin (nuclear DNA to which nonhistonic and histonic proteins are added), the mRNA transcribed by *in vitro* systems has a spectrum of sequences similar to the mRNA transcribed in the tissue from which the nonhistonic proteins were isolated. In this system, nonhistonic proteins must be added first, and histones afterwards: if this order is reversed the reconstituted chromatin will be inactive in transcription. For other details see the book of Freifelder[1] (cf. also Reference 3, Chapters IV.4 and X.7).

B. EXTENT OF GENE ACTIVATION IN ANIMAL CELLS

The most interesting quantitative feature of gene activation in eukaryotes is perhaps the existence of three abundance classes for cellular mRNA.[61-63] Studies in DNA-RNA hybridization-competition kinetics have demonstrated the existence of three classes of mRNA concerning the number of mRNA molecules per cell, namely: (1) the low copy number mRNA abundance class, with 0.01 to 15 molecules per cell; (2) the moderately prevalent class, with 10 to 300 molecules per cell and (3) the supervalent class, with 1000 to 10,000 molecules per cell.

There are several types of sequences corresponding to the low number class, namely 33,000 types in HeLa cells; possibly all inactive genes undergo some accidental transcription, probably during DNA replication; some authors indicate even 10^6 types of sequences for this class. For the moderately prevalent class, the number of reported sequences lies between 370 and 10,000, while for the supervalent class the number of reported sequences is small, 17 to 400.[61-63]

This clustering of mRNA molecules per sequence type in distinct domains suggests the existence of only three possible activation states for eukaryotic genes, which we shall call as inactive — "O", low activity — "I", and high activity — "II" states.[64] As we shall further suggest (see Section V.B), such a behavior would be a natural consequence of the cooperative nature of the interaction of activated proteins with gene control sequences. The problem to be elucidated is whether all three states of activation are possible for all genes.

These abundance classes should also be reflected in protein synthesis rates. It is not easy to measure synthesis rates per cell for individual proteins, such rates being also susceptible to post-translational controls. The protein quantities (enzyme activities) per cell will

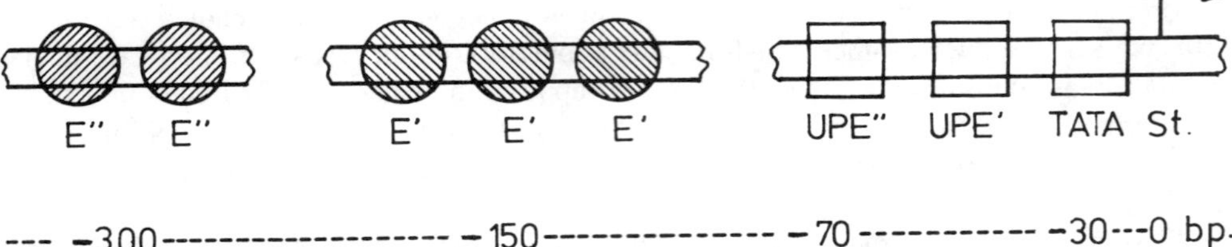

FIGURE 1.   Spatial organization of control sequences of the eukaryotic gene. St = RNA transcription startpoint; TATA = the TATA box; UPE′, UPE″ = upstream promoter elements; E′, E″ = different enhancer elements. Numbers indicate distances in base pairs, upstream from the transcription start.

also strongly depend upon decay rates. Gene amplification may additionally make things more complicated. Nevertheless, in cells committed to synthesizing large quantities of a certain protein, supervalent mRNA (state II) would correspond to this protein; this is the case for hemoglobin and the corresponding globin mRNA, in which case the corresponding genes are not amplified (quoted by Freifolder,[1] p. 510).

Small quantities of four histospecific mRNA transcripts were identified in each of the four different cell types investigated by the so called RAWTS-technique, favoring the idea of a low basal transcription rate for all genes in embryonic and adult tissues.[65]

Green, Goldberg and Todaro[66] measured the relative collagen synthesis rate (relative to the total protein rate) for 22 cell types in nongrowing dense cell cultures, based upon incorporation of radioactive amino acids, on the assumption that collagen contains 12.2% proline and the rest of proteins only 4.1%. They found three distinct domains for the relative collagen synthesis rates: 1.5 to 14% for all diploid fibroblast strains; 0.15 to 0.4% for a number of stabilized cell lines of nonfibroblastic origin (such as HeLa, KB, etc.); below the limit of detection (0.002%) for lymphocyte and reticulocyte-like cells. These three rate ranges might be explained by the three activation degrees for the collagen gene (100, 5 and 0%) — the variations within one range being due to different total gene activities in the different cell types.

Enzymatic activities in different tissues do not display distinct activity ranges, for instance dipeptidyl-peptidase-IV in 20 tissues,[67] adenylatedeaminase in 28 tissues[68] and a collection of 50 other enzymes in 17 tissues.[69] In contrast to relative collagen synthesis rates, enzymatic activities also depend upon the decay rates of the enzymes, and the stabilities of their mRNA-templates, i.e., processes which would ''smear out'' the distinct rate ranges for mRNA synthesis.

C. THE EUKARYOTIC GENE CONTROL ELEMENTS

The regulation of inducible and tissue — or cell — specific gene expression, comprising the organization of the control sequences was recently reviewed by Maniatis, Goodburn and Fischer.[70] Two types of control sequences are involved in the regulation of DNA transcription, namely promoters and enhancers. They are the sites of positive, activating regulation. Control sequences for negative, repressive regulation also exist for some genes — the so-called de-enhancers, attenuators or silencers.

The difference between promoters and enhancers is rather an operational one. Promoters act upstream and nearby the transcription start-point — typically 100 bp upstream, and are required for the exact and efficient initiation of transcription. Enhancers increase the transcription rate given by promoters; they act *cis*-linked to the promoters, but are situated in most cases upstream at longer distances from the transcription start-point and sometimes downstream from this starting point. Both control sequences act in the presence of the regulatory proteins by binding to these sequences. The typical spatial organization of these control sequences is depicted in Figure 1.

The promoter region consists of the so-called TATA-box, required for the exact initiation of transcription, and of one or several upstream promoter elements (UPEs), each of 8 to 12 bp length. Within an enhancer region, multiple binding sites can exist. The SV-40 early transcript gene enhancer comprises three DNA regions, each of them being required for functionality; first (upstream from the transcription start) a 5′ binding site for the SP_1-protein (a transcription enhancing factor) and afterwards a repeated B-A-B-A sequence binding two different proteins, A and B. For the integrated mouse mammary tumor virus (MMTV) gene, regulated by the glucocorticoid receptor protein (GRP), there is a group of three GRP binding sites at 150 bp upstream to the RNA start-point and another group of two GRP sites at about 300 bp. This multiple nature of control sequences seems to be common for the sites involved in the interaction of DNA with regulatory proteins and this interaction is required for active transcription of genes.[71,72]

Two mechanisms were put forward to explain the transcriptional stimulation of RNA polymerase II genes, by upstream promoter and enhancer elements. In the "looping model" the upstream enhancer element interacts directly, via the activating protein molecule, with the proximal promoter element. In the "scanning model" a transcription factor binds to the upstream element and scans along the DNA until it reaches the promoter. The discovery of stimulation of *in vitro* transcription by an SV-40 enhancer attached noncovalently to a β-globin promoter via a streptavidin molecule, favors the "looping model".[73]

Point mutations in enhancer sequences usually decrease the transcription rate of the active gene about 5 to 10 times. However, some point mutations do not decrease this rate, they even increase it (about 3 times). Mutations which increase the distance between the TATA-box and UPE-elements decrease transcription rates, especially if this distance corresponds to a semi-integer $(n + \frac{1}{2})$ of DNA turns. Possibly, both the activator protein (NHP) fixed at an upstream activator site (UAS) and TATA-box fixed protein, bind the RNA polymerase; the DNA chain between the UAS and the TATA-box is looped and it is thus available for transcription.[74]

The transcription of one gene is controlled by more than a single element. For instance, the regulation of the immunoglobulin gene requires at least three distinct types of control sequences; first, an enhancer characteristic of B cells (i.e., activated by a B-cell protein), a lymphoid-specific promoter and enhancer, and some intragenic sequences involved in post-translational control. The B-cell specific enhancer consists of five distinct binding sites (O, E1, E2, E3, E4), four of them binding the same B-cell specific factor. Deletion of any of these sites decreases the enhancer activity but does not abolish it. For *Drosophila* genes there are also several different enhancers controlling the same gene; in different tissues, different enhancers are active. For instance, the maximal expression of the alcohol dehydrogenase, Adh-1 gene, requires the activation of at least three DNA sites; lower levels of gene expression in other tissues require the activation of only two out of these three sites.[70]

The promoter of the mouse albumin gene has at least six binding sites for at least two different proteins.[75] For the rat albumin gene, at least four factors are known which interact with the activating sequences of this gene, one factor being similar or identical to the nuclear factor NF-1.[76] This gene seems to also be under the control of a negative factor,[76] as well as a yeast mating type gene, MAT-alpha, whose silencer binds the same RAP-1 protein which activates transcription when acting upon a UAS of the MAT-alpha gene.[77] An example of enhancers controlled by the same nuclear factor are the enhancers of the metallothioneine $hMT\text{-}II_A$ gene and SV-40 gene; the Ca^{2+} ion modulates the transcription of the two genes.[78]

To sum up, each gene of eukaryotic cells is controlled by several DNA elements (promoters, enhancers) responding to different activating factors. Enhancer elements have several binding sites, the maximal activating effect is obtained when the specific proteins are bound to all sites, while a lower number of bound proteins produces a lower activating effect. This modularity in promoters and enhancers was recently stressed by Dynan.[79] The importance of these features for regulation of gene activation and possible feedback loops for trigger action will be discussed in Sections V.A and V.B.

D. TRANSCRIPTION FACTOR (TFs)

This term (TF) is used for RNA polymerase and other proteins involved in the regulation of DNA-transcription. The cells of higher organisms have three types of RNA polymerases whose action requires several auxilliary proteins for gene recognition, as well as for other processes. The transcription factors have been recently reviewed by Wingender and Seifart[80] and Muramatsu.[81]

RNA polymerase I transcribes the 45 S rRNA precursor. RNA polymerase II transcribes the mRNAs. RNA polymerase III transcribes the small RNAs (t-RNAs, 5S RNA) and several viral RNAs.

Molecular mechanisms of transcription initiation by RNA polymerase I on the ribosomal RNA gene involve at least two factors. The binding of the factor termed TF ID to the promoter sequence is followed by the binding of a second factor, TF IA, and RNA polymerase I. Both factors remain bound to the ribosomal RNA promoter while RNA polymerase I repeats transcription several times. Using a human-mouse chimeric gene constructed by DNA-recombinant techniques, the TF ID recognition site on the promoter was determined. The results have shown that the -12 to -40 sequence was protected by partially purified TF ID against DN-ase I.

RNA polymerase II transcribes the mRNAs and has the most complicated regulation system. The transcription factors TF IIA, TF IIB, TF IID and TF IIE are required for an accurate and efficient initiation of the promoters of the adenovirus major late (AdML) gene, of the *Drosophila* heat shock protein (hsp) gene and the histone H4 and H2B genes. Fingerprinting analysis demonstrated that TF IID is in fact a TATA-box-binding factor, but from one gene to another the fingerprint appears to be different. In the case of the H4 gene, activation by TF IID required a downstream sequence.

For the RNA polymerase III system three factors were identified: the TF IIIA which is required only for initiation of 55 RNA, while TF IIIB and TF IIIC are necessary for all known polymerase III systems.

Recent studies[81] have indicated the existence of three hierarchies in transcriptional control: basic (common), species-specific and tissue-specific. These three modes of regulation were revealed in a fibroin gene system. For instance, using a HeLa extract, the fibroin gene was transcribed, and in this system only the TATA-box was necessary. This was proved using a mutant gene having a deletion up to -31 bp upstream which was still active in transcription. In order to have more efficient transcription of the fibroin gene in other extracts (ovarian tissue, middle silk gland, embryonic cell line, silkworm) another sequence (at -72 bp) is required. The increase in transcription was considered to be supported by species-specific and constitutive-type factors. For tissue-specific enhancement a further upstream region (at -238 bp) appears to be necessary. The sequence -73 to -238 bp could be a tissue-specific ''enhancer-like'' element.

The yeast transcription factor GAL-4 has 88 amino acid residues; the derivative of this protein with only the terminal 74 residues binds to upstream elements of the target gene without activating transcriptions.[82] The activating action of GAL-4 is inhibited by the GAL-80 factor, an inhibition which is reverted by the action of galactose.[83]

The hsp of *Drosophila*, which stimulates the transcription of the hsp 70 gene, has a molecular weight of 110,000 Da and binds specifically to the HSC sequence with a dissociation constant $K_D = 4 \times 10^{-12} M$ (mol/l). The protein also binds to *E. coli* DNA but with a reduced affinity ($K_D = 10^{-6} M$). The HSC sequence is found in one or more copies within the upstream control sequence of the heat shock response element, HSE, of the hsp 70 gene.[84]

Several authors use instead of the term ''transcription factors'' the term ''nuclear factors''

(NFs), like NF-A1, NF-A2, NF-kB. For instance, NF-kB exists in early pre-B cells, but it does not bind to the enhancer except after treatment with lipopolysaccharides (LPS) or phorbol esters (e.g., 13-β-O-tetradecanoylphorbol acetate, TPA), which induce the expression of the k-gene through pretranscriptional modification. In B, T or even HeLa cells treated with TPA, NF-kB appears to be activated, suggesting that the phosphorylation by PKC could be involved in this process. The regulation of the *myc* gene is also relevant; a negative control element (or silencer) between -100 and -353 bp and also a positive control sequence having two NF-1 binding sites were identified, both located near DN-ase hypersensitive sites.[81]

As a conclusion, multiple regulation regions of a gene could be under the control of multiple trans-acting factors. Under some conditions these regions bind different factors, or a factor can be bound at different regulatory regions. Evidence is available for the cooperative binding of transcription factors to such control sites,[70] for instance the binding of the heat shock transcription factor (HSTF) to the heat shock response element (HSE) in *Drosophila*. The binding of two dimeric HSTF molecules to both HSEs of the hsp 70-promoter are required to activate the transcription of the heat shock gene. For the B-cell enhancer elements discussed in the previous paragraph, protein factors binding to three out of the five sites exist also in other cells, but their action is not sufficient for activation; the sites may be inaccessible in other cells or the protein factors must be activated before binding to the sites. The HeLa cell protein TEF-1 binds specifically and cooperatively to two enhancer motifs of SV-40.[85] The GRE/PRE DNA-minisequence, responsible for gene induction by glucocorticoids in rats and by progesterone in chicken, binds in a cooperative manner two receptor-protein molecules.[86] The AP-1 DNA sequence binds either a dimerized c-Jun protein or a complex of one c-Jun and one c-Fos protein molecules.[87] The human estrogen receptor protein, in the presence of estrogen, also binds as a dimer to its specific DNA-binding sequence.[88]

E. NEGATIVE TRANSCRIPTIONAL CONTROLS

Several mechanisms are known for negative transcriptional control (downregulation of transcription). One mechanism consists of binding of the inhibiting protein to an activating transcription factor. The transcriptional inhibitor GAL-80 of the GAL-4 activator binds to this activator and not directly to the DNA.[89] Proteins coded by antioncogenes, for example the one coded by the retinoblastoma gene, act by combining the activating proteins coded by oncogenes.[40-94] A complex of one c-Fos and one c-Jun protein is quoted[93] to bind to the *fos* promoter and to stop the transcription of *fos*. A glucocorticoid receptor, binding the hsp 90, instead of the hormone, is inhibited in its specific transcription activating function.[90]

Another mechanism is the competition of the inhibitor and activator protein for the DNA control sequence. The thyroid receptor protein T_3 binds to the vitellogenin gene A-2 estrogen response element, in competition with the estrogen receptor protein and inhibits the vitellogenin gene transcription.[91] The engrailed gene protein competes with the *ftr* gene protein for transcriptional enhancers specific for the Ft-protein and counteracts ftr-activation.[92]

The *Drosophila eve* gene protein is a repressor for *ubk, ftr* and *wg* genes, but the repression does not seem to be due to competition with an activator protein.[95] The negative regulator of T-cells, responsible for downregulation of the IgA-enhancer action, also seems to interact more directly with the IgA-coding genes.[96] Interaction with a ''silencer'' DNA sequence could be the mechanism for these cases.

Competitive downregulation of the transcription activated by a steroid hormone receptor, by the presence of receptor proteins for other steroid hormones (and by these hormones) implies an intricate mechanism. Competition for a common, limitative, additional transcription factor could be the mechanism for this competitive inhibition.[97]

F. EFFECT OF DNA REPLICATION AND OTHER MECHANISMS ON THE REGULATION OF GENE ACTIVITY

The DNA replication process must produce a temporary dissociation or relaxation of the nucleoproteic complex in order to synthesize the new strand on the template parent strands. This should be a good opportunity for binding new regulator proteins to the DNA control sequences and this occurs in agreement with the "quantal mitosis" — mechanism of Holzer and Rubinstein:[98] a differentiation process is started by a mitosis which produces one daughter cell retaining the characteristics of the parent cell (unmodified DNA-regulator proteins pattern), while the second is committed toward differentiation (new pattern). During mitosis, inactive genes may become available for accidental transcription and this could explain the low but non-zero number of mRNA molecules for the low copy number abundance class (see Section III.B).

The possibility of an "inheritance" of gene superstructure was also considered.[99,100] According to this, both daughter chromatids should inherit the superstructure and the activation pattern of the parent chromatid (by a cooperational binding of the corresponding regulator proteins immediately after DNA replication). Once fixed, a chromatid superstructure (and the corresponding gene activation degree) does not require the maintenance of the mechanism which created it. This would give a straightforward explanation for the maintenance of allelic exclusion (of the X-chromosome, for instance) and of gene activation degrees. Nevertheless, it is not easy to imagine a molecular mechanism by which, during DNA replication, the regulator proteins would recognize and bind to the same type of regulator proteins out of a great number of available proteins. The stable propagation of the active transcriptional state of an immunoglobulin μ-gene, considered as a possible example for the gene superstructure inheritance-mechanism,[100] was recently demonstrated to require the continuous enhancer function.[101]

Alternative explanations for allelic exclusion are also possible. Crossing-over, with formation of a productive and nonproductive rearrangement in the two alleles, was also considered (see p. 653 of Lewin's treatise[2]). An explanation based upon specific repressors could furnish another mechanism. Two alleles (groups of genes) are under the control of the same specific repressor, R, synthesized by both alleles, but an activator, A, binds in the absence of R to the R-control site and makes the allele unresponsive to the action of R. The repressor R is supposed to have a short life and to not be synthesized during a period of time before the replication of the chromosome regions containing the respective alleles. During the S (DNA-replication) period, the active euchromatin is replicated earlier than the inactive heterochromatin. If an allele is situated into an active euchromatin domain, it is replicated first and A (in the absence of R) makes the allele unresponsive to the inhibiting action of R, now synthesized (after some lag for transcription — RNA maturation-translation) by the allele. When the second (inactive) allele, situated in a heterochromatin domain divides, R is present and maintains the inactive state of the resulting pair of alleles. The parent's sex may also affect gene expression, due to different degrees of methylation for the maternal and, respectively, paternal allele.[102] Control of splicing intervenes in *Drosophila* sex determination[103] and in expression of *H-ras* proto-oncogenes.[104] The *H-ras* proto-oncogene transcript contains a negative-acting element. A point mutation in the last intron excludes this element and increases the abundance of the transcript, possibly by increasing the stability of the message.

A blockage of transcriptional elongation was found to produce a 10 to 100 times decrease of the *c-myb*-mRNA levels which accompanies the differentiation of pre-B cells to differentiated B cells in a murine lymphoid tumor.[105] The protein beta-tubulin modulates the stability of its own mRNA, an interesting case of self-regulation in animal cells.[106]

An important mechanism for gene regulation is gene alteration, due especially to transpositions which couple genes to non-neighbor activating enhancer elements (Reference 1,

Chapter 16). This mechanism is involved in the regulation of immunoglobulin synthesis.[107] A transposition of a "mating type" gene, removing it from the neighborhood of a silencer element, is involved in the transition from haploid to diploid state in homothalic yeast.[108]

According to studies upon gene activation in Chinese hamster ovary cells, the cytoskeleton could be implied in gene regulation. The assumed mechanism should be the following: hormonal signals acting upon cell membrane receptors produce changes within cytoskeleton, which extends to the nuclear membrane, where parts of some chromosomes are attached.[109] The possible importance of mechanochemistry, of intra- and intercellular bonds via the matrix system was stressed in a recent *Perspectives in Cancer Research* review.[110] Active genes and their regulatory sequences seem to be attached to the nuclear matrix. This system of microtubules and microfilaments spans like a net in the cytoplasm and penetrates neighboring cells. Disruptions in this mechanical system of information transfer are seen in cancer cells and are correlated to the increased mobility of these cells. Such a mechanism could explain a general control of membrane characteristics, but more specific controls, such as couplings between certain genes and their maintenance during cell proliferation would be much more difficult to explain. DNA-methylation is also considered as a general mechanism for transcriptional repression.[111]

G. GENE REGULATION AND THE RECOGNITION PROBLEM

Gene regulation within the eukaryotic genome involves rather stringent requirements of specificity. The mammalian cell genome corresponds to a DNA-length of approximately 10^9 bp (haploid genome) and almost the same number of short overlapping nucleotidic sequences, among which the regulator proteins must recognize the correct one. Since binding to DNA sequences other than the control sequences may have no influence, this number could be reduced to 10^8 or even 10^7. Such a recognition problem is not trivial:[112] small structural modifications produce only small variations in the effector-receptor affinity and the recognition site of this pair must be large enough in order that all the 10^8 incorrect DNA-sequence-protein pairs have a sufficiently reduced affinity in comparison to the correct regulatory DNA-sequence-protein pair. Evaluations of the required size for the recognition site in the repressor-operator gene interaction in *E. coli* indicate about 20 to 30 bp;[113,114] for the 10^3 times longer mammalian genome, the required size would be about 5 bp larger. The typical size of a regulatory binding site in eukaryotes is 8 to 12 bp; repeated three times[70] since enhancer and promoter elements have a multiple structure, this yields the required size. This multiple structure is considered by Echols[71] to be required by the high specificity of the DNA-regulator protein interactions.

The investigations of the spatial structure of regulatory proteins and of their complexes with DNA sequences, especially for the *E. coli* CAP-protein, cro-protein and lambda-phage repressor explain the specificity of DNA-regulator protein interactions. Molecular framework models demonstrate the formation of a large number of hydrogen bonds and the involvement of other intermolecular forces (e.g., hydrophobic interactions) in such complexes.[115] For the interaction of transcription factors with DNA control elements, similar mechanisms could operate.[116] The DNA binding proteins of eukaryotes (the NHPs) consist of a domain with a well-defined conformation, often dimeric, and a region with poorly defined conformation and an excess of negative charges (acid blob or negative noodles). The specific DNA recognition is based upon a finger structure of the corresponding domain, due to a complex of a Zn^{2+} ion and four cysteine and histidine residues (zinc finger).[117-120] The superfamily of steroid hormone receptors also have Zn^{2+} finger-binding domains consisting of nine Cys residues interspersed with sequences of various lengths (2 to 17) of other amino acidic residues. These domains present a high similarity;[121] small changes in the 13 residues between the second pair of Cys residues seem responsible for the specificity (vs. enhancers) within this family. The exchange of a Gly-Ser sequence in the GRE (glucocorticoid)-receptor produces a protein that activates transcription governed by the ERE (estrogenic) receptor.[122] The DNA-responsive elements (enhancers) for the GRE, ERE and TRE (thyroid hormone) receptors also present similar, palindromic consensus sequences, suggesting that each DNA-element is recognized by a receptor site with a binary symmetry (dimeric receptor).[123] Another type of binding domain with the α-helix-tight turn-α-helix motif is also common for several DNA-binding proteins in prokaryotes and eukaryotes.[121]

This recognition problem also exists for all the other gene regulation mechanisms. Gene transposition requires the recognition and excision of the correct gene by the transposition complex and also the recognition of the new site into which the gene must be located. The hypothetic transmission of chromatin superstructure during DNA replication would require the combination of the evolving, new DNA helixes with the proper "old-type" regulatory proteins, assisted by the existent old-type-proteins of the parent strand. A crystallization-type mechanism favoring the increase of the "active-type" or "inactive-type" nucleoprotein crystal was proposed.[100] Nuclear RNAs as regulators, as in the model of Britten and Davidson,[13,63] could recognize specific sites in DNA through the complementary base pairing mechanism, but the hormone-receptor protein complex should also have to recognize the correct nuclear RNA.

H. GENE CONTROL SYSTEMS AND THEIR MODIFICATION IN MALIGNANT CELLS; ONCOGENES

The knowledge of the control systems for the genes involved in growth and differentiation would help in understanding carcinogenesis. Until now, only a few gene control systems were studied, and even these are not completely understood. Such a system is the control of the yeast cell cycle.[108] This control consists in a hierarchical sequence of gene activation and deactivation processes in which the product of a gene activates or deactivates other genes. A gene transposition is also involved in this control. In order to obtain the correct pattern of the so called "mating-type" switches in this cycle, an accurate timing of the various activations of transcriptions is required and the regulatory products, coded by the genes, must have short lifetimes.

The homeobox, where the genes involved in the control of development in higher organisms are located, was also studied from the viewpoint of gene control, especially in *Drosophila*.[124] The homeobox proteins are sequence-specific transcription factors which control the timing of gene activation in different segments of the developing embryo.[125] Several cases of autoregulation were recently discovered for homeobox genes. The engrailed protein binds specifically to DNA sequences upstream of several genes, including its own coding gene.[125] A self-regulatory function of the engrailed protein is probable, as well as for the product of one of the *eve* genes.[126] The Dfd protein also autoactivates its expression from the *dfd*-locus, a self-regulation circuit which supplies a simple mechanism for the stability of the determination state controlled by *dfd*.[127]

An interesting point in molecular oncology was the discovery that more than 50 normal genes (proto-oncogenes) have the potential to induce cancer when they become activated (oncogenes).[128] We have discussed (Section II.C) that many of these genes (especially *ras* family genes) are considered to be targets for mutations that are responsible for cell transformation. Many of these genes are believed to be involved in the regulation processes of normal growth and development. The oncogenes were first identified in retroviruses. It has been established that these genes have been acquired by the viruses from the genome of mammalian normal cells. In normal cells the proto-oncogenes are silent or only temporarily transcribed.

The *c-fos* gene — a multifaceted proto-oncogene — belongs to this class, and this gene is homologous with the *v-fos* oncogene found in two related murine viruses (FBJ-MSV and FBR-MSV) which produce osteogenic sarcoma.[129-130] The elucidation of the molecular structure of the *fos* oncogene casts light on the system of complex regulation of its expression

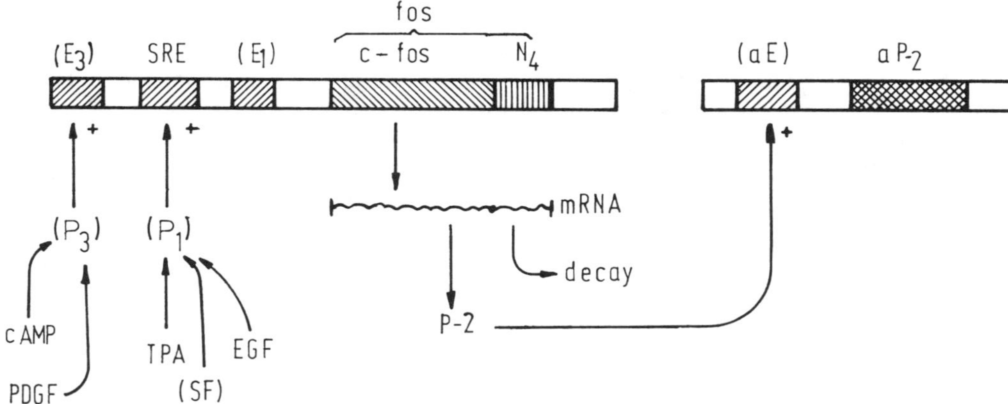

FIGURE 2.   Control processes of the *c-fos* gene. E-1, SRE, E-3-activating sequences of the *c-fos* gene, aE-of the aP2 gene (adipocyte gene), aE′ of the *c-jun* gene. The N-4 sequence of the *c-fos* gene encodes a nucleotidic sequence enhancing the degradation of the *c-fos*-mRNA. The proteins coded by the genes *c-fos* and *c-jun* are c-Fos and c-Jun, respectively. P-1-protein implied in the *c-fos* activation by TPA (phorbol esters), SF (serum factor) and EGF (epidermal growth factor) activate the *c-fos* gene via the E-3 sequence. The *c-jun* gene is activated by a c-Fos-c-Jun heterodimer.

in a variety of cell types. Figure 2 summarizes the control processes studied for this gene. The following regulatory sites of the *fos* gene were discovered: (1) a site (marked E_1 in Figure 2), 100 bp upstream the transcription start; (2) the SRE-site and (3) a negative control site (N_4) located after the transcription terminator site. SRE is activated by a specific protein (P_1) which probably mediates the effect of the epidermal growth factor, EGF, serum factor (SF) and of phorbol esters (TPA). The SRE-sequence and the c-Fos protein coded by the *c-fos* gene are strongly conserved during evolution; similar elements are found in *Xenopus laevis*. The E_3-sequence is involved in the induction of the *c-fos* gene by platelet-derived growth factor (PDGF) and by c-AMP. The deletion of the (N_4) chromosomal sequence increases the stability of the transcribed *fos*-mRNA and is implied in the conversion of the normal proto-oncogene into the corresponding oncogene. The c-Fos protein binds to a control sequence (aE) of the adipocyte gene aP2, activating it during the adipocyte differentiation. The serum growth factors and the other inducers of the *c-fos* gene activate cellular kinases which produce protein phosphorylation. Factors which bind specifically to *c-fos* enhancers are found in HeLa cells, but in A 431 and BALB/3T3 mouse cells such factors appear only after the cell cultures were treated with EGF or PDGF, respectively.

The recently discovered *v-jun* oncogene in avian sarcoma virus has been shown to encode a protein with homology to a protein (GCN4) from yeast that regulates DNA transcription. It was found that, using DNA-recombinant technique for making chimeres of GCN4 in yeast by substituting the *jun* sequences which encodes GCN4, the yeast still makes a product that functions like GCN4.[131] The *v-jun* oncogene and the human proto-oncogene *c-jun* encode DNA-binding proteins similar, as structure and DNA-binding specificities, to the human transcription factor AP-1 (isolated from HeLa cells).[132] The AP-1 factor was shown to bind to DNA sequences identical to those of GCN4.[134] The product of the *c-jun* gene and AP-1 have common antigenic and enhancer-binding properties suggesting that these proteins are closely related, if not even identical.[133] Actually, the human DNA sequence *c-jun* encodes one of the polypeptides present in affinity-purified preparations of AP-1. The *c-fos* proto-oncogene is also associated with the AP-1 recognition sequence, the protein p 39, which was demonstrated to be the product of *c-jun*.[135,136]

These proteins are products of families of inducible genes and could play an important role in modulating gene expression at the end of a cascade of signals transduced directly from the cell surface. For example, the cotranslated c-Jun and c-Fos proteins bind (together, one molecule of each) 25 times more efficiently to the AP-1 DNA-binding site (of *c-jun*) than the c-Jun homodimer.[87] The gene product enhances *c-jun* activation function of TPA, probably also via the c-Jun-c-Fos protein complex. The formation of this complex is stabilized by a heptad repeat of leucine residues, the so called leucine zipper (hydrophobic interaction).[136-138] This c-Fos-c-Jun complex is quoted to inhibit the transcription of the *c-fos* gene and to be responsible for the only transient activation of this gene in response to TPA induction.[93] The *c-jun* proto-oncogene is also positively autoregulated by its product, c-Jun and this positive loop is probably responsible for the prolongation of transient signals generated by the activation of protein kinase C.[139]

The transcription factor Sp1 and NK-1 kB-like factor are implied in the activation of HIV (AIDS retrovirus).[142,143] An array of regulatory genes enables HIV to remain latent or replicate at various rates. The *tat* gene increases the production of viral proteins indiscriminantly. The *rev* gene has differential effects: if, due to splicing, the CAR-sequence is eliminated out of the transcribed mRNA, a repressor results, but if the whole mRNA (with CAR-sequence) is transcribed, the rev-protein overrides the repressive effects and viral growth is switched on. The *nef* gene protein is, probably, attached to the inside of the cell membrane and exerts inhibitory effects via some cellular second messenger. Modulation of selective mRNA transport could play a role in this regulation.[144,145] Tumor necrosis factor α stimulates HIV-1 gene expression. Cytokines are also involved. These results support the idea that infection and immunologic stimulation may trigger the development of the latent virus.[146]

An adenovirus *E1A* gene promoter, which probably also exists in normal mammalian cells, is activated by a factor E2F found in F-9 teratocarcinoma cells and in HeLa cells.[147] When the F-9 cells differentiate under the effect of retinoic acid and c-AMP, both the E2F-factor and the *E1A* gene product decrease below the detection limit. These two factors increase when the gene is introduced in differentiated cells through adenovirus infection. The activation of the E1A gene by the E2F factor seems to require the activity of the gene itself, suggesting a positive, autoactivating feedback.

Viral promoters and enhancers, such as those of SV-40 and adenovirus, are active in most cell types.[70,148] Their activity level seems to be regulated by some cellular or viral products which act upon other transcription factors. Immediate early viral proteins, IE, promote the activity of various RNA polymerases of type II and III. Such promotion is absent in virus mutants for the corresponding EI gene. Even in absence of viral infection, nondifferentiated embryocarcinoma cells contain an IE-like factor which disappears when these cells differentiate.

Not all oncogene products are necessarily transcription factors only. A large family of genes, including several proto-oncogenes, code for proteins with tyrosine-kinase activity in various organisms, including *Saccharomyces, Drosophila* and mammals. A many-fold increase of *src* expression was observed during differentiation of HL-60 cells. The proto-oncogenes *src, fms, lck, fes, fos* are preferentially activated in brain cells. The *ras* oncogene also belongs to this family. These kinases also phosphorylate other proteins with a role in differentiation and malignant transformation.[81,149]

The product of the *c-myc* oncogene as a role in the DNA replication complex; it is involved in breast cancer.[150] Rearrangement of *c-myc* juxtaposing it to the heavy chain immunoglobulin enhancer was found in DNA from acute lymphoblastic leukemia cells.[151]

Tumor promoters are also implied in transcription activation, for example they induce increased levels of m-RNA transforming growth factor (TGF-beta) in epidermal cells when applied upon mouse skin.[152] A review on regulation of gene expression by tumor promoters was recently written by Carter.[153] DNA methylation is also supposed to play a role in regulating gene expression, differentiation and carcinogenesis.[154] Chemical carcinogens perturb DNA methylation: altered 5-methyl-cytosine DNA levels are found in various natural

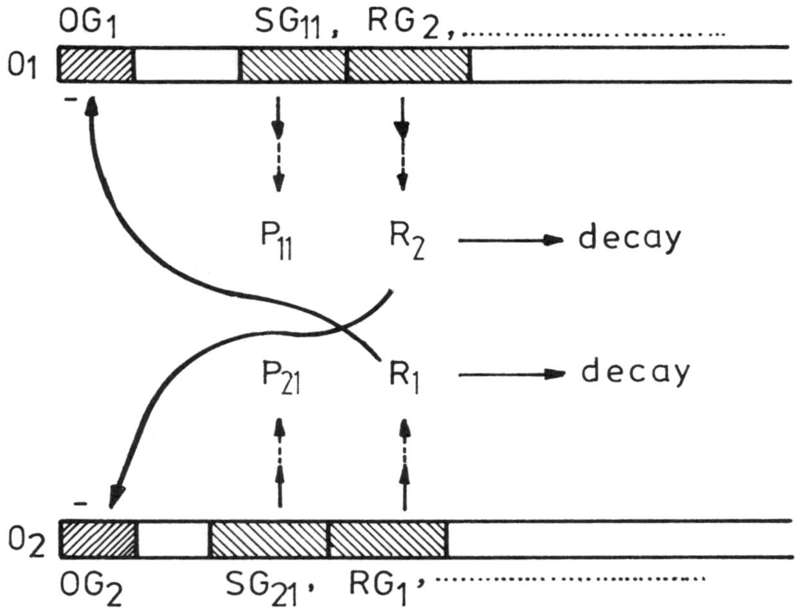

FIGURE 3. The Monod-Jacob trigger. O_1, O_2 = operons; SG_{11}, SG_{12} . . . synthesis genes; RG_1, RG_2 = regulator genes, R_1, R_2 = repressors; P_{11}, P_{21} . . . = products.

and experimental tumors, processes which could be related to various malignant transformation of the cells. One should mention that nongenotoxic substances can also play a role in carcinogenesis.[155]

Let us remind here that qualitative models also implying positive regulation of translation were set up for the "mating-type" switch in homothalic yeast[108] (see also Section III.F) and for viral infections, especially for the latency-pathogenic switch of the HIV-virus[144] (see also Section III.H).

IV. MATHEMATICAL MODELS FOR NEGATIVE GENE CONTROL

A. GENERAL PRINCIPLES

The differentiation process in higher organisms requires a mechanism by which stable active and inactive states for the transcription of various genes are maintained, but also allowing switches between such states. A model for such a mechanism was already given by Monod and Jacob,[6] i.e., the trigger of cross and feedback interrelated operons by repressors (Figure 3).

Several mathematical models based upon this hypothetical trigger appeared in the 1960s and early 1970s.[156-160] Although the Monod and Jacob regulation is not operative, or at least not dominant in higher cells, we shall discuss here some aspects of this model. Several of the developed ideas are pertinent for the positive control, as well as for the integration problem of triggers into the entire cell regulation. Negative control elements (silencers, dehancers) were also observed among the control elements of eukaryotic genes (see Section III.C). Some models for oscillatory gene activities will also be discussed here.

These models are based upon a simplified usual scheme of reaction involving transcription, translation, decay process, effector-receptor equilibria, etc. The kinetics of these processes are described by a set of differential equations, with protein and RNA concentrations as time-dependent variables. The system of equations is studied analytically or by computer simulation, in search of conditions producing stable steady-states or oscillatory behavior. Eventually the trigger is simplified as a Boolean element and integrated into a molecular automaton model of a more complex regulatory system.

B. POLY-STEADY-STATE TRIGGERS WITH NEGATIVE CONTROL

Consider the Monod-Jacob trigger of Figure 3. If the operon O_1 is transcribed, the repressor R_2 is synthesized and operon O_2 is repressed: on the contrary, if O_2 is transcribed, O_1 must be repressed. This trigger should thus have two steady-states. The switch could be achieved by the temporary effect of an inducer-type substance which combines with R_2 and inactivates it. The operator gene OG_2 will dissociate the bound R_2-molecule, operon O_2 will be transcribed, producing R_1 which represses operon O_2. Some time thereafter the inactivated R_2-molecules will disappear through enzymatic lysis and the new state, O_2-active, O_1-inactive, remains stable even if the inducer is withdrawn.

Let us write down the equations describing the kinetics of this trigger. With y denoting the protein concentration, x the concentration of mRNA, the transcription, translation and decay processes are described by:

$$\frac{dx}{dt} = \frac{1}{V}\,\varphi A - \lambda_N x \tag{1a}$$

$$\frac{dy}{dt} = \Psi x - \lambda_P y \tag{1b}$$

V is the cell volume (or perhaps the nucleus volume), φ and Ψ are transcription and translation rates, respectively, λ_N and λ_P are decay rates for mRNA and protein, and A is the gene activation degree. Consider a simple association-dissociation equilibrium for the repressor-operator gene interaction, as in Figure 3.

$$OG + R \rightleftharpoons OG_{rep} \qquad \frac{[OG]y}{[OG_{rep}]} = K \tag{2}$$

the gene activation degree will be:

$$A = \frac{[OG]}{[OG] + [OG_{rep}]} = \frac{K}{K + y} \tag{3}$$

$[OG]$ and $[OG_{rep}]$ represent the concentration of free and repressed operator gene, respectively, A is the probability that the operator gene is not repressed at the given repressor concentration, y.

If the mRNA has a relatively short life ($\lambda_N \gg \lambda_P$) the steady-state assumption can be adopted for its concentration ($dx/dt = 0$), and one can use a single equation for the kinetics of the protein synthesis and decay:

$$\frac{dy}{dt} = kA - \lambda_P y; \qquad k = \frac{\Psi\varphi}{V\lambda_n} \tag{4}$$

With these assumptions, the equations describing the Monod-Jacob trigger are:

$$\frac{dy_1}{dt} = \frac{k_1 K_1}{K_1 + y_2} - \lambda_1 y_1 \tag{5a}$$

$$\frac{dy_2}{dt} = \frac{k_2 K_2}{K_2 + y_1} - \lambda_2 y_2 \tag{5b}$$

Heinmets[156] studied such a trigger by using computer simulation. His system was actually more complicated, also considering other processes which take place during enzyme synthesis in bacterial systems, but all these processes were described by simple, noncooperative kinetic and equilibrium equations. His model was successful in simulating several processes, such as substrate induction and product inhibition, but did not succeed in finding a trigger behavior for two interrelated operons. Instead, both operons were transcribed at a submaximal rate.

An analytical study of the system (Equations 5a,b), showed that the Monod-Jacob trigger had a single steady-state if the R-OG-interaction is based upon a simple, type 2 equilibrium.[157] Two stable states can be obtained in somewhat more complicated systems, for example, if transcription can be interrupted by collision with the repressor molecule before the mRNA chain has reached a certain length,[157] or if R_2 has a protease action and increases the decay rate of R_1.[158] The most realistic solution is to consider a cooperational character for the R-OG-interaction, i.e., at least two molecules of R, ($n \geq 2$) must combine with the OG to produce repression:[159]

$$OG + nR \rightleftharpoons OG_{rep}; \qquad K = \frac{[OG]y^n}{[OG_{rep}]}; \quad n \geq 2 \tag{6}$$

and the system of equations becomes:

$$\frac{dy_1}{dt} = \frac{kK_1}{K_1 + y_2^n} - \lambda_1 y_1 \tag{7a}$$

$$\frac{dy_2}{dt} = \frac{kK_2}{K_2 + y_1^n} - \lambda_2 y_2 \tag{7b}$$

This system was studied by computer simulation and two stable steady-states were indeed obtained, one corresponding to almost maximal transcription of O_1 and almost complete repression of O_2 and the second to the reverse situation.

The Monod-Jacob triggers were studied also in the framework of Prigogine's theory of dissipative instabilities.[160] The existence of a stable steady-state, within well-defined ranges of parameter values, was proved.

The existence of stable steady-states for the system of Equations (5a,b) and (7a,b) is proved in Appendix 1.

C. MODELS FOR OSCILLATORY BEHAVIOR

The models for an oscillating system in which the concentration of certain substances undergo periodic variations are of obvious interest for cell cycle and growth control. Such models were given by Goodwin[161] and are based upon negative feedback with several retarding links (Figure 4). The functioning of such models is described by a system of equations of the types:

$$\frac{dX_1}{dt} = \frac{K}{K + X_m^n} \Psi - \lambda_1 X_1 \tag{8a}$$

$$\frac{dX_2}{dt} = k_1 L X_1 - \lambda_2 X_2 \tag{8b}$$

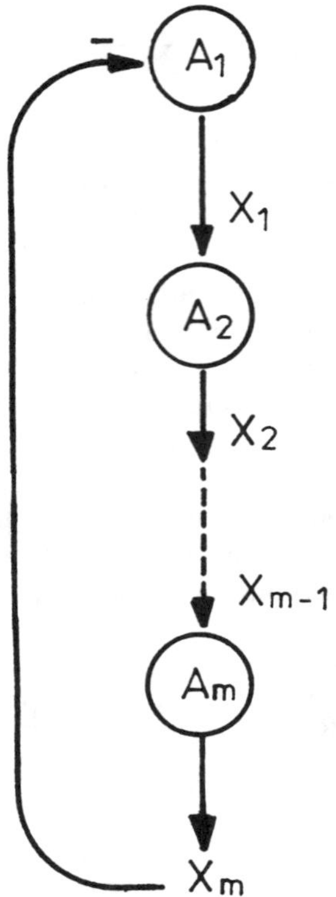

FIGURE 4.   Model for cyclic behavior: X_1, X_2 . . . , are substrates for reactions A_2, A_3 . . . , X_m is an inhibitor of reaction A_1.

$$\frac{dX_m}{dt} = k_{n-1}X_{n-1} - \lambda_n X_n \tag{8c}$$

Simulations on analogic computers have demonstrated the possibility of undamped oscillations, although these occur in a seemingly narrow range of parameter values.[162] The problem is that such systems are analogous to mechanical systems with friction, in which all oscillations are damped. Analogic computers introduce some stochastic components in the concentrations (X_is) and this maintains oscillations as well as the doubling of the genetic material, as in a model for self-maintained oscillations for beta-galactosidase activity in *E. coli*.[163]

More complicated systems of such oscillators, coupled by some of their products, were simulated on digital computers by Fraser, Tivari and Beckman[164,165] with and without specially introduced stochastic components. They conclude that loops consisting of a single gene without stochastic components present undamped oscillations only is very restrictive, unrealistic conditions. If stochastic components are introduced, undamped oscillations appear, but they are of an irregular nature. Cyclic systems consisting of an uneven number of genes with a feedback loop present undamped oscillations also in the absence of stochastic components if the efficiency of feedback repression, and the translations rates, are high enough. The period of oscillations is determined by the lifetimes of proteins. Allowance for stochastic components reduce the requirements for the appearance of undamped oscillations. A recent study concerning oscillations and multiple steady-states in cyclic genome models is also to be mentioned[166] as well as a general study concerning stability of oscillating chemical reactions.[167]

The interest of such systems for cell cycle models is obvious. A system of two operons with feedback cycle controlled by their proteins was used as a model for regulation of a phage replication.[168]

D. INTERCONNECTED GENES AS CELL REGULATION MODELS

A model for the self-regulation of mitotic and functional cell activity was devised by Tsanev and Sendov[169] based upon the Monod-Jacob trigger and the model of Bullough for growth regulation (see Section II.B). In this model the mitotic operon and the "histospecific operon" are cross and feedback interconnected by their repressor and form a trigger which controls DNA replication and cell division via a mitotic protein. Diffusion of a regulating substance — the chalone, among a subset of cells is also considered. This model, described by about 20 differential equations, with all or none conditions for gene activation, allows the description of (by computer simulation) cell division and synthesis of a histospecific protein as expected for the Bullough model. The same type of model, but with several individual elements, was used for simulating the carcinogenesis process of the liver.[170,171] Differentiation processes were simulated by the same authors[172] using the above mentioned model in which irreversible blockage of genes by histone (chromatin superstructure inherited through DNA replication — see Section III.E) is also considered. A mathematical model for the trigger mechanism for temperature activation of a *src* oncogene mutant was set up by Kovarski and Porfir,[173] based upon negative transcriptional control.

If large numbers of interconnected genes are considered, one has to adopt simplifying assumptions. The genes are considered to be bistable Boolean elements with two states: 0 for inactive and 1 for active. The state of one gene at a given moment is a function of all the gene states one step before, due to the absence or presence of an effector (repressor, activator) synthesized by these genes. The cell regulation system is thus considered as a molecular automaton.[174] Such networks of randomly connected Boolean elements, as models for gene regulation, homeostasis, metabolism, differentiation, were devised by Kauffman.[175] In a more realistic version, the networks are buffered, i.e., the gene products acting upon the gene inputs, according to a threshold concentration rule, are continuously synthesized and allowed to accumulate in time.[176] The time evolution in the gene activation phase space was studied for networks of up to 80 elements. After an initial period, either a stable state or a periodic behavior is attained, i.e., a point or a closed curve in the phase space. For all simulations, the number of states actually obtained is much lower than the one theoretically possible for the network. Transitions between stable states are also possible by temporal modifications in concentrations of "critical" effectors, but even for dramatic modifications in "noncritical" effectors, the system retains the previous stable state after a readjustment period.

V. POSITIVE FEEDBACK TRIGGER FOR GENE REGULATION

A. EXPERIMENTAL EVIDENCE AND SPECIFIC REQUIREMENTS

Gene activation by specific NHPs has suggested a trigger with positive feedback, in which the NHP activates its own gene.[5,11,12] Such a trigger could exist in an inactive or active state and the NHP coded by it could also control (activate) other genes with a common control element, which is responsive to the same NHP. A simple and attractive model results in the differential activation of genes in the cells of different tissues.[177] We have proved, by analytical and computer simulation studies, that with reasonable assumptions for kinetic and equilibrium parameters, this trigger explains a series of features of gene regulation in eukaryotes.[178,179]

Evidence for the existence of such triggers appeared recently. The engrailed protein, coded by *Drosophila* homeobox gene, binds to an upstream DNA sequence of its own gene.[125] The activation of the E1A gene of F-9 and HeLa cells by the E2F factor also seems to imply an autoactivation mechanism.[147] Other cases of gene self-regulation were found for the *eve* gene[126] and the *dfd* gene in *Drosophila*[127] and for the *c-jun* proto-oncogene[139] (see also Section III.H). Positive autoregulation seems to exist also for the myogenic determination gene *myoD1*[140] and for the *ftr* gene of *Drosophila*.[141] There are several data concerning the features of NHP-control element interactions.[70] Each gene seems to have more than a single activating element (promoter, enhancer), responding to different NHPs. The control elements have a multiple nature, binding more than a single NHP molecule (usually two). Binding of NHPs to all control elements allows a maximal transcription rate, while a reduced transcription rate is obtained if only a part of the control elements binds NHPs (see also Sections III.C and III.D).

The following gene regulation features must be explained and reproduced by simulation by the trigger with positive feedback:

1. The trigger must have two (or better three) stable steady-states corresponding to the three mRNA abundance classes (see Section III.B): the inactive "O"-state for the low number class; a low activity "I" — state for the moderately prevalent class; a high activity "II" — state for the supervalent class.
2. The trigger states should be stable within reasonable ranges of parameter values and of concentrations for the NHP and its mRNA. For example, the "O"-state must be stable for the concentrations of NHP and its mRNA corresponding to the low number abundance class.
3. Transitions between trigger states should be possible under the temporary action of external effectors inducing cell differentiation (hormones, growth factors, morphogens).
4. The kinetics of the trigger, and the time for switches and for reaching stable-states, should be in the range of hours, as required by hormonal induction and differentiation processes.
5. For a sufficient functional reliability a single mutation in pertinent genes and control elements in diploid cells should not dramatically affect the stability of trigger states and the characteristics of switches between states.
6. An interpretation must be given for the fact that some cells are competent for induction of differentiation processes and for the synthesis of certain proteins, while others are not.

B. TRIGGER WITH POSITIVE FEEDBACK MODEL

The idea of a trigger with positive feedback is the following:[177,178] the synthesis gene, SG, for the activating NHP, is activated by a combination of the control elements (promoter, enhancer) with two molecules of NHP. The resulting mRNA transcription rate yields a NHP-concentration sufficient to maintain the gene activation. For higher NHP-concentration, two further molecules of NHP combine with the control elements, and a higher activation degree of the SG results, yielding a higher NHP-concentration able to maintain the second activation degree (Figure 5). The combination of control elements with more than one molecule of NHP is required by the mathematics of the model and agrees with the above-mentioned multiple nature of control elements (enhancers; see also Section III.C).

The system of equations describing our trigger model is:

$$\frac{dx}{dt} = \frac{\varphi_1}{V} A_1 + \frac{\varphi_2}{V} A_2 - \lambda_N x \qquad (9a)$$

$$\frac{dy}{dt} = \Psi x - \lambda_p y \qquad (9b)$$

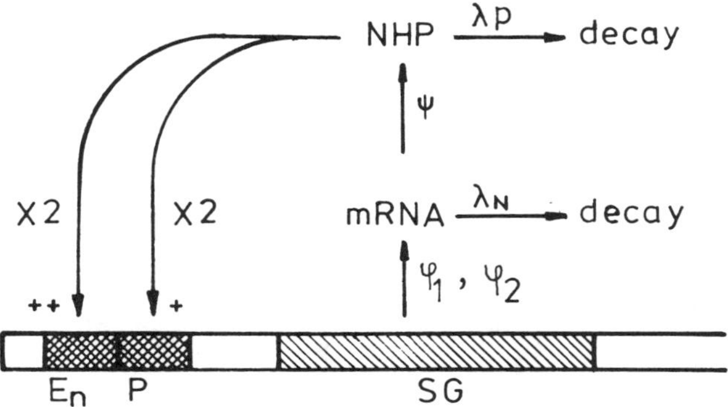

FIGURE 5.   Trigger with positive control and three stable steady-states. NHP — activator protein; mRNA its messenger; λ_P, λ_N — decay rates. φ_1, φ_2 — low and high activity transcription rates, Ψ — translation rate; Pr, En — promoter, enhancer; SG — synthesis gene for the NHP.

$$A_1 = \frac{y^n}{K_1 + y^n}; \qquad A_2 = \frac{y^n}{K_2 + y^n} \tag{9c}$$

$$n \geq 2; \quad K_1 \ll K_2; \quad \varphi_1 \ll \varphi_2 \tag{9d}$$

The mRNA-concentration is x, the NHP-concentration is y, the transcription rates for low and high gene activity are φ_1 and φ_2, the translation rate of mRNA is Ψ, and the mRNA- and NHP-decay rates are λ_N and λ_P; the cell volume is V.

The already mentioned assumption of cooperativity for promoter (enhancer)-NHP interaction (n $\geq$2) gives a natural explanation for a discontinuous range for gene activation degrees A_1 and A_2. Consider the equilibrium:

$$Pr + nNHP \rightleftharpoons Pr_{act}; \quad \frac{[Pr]y^n}{[Pr_{act}]} = K_1 \tag{10}$$

with the corresponding gene activation degree

$$A_1 = \frac{[Pr_{act}]}{[Pr] + [Pr_{act}]} = \frac{y^n}{K_1 + y^n} \tag{11}$$

[Pr] and [Pr$_{act}$] are the concentrations of the promoter in the inactive transcription state and of the activated promoter (by combination with NHPs), respectively. The gene activation degree A_1 (for low transcription rate) is equal to the probability of binding the promoter in the active state at the given NHP-concentration, y. For the high transcription rate the corresponding equations refer to the activation degree A_2, with [En] and [En$_{act}$] for the concentrations of the inactive and activated enhancer, respectively, and with the higher enhancer-NHP-dissociation-constant K_2. In Figure 6, the $A_1 = A_1(y)$ — function is depicted for n = 1 (broken curve) and the n = 3 (full curve). While for n = 1, A_1 increases from 0 to 1 in a large interval of y-concentration, for n = 3 this interval becomes much narrower. For a high degree of cooperativity (n $\gg$1), A_1 will be a step function of y, with $A_1 = 1$ for y $> K_1^{1/n}$ and A = 0 for y $< K_1^{1/n}$ and no intermediate gene activation degrees are possible.

As proved by computer simulations,[179] there are really three stable steady-state solutions for the system (Equations 9a to d). If a high degree of cooperativity is assumed, these solutions (A, C, E) together with the two unstable steady-state solutions (B, D) are:

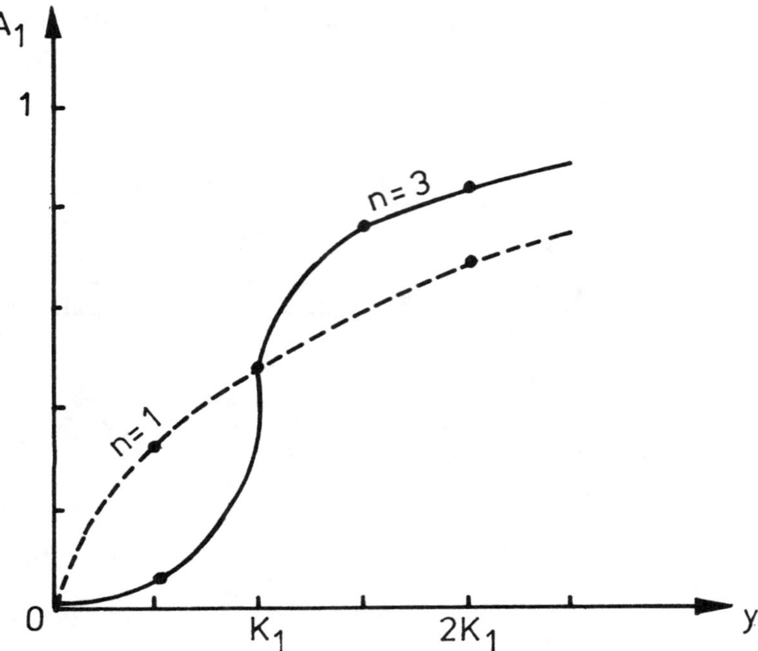

FIGURE 6. The $A_1 = A_1(y)$ dependence for $n = 1$ and $n = 3$; A_1 — gene activation degree; y — NHP — concentration; $n = 1$ — noncooperative, $n = 3$ — cooperative behavior.

A: stable, "O"-inactive state:

$$x_O = 0, \qquad y_O = 0 \tag{12a}$$

B: instable (O-I transition):

$$x_B = \frac{\lambda_P}{\Psi} K_1^{1/n}, \qquad y_B = K_1^{1/n} \tag{12b}$$

C: stable, "I"-low activity state:

$$x_I = \frac{\varphi_1}{V\lambda_N}, \qquad y_1 = \frac{\varphi_1}{V\lambda_N\lambda_P} \tag{12c}$$

D: instable (I-II transition):

$$x_D = \frac{\lambda_P}{\Psi} K_2^{1/n} \quad y = K_2^{1/n} \tag{12d}$$

E: stable, "I"-high activity state:

$$x_{II} = \frac{\varphi_2}{V\lambda_N}, \qquad y_{II} = \frac{\varphi_2}{V\lambda_N\lambda_P} \tag{12e}$$

These solutions and their stability are discussed in Appendix 2 where it is also demonstrated that in order to obtain all three stable-state solutions, the following inequalities must be satisfied:

$$K_1^{1/n} \ll \frac{\varphi_1 \Psi}{V \lambda_N \lambda_P} \ll K_2^{1/n} \ll \frac{\varphi_2 \Psi}{V \lambda_N \lambda_P} \tag{13}$$

Transition between the stable steady-states are supposed to be produced by the temporary presence of external effectors which combine with the NHP and increase or decrease its affinity for the DNA control element (promoter, enhancer). In our model, the NHP-promoter (or enhancer) dissociation constant K_1 (or K_2) is decreased or, respectively, increased to a new value K_{1N} (or K_{2N}), for a certain time interval. For instance, for an activating $I \rightarrow II$ transition, the initial steady-state concentrations are x_I, y_I; K_2 is decreased to K_{2N} such that $y_I^n > K_{2N}$. The second set of NHP-molecules combines with the enhancer and the high gene activation results ($A_2 = 1$). The NHP-concentration increases; when a sufficiently high concentration is reached, $y > K_2^{1/n}$, the system will evolve toward the II state, even if the old K_2-value is restored.

The $f(x,y)$-curves which separate stability domains of the O, I and II states cannot be obtained by analytical methods; all that one can say is that the unstable solutions, x_B, y_B and, respectively, x_D, y_D (Equations 12b, d) must be situated upon these curves.

For other genes controlled by the same NHP ("slave genes" in terms of hierarchical models[13]) and the activation degree will be the same as for the trigger ("master gene") which controls them.

A discussion of the steady-state solutions of Equations 9a to d and of their stability is given in Appendix 2.

C. COMPUTER SIMULATION

The system of Equations 9a to d was studied by computer simulations, concerning the time dependence of the mRNA- and NHP-concentrations, the stability of the steady-states and switches between steady-states.[179] The program for these simulations and for the corresponding graphics is described in Appendix 3.

For most runs, the following set of parameters was used:

$$V = 1; \varphi_1 = 1; \varphi_2 = 100; \Psi = 1; K_1 = 0.01; K_2 = 100; \lambda_N = 4; \lambda_P = 1 \tag{14}$$

The duration of each run was fixed, usually, to 10 time units, and the time step was usually fixed to 0.1 time units. For the parameter set (Equation 14) the steady-state values obtained in the simulations were:

$$x_o = y_o = 0; \quad x_1 = y_1 = 0.22; \quad x_{II} = y_{II} = 20.4 \tag{15}$$

rather close to the approximate solutions (Equations 12a to e):

$$x_o = y_o = 0; \quad x_I = y_I = 0.25; \quad x_{II} = y_{II} = 25 \tag{15a}$$

The approximate values for the unstable solutions B and D (Equations 12b, d):

$$x_B = y_B = 0.10; \quad x_D = y_D = 10$$

should also represent separating values between the "O" and "I" states and, respectively, between "I" and "II" states. This may be compared to the final concentration values x_f, y_f — obtained for different initial $x(O)$, $y(O)$ concentrations in a series of runs listed in

TABLE 1

Time Evolution of System (9a to d)

Set of parameters	Initial conc.		Final conc		
	x(0)	y(0)	xf	yf	State
(14) $V = 1$, $\varphi_1 = 1$,	0.030	0.030	0.00	0.00	0
$\varphi_2 = 100$, $\Psi = 1$,	0.060	0.100	0.22	0.22	I
	0.950	2.00	0.22	0.22	I
$K_1 = 0.01$; $K_2 = 100$	1.00	2.00	0.22	0.22	I
$\lambda_N = 4$, $\lambda_P = 1$	4.00	5.00	20.4	20.4	II
	16.00	4.00	20.4	20.4	II
	22.00	21.00	20.4	20.4	II
(14) $V = 1$, $\varphi_1 = 1$,	0.030	0.030	0.00	0.00	0
$\varphi_2 = 100$, $\Psi = 1$,	0.060	0.030	0.00	0.00	0
	0.060	0.100	0.44	0.22	I
$K_1 = 0.01$, $K_2 = 100$	0.200	0.100	0.44	0.22	I
$\lambda_N = 2$, $\lambda_P = 2$	20.50	4.00	40.8	20.4	II
	22.00	4.00	40.8	20.4	II
(14b) $V = 1$, $\varphi_1 = 1$,	0.030	0.030	0.00	0.00	0
$\varphi_2 = 100$, $\Psi = 1$,	0.120	0.030	0.00	0.00	0
$K_1 = 0.01$, $K_2 = 100$,	0.060	0.100	0.875	0.22	I
	28.50	4.00	81.6	20.4	II
$\lambda_N = 1$, $\lambda_P = 4$	48.8	11.6	81.6	20.4	II
(14c) $V = 1$, $\varphi_1 = 1$,	0.150	0.300	5.10	10.20	II
$\varphi_2 = 100$, $\Psi = 1$,	0.300	0.600	5.10	10.20	II
	1.00	2.00	5.10	10.20	II
$K_1 = 0.25$, $K_2 = 9$,	2.00	4.00	5.10	10.20	II
$\lambda_N = 2$, $\lambda_P = 0.5$	7.50	15.00	5.10	10.20	II

Table 1. For three of the parameter sets, three stable steady-states are obtained, except the last one (14c), in which all the runs finally yielded the high activation x_{II}, y_{II} values. This is because of a less drastic fulfillment of inequalities (13) by the set of parameters (14c, Table 1) where:

$$K_1^{1/2} = 0.5; \quad \varphi_1\Psi/V\lambda_N\lambda_P = 1; \quad K_2^{1/2} = 3; \quad \varphi_2\Psi/V\lambda_N\lambda_P = 10$$

Different runs with parameters (14) are illustrated in Figure 7a to e and for increased protein synthesis rates in Figure 8a,b. The steady-state values are reached after about 5 to 10 time units, in a time interval about 10 times larger than the slowest decay time (λ_N^{-1} or λ_P^{-1}).

Activating I → II switches were simulated by decreasing K_2 to $K_{2N} = 1$ from $t = 0$ until a threshold $y_o \geq 5.0$ was reached, for the parameter set (14) in Figure 9a, and for the set with $\lambda_N = 2$, $\lambda_P = 2$ in Figure 9c. A deactivating II → I switch was simulated by the increase of K_2 to $K_{2N} = 200$ until y decreased below a threshold $y_o \leq 2.0$ (Figure 9b, parameter set [14]). The time required for the activating switches was about one time unit, for the deactivating switch about 12 time units.

The simulations prove the general validity of the qualitative analysis of the trigger behavior given in the previous paragraph. The following general requirements for models of gene regulation and differentiation are also met: (1) more than a single stable steady-state solution; (2) stability of these solutions in a reasonable range of initial concentrations and parameters and (3) the possibility of switch between states of different gene activation degrees.

D. EVALUATION OF PER-CELL VALUES FOR THE STEADY-STATES

Mammalian cells have volumes V roughly 10^{-12} 1.[180] For maximal RNA synthesis rates, e.g., for HeLa cells with several thousands of rRNA molecules per ribosomal cistron and

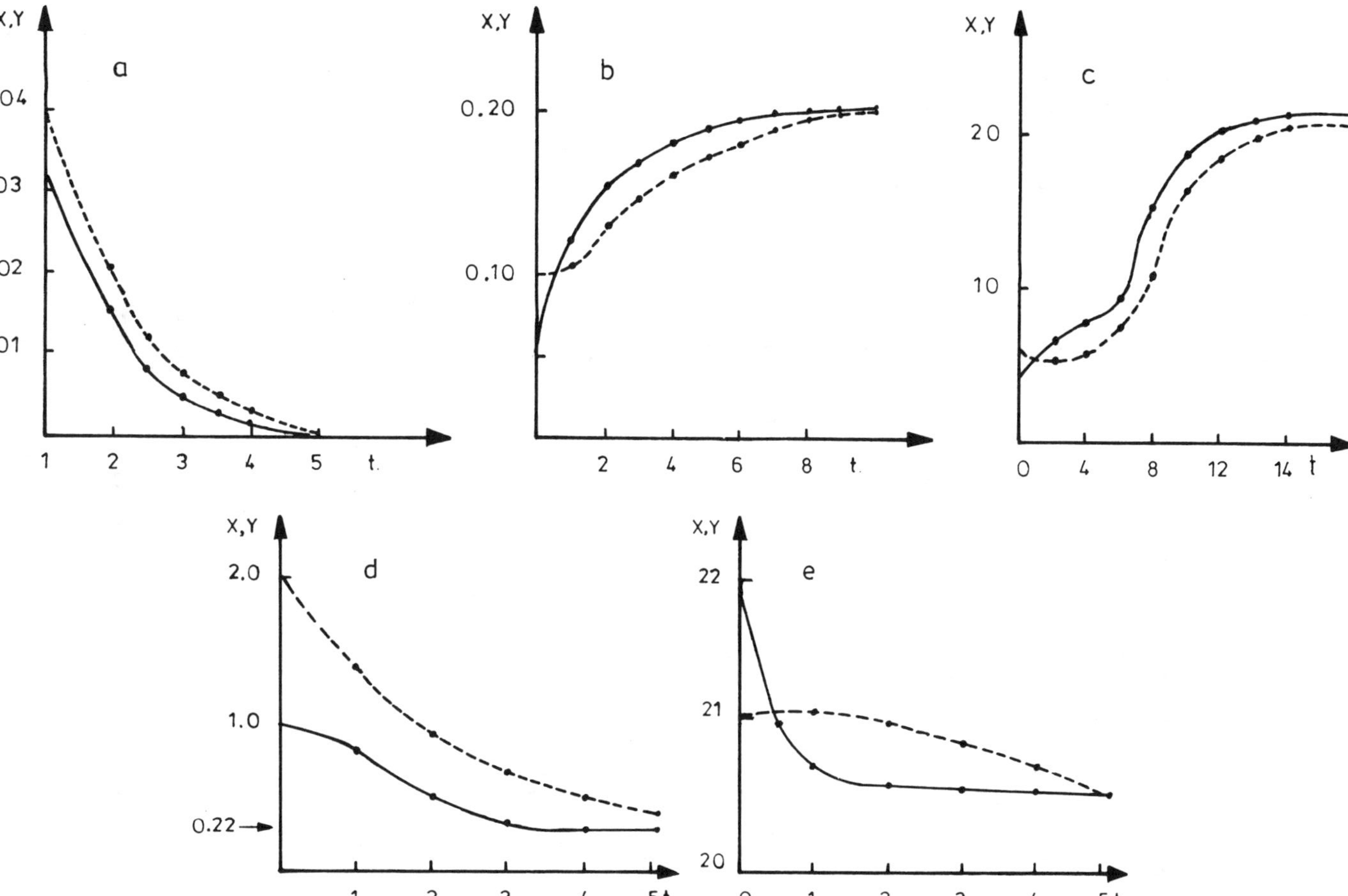

FIGURE 7.   Computer simulation for the set of parameters. Unbroken line = mRNA concentration, x; broken line = NHP concentration, y; t = time; "O" — type steady-state is reached; in b, c and d, "I" — type steady-state is reached and in e, "II" — type steady-state is reached; K_1 and K_2-NHP-enhancer dissociation constants. Other notation — see legend of Figure 5.

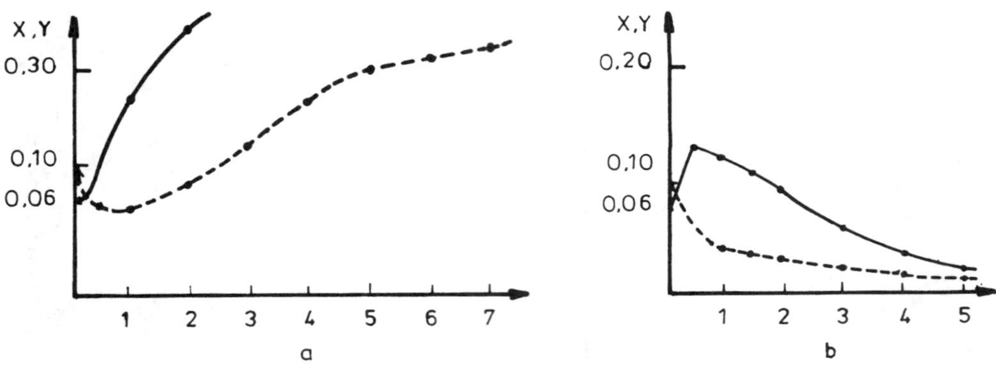

FIGURE 8.   Computer simulations for increased protein decay rates. Modifications in the set of parameters; (A) $\lambda_N = 2$, $\lambda_P = 2$ (B) $\lambda_N = 1$, $\lambda_P = 4$.

a maximal growth rate of 12 h cell cycle,[181] a maximal transcription rate of about 200 molecules/h and cistron results, but synthesis rates of up to 3000 molecules per gene and h are indicated for hemoglobin mRNAs in mouse erythroid cells,[182] which could be taken as an upper limit for φ_2. Very different decay rates are indicated for mRNA and protein in mammalian cells;[183] turnover times in the range from less than 1 to several hours are quite reasonable.

With a cell volume $V = 1 \times 10^{-12}$ L and $\varphi_2 = 6000$ mol/cell and h, or 10×10^{-21} mol/cell and h, a quotient of $\varphi_2/V = 1000 \times 10^{-11}$ M/h results. (M stands for moles/liter). To bring this quotient to the value $\varphi_2/V = 100$ of the set (14), all concentration-dependent parameters are to be multiplied by 10×10^{-11}. The correspondence with the set of parameters (14) thus becomes:

$$\varphi_2/V = 1000 \times 10^{-11} M/\text{h}; \quad \varphi_1/V = 10 \times 10^{-11} M\text{h}; \quad \Psi = 1\text{h}^{-1}$$

$$K_1^{1/2} = 1 \times 10^{-11} M; \quad K_2^{1/2} = 1 \times 10^{-9} M; \quad \lambda_N = \text{h}^{-1}; \quad \lambda_P = 1\text{h}^{-1} \tag{16}$$

and the corresponding steady-state concentrations are:

$$x_I = 2.2 \times 10^{-11} M, \text{ corresponding to 13 mRNA molecules/cell}$$

$$y_I = 2.2 \times 10^{-11} M, \text{ i.e., 13 NHP molecules/cell} \tag{17a}$$

and, respectively:

$$x_{II} = 20.4 \times 10^{-10} M, \text{ i.e., 1200 mRNA molecules cell}$$

$$y_{II} = 20.4 \times 10^{-10} M, \text{ i.e., 1200 NHP molecules/cell} \tag{17b}$$

The unstable "B" steady-state solution which separates the inactive state "O" from the low active state "I" would correspond to:

$$y_B \cong K_1^{1/2} = 1 \times 10^{-11} M, \text{ corresponding to 6 NHP molecules/cell}$$

$$x_B = \frac{\lambda_P}{\Psi} y_B = 1 \times 10^{-11} M, \text{ i.e., 6 mRNA molecules/cell} \tag{18}$$

which would give the inactive "O" state a sufficient stability against accidental transcription of the inactive trigger-gene.

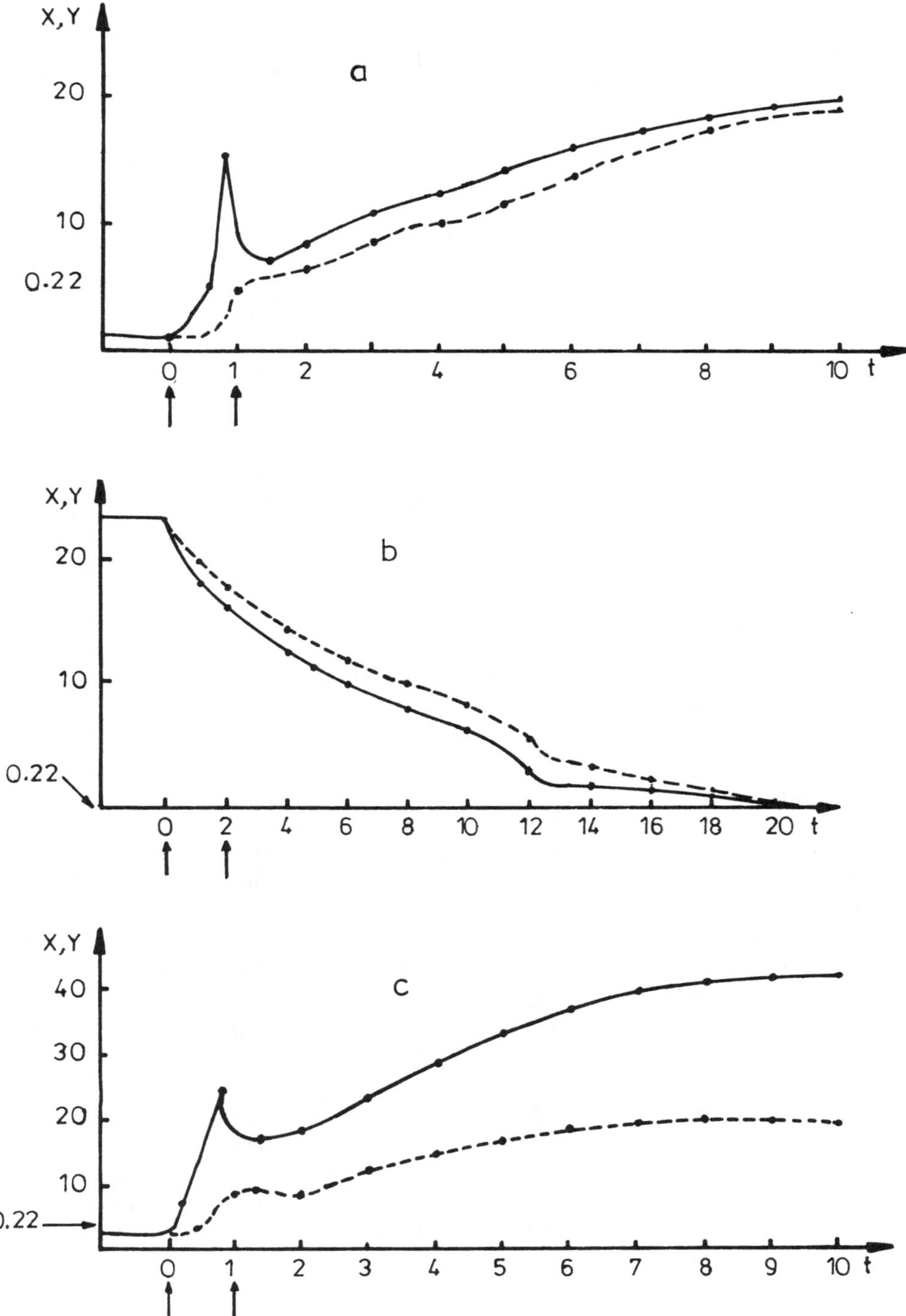

FIGURE 9. Computer simulations of transitions between stable states. In a and b, switches I → II and II → I are simulated by decreasing K_2 to $K_{2N} = 1$ in the time interval between the two bolts, and by increasing K_2 to $K_{2N} = 200$ (parameter set — **14**), respectively. In c, the I → II switch is simulated by decreasing K_2, for increased protein decay rate ($\lambda_N = 2$, $\lambda_P = 2$).

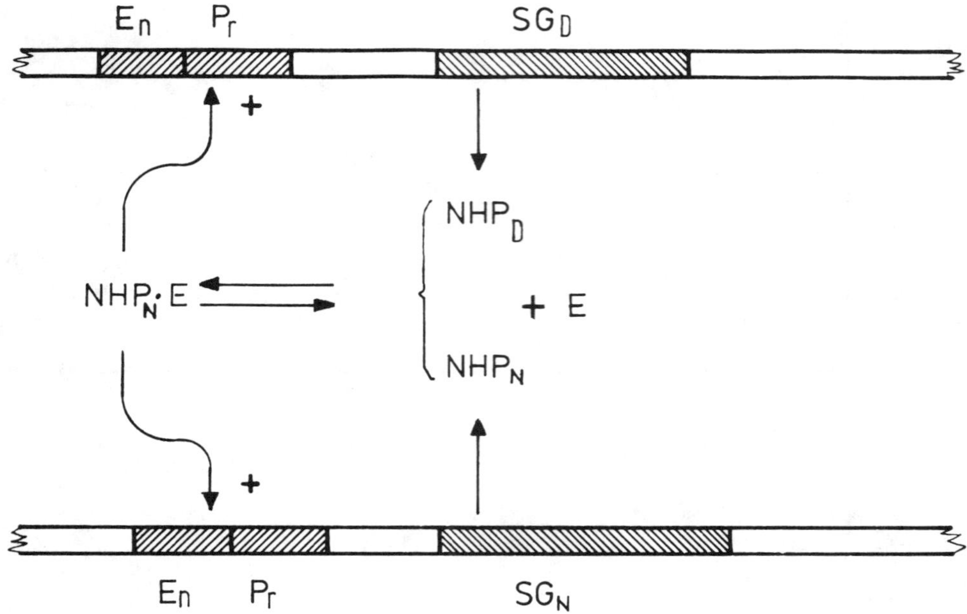

FIGURE 10.   Regulation of deactivating transition in a mutated diploid cell.

All solutions (Equations 17a,b and 18) generally meet the requirements of Section V.A., for the functioning of such triggers.

E. STABILITY TOWARD MUTATIONS IN DIPLOID CELLS

As discussed in Section II.C, irreversible activation of proto-oncogenes could be involved in the initiation, evolution and maintenance of malignancy. In the negative Monod-Jacob control, a mutation inactivating the operator gene produces an irreversible activation for the transcription of all the operon's genes. Diploidy, which assures a higher reliability for enzyme synthesis (both alleles must be altered) is of no use here.

We have proved[184] that our positive feedback trigger requires mutations in both alleles in order to give irreversible gene activation, assuming that the parameters of the trigger are within a favorable range (which could be achieved during the evolutionary process). The effect of most mutations is to produce defects, and only very rarely, could it improve a function of a protein (evolutionary event). A mutation in the NHP-synthesis gene, making the activating protein insensible toward the external effector E, (which increases the K_1 or K_2 dissociation constant) would produce a lack of sensitivity towards deactivating switches. This requires mutations in both alleles in diploid cells, as we shall show further on.

Consider the two trigger genes of which one allele, SG_D, is mutated, and the other, SG_N is normal (wild type) (Figure 10). Half of the activator protein, NHP_D will be mutated, and half will be normal, NHP_N. In the presence of the deactivating effector E, the NHP-enhancer equilibrium will be (for the II $\rightarrow$ I transition):

$$\frac{y_D^2[En]}{[En_{act}]} = K_2; \qquad \frac{y_N^2[En]}{[En_{act}]} = K_{2N}$$

$$y_N = y_D = \frac{y}{2}, \ K_{2N} \gg K_2 \tag{19}$$

and the activation degree will be:

$$A_2 = \frac{[En_{act}] + [En'_{act}]}{[En] \neq [En_{act}] + [En'_{act}]} = \frac{y^2}{\dfrac{2K_2K_{2N}}{K_2 + K_{2N}} + y^2} \tag{20}$$

The fact that half of the total NHP is sensible to the action of the deactivating effector E, produces an increase of K_2 only to the new, apparent dissociation constant:

$$K_{2N}^{app} = \frac{2K_2K_{2N}}{K_2 + K_{2N}} \tag{21}$$

which is, at most, the double of K_2 instead of the increase to K_{2N}. This is, nevertheless, sufficient to produce the deactivating II $\rightarrow$ I switch.

We simulated[184] a II $\rightarrow$ I transition for our trigger (Equation 9d) with the set of parameters (14). At $t = 0$, $x_o = y_o = 20.4$, and K_2 increased from $K_2 = 100$ to $K_{2N} = 1000$, until the threshold $y_o \leq 2.0$ is reached. For the wild-type diploid cell, this takes place after 3.6 time units (Figure 11a).

For the mutated cell (Figure 11b) K_2 is increased only up to $K_2^{app} = 182$. The deactivating II $\rightarrow$ I switch takes place, but about 25 time units of effector action are required in order to reach the $y_o \leq 2.0$ threshold.

A deactivating I $\rightarrow$ 0 switch was also simulated for the same system with $x_I = y_I = 0.22$ for $t = 0$, $K_{1N} = 1$ for the wild type and $K_{1N}^{app} = 0.02$ (instead of $K_1 = 0.01$) for the mutant. In both cases the switch takes place, but while for the wild type only 2.4 time units effector action are required to reach $y_o \leq 0.03$ (Figure 12a), for the mutant almost 15 time units are required (Figure 12b).

The deactivating switch also takes place for the mutant, but more drastic conditions are required: a longer time for the deactivating effector action, a higher K_{2N} value; for example with $K_{2N} = 200$, $K_{2N}^{app} = 133$, the II $\rightarrow$ I switch in the mutant is not possible.

A single mutation, of the type that causes a membrane receptor to transduce a growth signal into the interior, in the absence of the growth factor[45] (see Section II.C), would be sufficient to produce an irreversible activation. But such function-enhancing mutations, which fix the active protein conformation out of a multitude of inactive ones, are certainly very rare events.

F. TRIGGER MODEL FOR GENE REGULATION BY STEROID HORMONES

Most available data established the capacity of steroid hormones to induce or promote carcinogenesis. Estrogens, per se, are not mutagenic. They may act by epigenetic mechanisms, stimulating cell proliferation in the estrogen dependent target tissue. It is also possible that mutations are also produced by the products of metabolic activation of such hormones. The complexity of the implications of steroid hormones in the induction and evolution of malignancy is obvious.[31]

We will discuss gene regulation by steroid hormones which is a relatively well-studied process.[86,88,185-192] The experimental evidence concerning the interaction of the steroid hormone receptor protein with chromatin suggests the following processes to be considered for the trigger[193] (depicted in Figure 13): (1) transcription of the activated SG (rate φ); (2) degradation of the corresponding mRNA (rate λ_N, concentration x); (3) translation with synthesis of the NHP-monomer (rate Ψ, concentration y); (4) degradation of the NHP-monomer (rate λ_P); (5) dimerization to the NHP-dimer (concentration z, dissociation constant K_2); (6) unspecific absorption of the dimer on the chromatin (chromatin saturation degree, u, absorbed quantity uVC, dissociation constant K_3); (7) activation of the SG, by migration

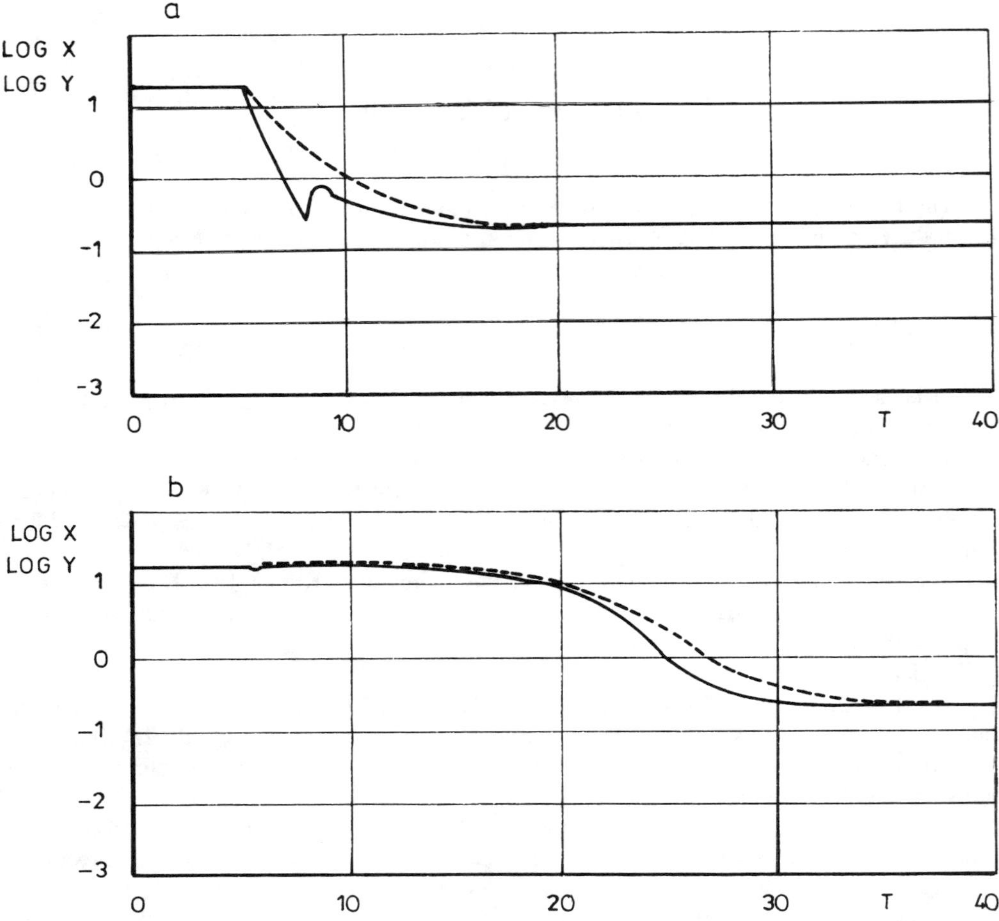

FIGURE 11.   (a) Computer simulation of a deactivating II → I switch. Normal diploid cell (wild type). Set of parameters, initial x_o, y_o concentrations and times T of switches K_1 and K_2 — constants: T = 0.00, 5.00, 8.60; K_1 = 0.01, 0.01, 0.01; K_2 = 100, 1000, 100; φ_1 = 1.00; φ_2 = 100; Ψ = 1.00; λ_N = 4.00; λ_P = 1.00; x_o = 20.40 and y_o = 20.40. (b) Computer simulation of a deactivating II → I switch. Mutant. Set of parameters and times T for switches: T = 0.00, 5.00, 24.90; K_1 = 0.01, 0.01, 0.01; K_2 = 100.000, 182.00, 100.00; φ_1 = 1.00; φ_2 = 100; Ψ = 1.00; λ_N = 4.00; λ_P = 1.00; x_o = 20.40 and y_o = 20.40.

of the absorbed NHP-dimer to the enhancer, En, i.e., specific absorption (degree of activation v; dissociation constant from unspecific to specific sites: K_4); VC is the NHP quantity adsorbed per saturated chromatin. In addition to processes demonstrated by the experimental evidence, there is the assumption that the hormone receptor protein also plays the role of an activator protein (NHP) for its own SG, and that the receptor degradation takes place mainly at the monomer level.

We could not find the required parameters for a single system, but the steroid hormone receptor proteins are stated to have rather similar characteristics.[186] At a total concentration of about 10^{-8} M (mol/L) in hormone stimulated target cells, these receptor proteins are found mostly as dimers (i.e., $K_2 \lesssim 10^{-8}$ M) consisting of identical or different polypeptide chains.[88,185,189] The receptor binds first to nonspecific chromatin sites, and only afterwards to a specific site.[185] For the specific factor which activates the adult chicken globin gene,[194] the dissociation constants for the factor adsorbed at nonspecific and specific chromatin sites are 4.10^{-8} M and 1.5×10^{-12} M, respectively; these figures should correspond to K_3 and K_3K_4, respectively.

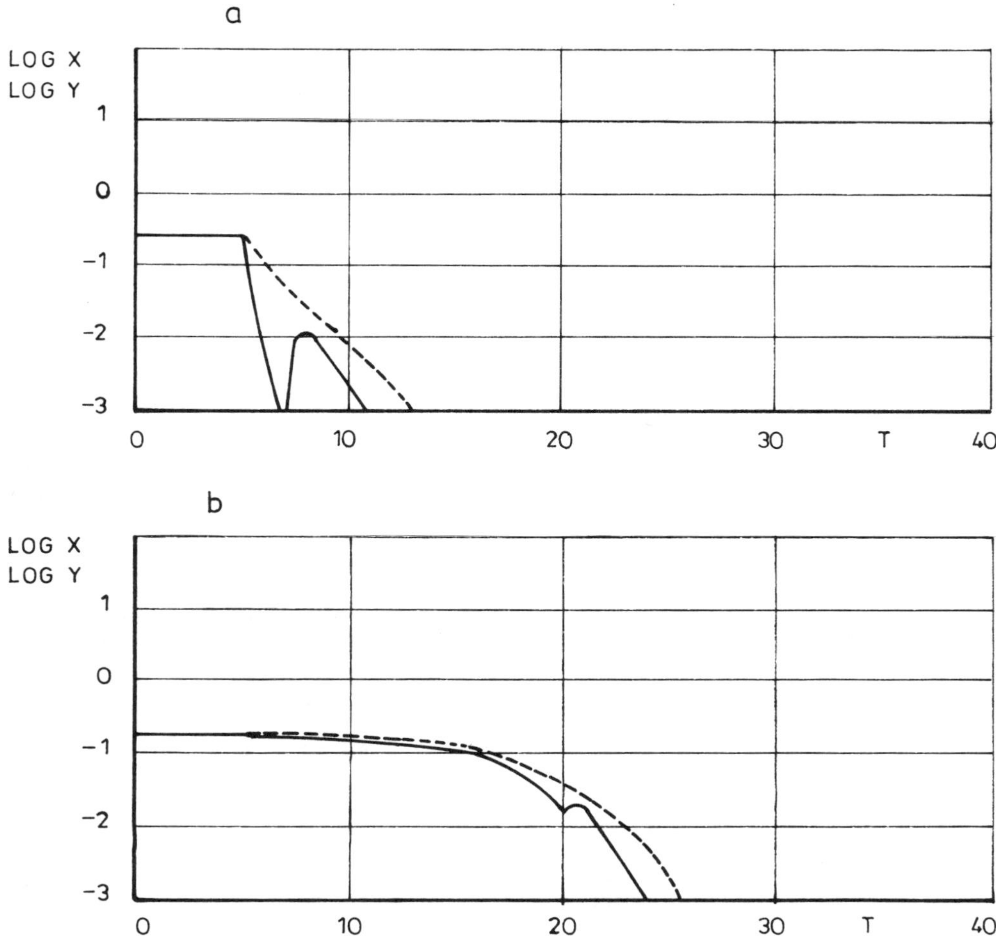

FIGURE 12. (a) Computer simulation of a deactivating I → O switch. Wild type. Set of parameters and times for switches: T = 0.00, 5.00, 7.40; K_1 = 0.01, 2.00, 0.01; K_2 = 100.00, 100.00, 100.00; φ_1 = 1.00; φ_2 = 100.00, Ψ = 1.00; λ_N = 4.00; λ_P = 1.00; x_o = 0.22 and y_o = 0.22. (b) Computer simulation of a deactivating I → O switch. Mutant. Set of parameters and times for switches: T = 0.00, 5.00, 19.80; K_1 = 0.01, 0.02, 0.01; φ_1 = 1.00; φ_2 = 100.00; Ψ = 1.00; λ_N = 4.00; λ_P = 1.00; x_o = 0.22 and y_o = 0.22.

The inverse of decay constants, λ_N^{-1} and λ_P^{-1}, should approximately correspond to the time lags for hormonal induction of the specific cell differentiation. For induction of chick uterine differentiation by estrogens, this lag is about 6 h,[187,188] during gene induction by glucocorticoids the half-life of tyrosine-aminotransferase mRNA is 1.5 h.[186,195]

Concerning cytoplasmic or nuclear localization of steroid hormone receptors, for the progesterone receptor cytoplasmic monomers which bind progesterone interact at the nuclear membrane with nuclear monomers and the receptor dimer is transferred hereby in the nucleus.[196] The estrogen receptor is located exclusively in the nucleus.[198] For simplification, we consider a unique, cellular localization of the receptor in our model.

The stable maturation of chick oviduct is induced by estrogens; after withdrawing the estrogen, there remains about 10 ovalbumin mRNA molecules per cell. Intense ovalbumin synthesis, corresponding to a quantity of about 5000 mRNA molecules per cell, is induced only transiently, under progesterone or estrogen action.[185] Other per cell quantities — about 32,000 estrogen receptor molecules[198] and 63,000 progesterone receptor molecules are found in GH_3 cells. Twelve hundred estrogen receptor molecules are reported in estradiol-induced

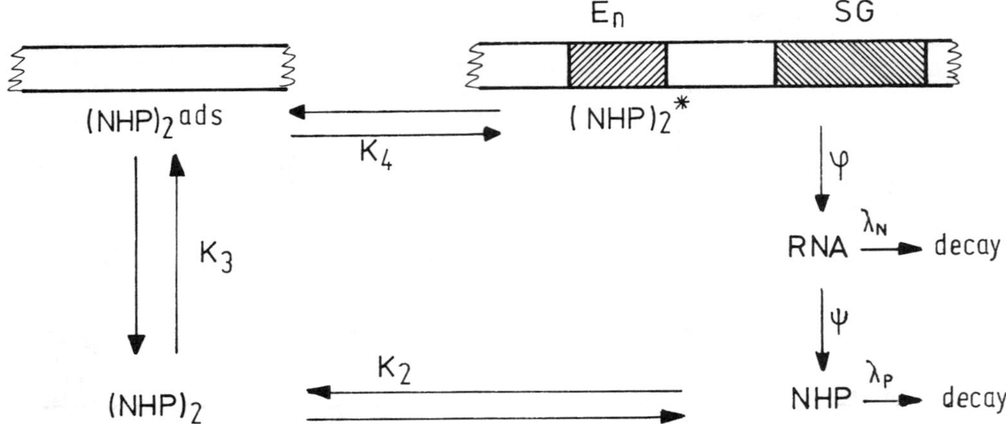

FIGURE 13.   Trigger model for gene regulation by steroid hormones. NHP-activating protein, monomer; $(NHP)_2$- dimer; $(NHP)_2^x$ — adsorbed on unspecific chromatin sites; $(NHP)_2^+$ — specifically adsorbed upon the enhancer, E_n, of its own synthesis gene; y, z, u — corresponding concentrations; V — gene activation degree; K_2, K_3, K_4 — equilibrium constants; φ, Ψ, λ_N, λ_P — rates.

Xenopus laevis hepatocytes.[199] In the same induced hepatocytes, the absolute transcription rates for the four vitellogenin mRNAs (A1, A2, B1, B2) range between 100 and 700 mRNA molecules per cell and h.[199] Therefore, the trigger of Figure 13 was devised for only two states: inactive, ''O'' and low activity, ''I''. The equations describing this trigger are:[193]

$$\frac{dx}{dt} = \frac{\varphi}{V} v - \lambda_N x \tag{22a}$$

$$\frac{dp}{dt} = \Psi x - \lambda_P y \tag{22b}$$

$$z = \frac{y^2}{K_2} \tag{22c}$$

$$u = \frac{z}{z + K_3} \tag{22d}$$

$$v = \frac{u}{u + K_4} \tag{22e}$$

$$p = y + 2z + uC \tag{22f}$$

According to the experimental evidence mentioned above, the following set of parameters were used:

$$V = 3.10^{-12} \text{ L}; \quad \varphi = 18 \text{ molecules/cell h} = 3.10^{-23} M \text{ h}; \quad \Psi = 10 \text{ h}^{-1};$$

$$\lambda_N = 0.8 \text{ h}^{-1}; \quad \lambda_P = 0.3 \text{ h}^{-1}; \quad C = 10^{-8} M; \quad K_2 = K_3 = 10^{-8} M \text{ and } K_4 = 10^{-4} \tag{23}$$

We remind that L stands for liter (volume), h for hour and M for mol/L (concentration). Constant K_4 is adimensional, while the product CV represents the total adsorbtive capacity of the chromatine for the steroid receptor protein (NHP).

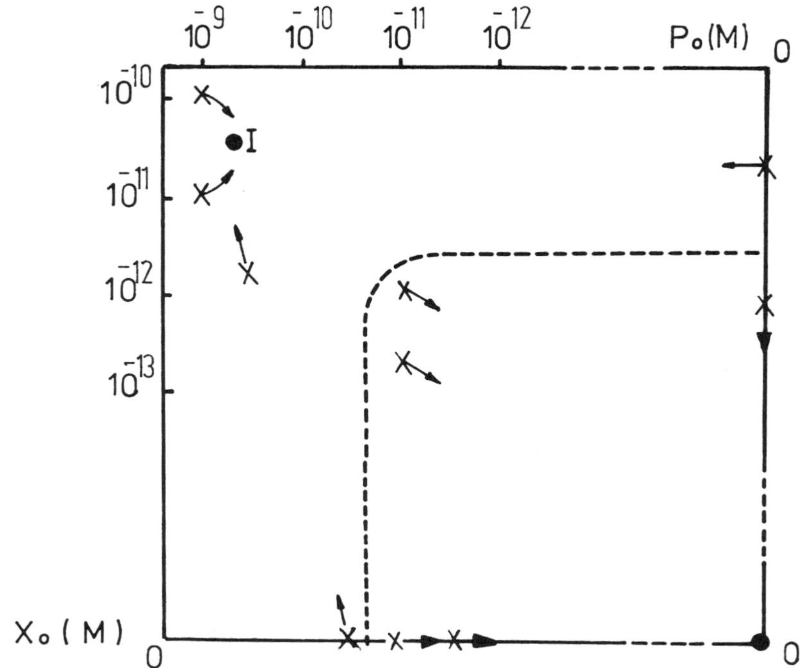

FIGURE 14.   Evolution toward the steady-states (●) O or I of different pairs (x) of initial concentrations of mRNA (x_o) and NHP protein (p_0). The dotted line marks the threshold domain. M stands for mol/L.

The stable states of this system are (Appendix 4):

$$\text{``O'': } x_o = 0, \ y_o = 0; \quad \text{``I'': } x_1 \cong \frac{\varphi}{V\lambda_N}; \quad y_1 \cong \frac{\varphi\Psi}{V\lambda_N\lambda_P} \tag{24}$$

while the separating values, corresponding to an intermediate unstable steady-state, are:

$$y_{int} \cong (K_2K_3K_4)^{1/2}; \quad x_{int} = \frac{\lambda_P}{\Psi}(K_2K_3K_4)^{1/2} \tag{25}$$

Transitions between the two stable-states are simulated by a temporary increase or decrease of K_4 to K_{4N}. Binding of progesterone or estrogen to the corresponding receptor protein really increases its affinity for chromatin.[88,190] For activating O → I switches and deactivating I → O switches, $K_{4N} = 10^{-8}$ and $K_{4N} = 1$, respectively, are considered.

Several runs, starting from different initial mRNA and total protein concentrations x(O), p(O) were performed. The results are listed in Figure 14. All runs end in one steady-state:

$$\text{``O'': } x_o = 0; \ y_o = 0 \text{ and ``I''} x_I = 1.17 \times 10^{-11} \ M; \ y_I = 4.52 \times 10^{-10} \ M \tag{26}$$

fairly close to the approximate solutions (Equation 24) of about $1.25 \times 10^{-11} \ M$ and $4.1 \times 10^{-10} \ M$, for x_I and y_I, respectively.

Two runs ending into the active state "I" are illustrated in Figure 15, one run ending in the inactive state "O", in Figure 16 and a deactivating switch in Figure 17. The time required for a I → O switch is of about 20 h, and for a O → I switch, about 5 h.

The steady-state values (Equation 26) correspond to about 20 mRNA molecules per cell

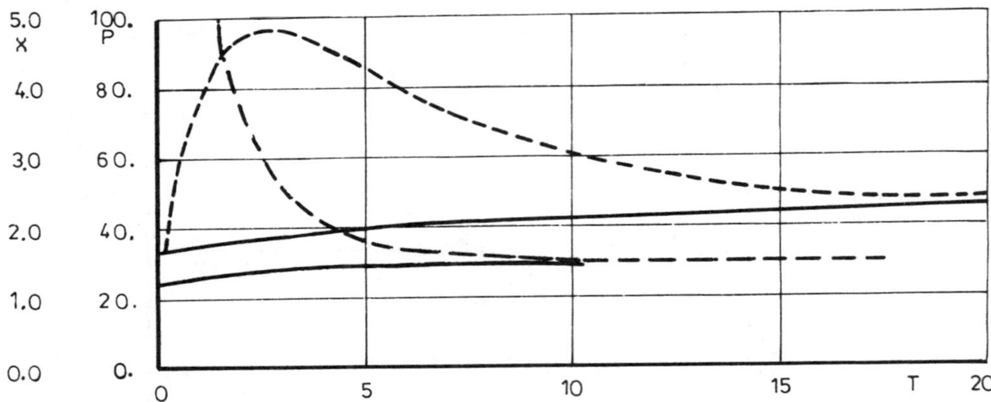

FIGURE 15.   Simulation of a steroid hormone trigger. Two runs ending into the active state I. Rate and equilibrium constants (see Figure 13) — relative values (concentrations dependent values are to be multiplied by 10^{-8}): φ/V = 0.001, Ψ = 10 h^{-1}, λ_N = 0.8 h^{-1}, λ_P = 0.3 h^{-1} C = 1; K_2 = 1; K_3 = 1; K_4 = 0.0001; V — cell volume; initial concentrations: x_{oa} = 0.01, y_{oa} = 0.01; x_{ob} = 0.001, y_{ob} = 0.001. X indicates mRNA and P indicates total NHP — concentration. Scale values are to be multiplied by 10^3. Broken and full lines as in Figure 7.

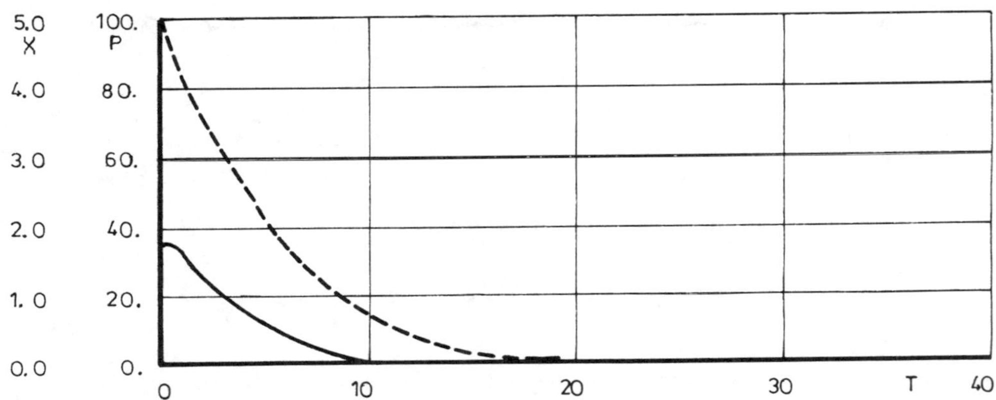

FIGURE 16.   Simulation of a steroid hormone trigger. Run ending into the inactive state O. Rate and equilibrium constants as in Figure 15. Initial concentration: x_o = 0.15 $\times$ 10^{-4}, y_o = 0.1 $\times$ 10^{-2}. Scale values to be multiplied by 10^5. Broken and full lines as in Figure 7.

and 800 NHP molecules per cell. The unstable approximate solution (Equation 25) corresponds to about 1 $\times$ 10^{-10} M or 180 NHP molecules per cell and 3 $\times$ 10^{-12} M or 5 mRNA molecules per cell. They are in satisfactory agreement with the above quoted experimental evidence and allow for a certain stability of the inactive ''O''-state against accidental transcription of this mRNA. For the glucocorticoid receptor, binding at the DNA response element (enhancer) of one receptor, dimer increases 100 times the binding constant for a second receptor dimer.[197] The synergism is stronger than in our model (n = 4 instead of n = 2), but the steady-state concentrations given by our computer simulation are, anyhow, near the approximative solutions (Equation 24) which correspond to a very strong synergism (n $\rightarrow$ ∞).

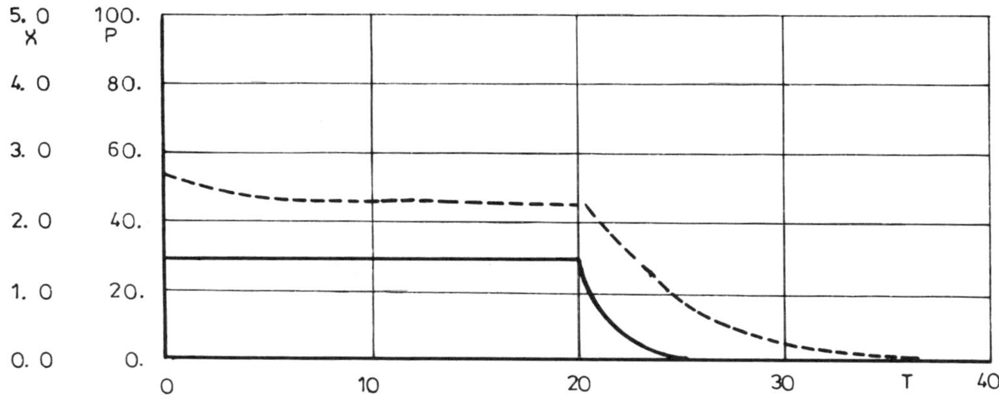

FIGURE 17. Stimulation of a steroid hormone trigger. Deactivating switch. Rate and equilibrium constants as in Figure 15. Initial concentrations: $x_o = 0.0012$, $y_o = 0.045$. At $T = 20$, $K_4 = 10^{-4}$ is switched to $K_{4N} = 1$ until $T = 25$. Scale values to be multiplied by 10^3. Broken and full lines as in Figure 7.

VI. CELL REGULATION AND THE CARCINOGENESIS PROCESS

A. INTEGRATION OF THE POSITIVE CONTROL TRIGGER INTO CELL REGULATION

The positive control trigger discussed in the previous sections (V.A to V.E) gives a reasonable explanation for a series of features of gene regulation in eukaryotes. The evidence for the existence of such triggers is only beginning to accumulate (see Section V.A) and the existence of other types of mechanisms for gene regulation (see Section III.E) must not be overlooked. Nevertheless, this type of positive control for differentiated gene expression is very simple and straightforward and it is likely that it is used on a wide scale.

The integration of this trigger into the cellular regulation of gene activity should take place along the line of hierarchical models (Britten and Davidson,[13] Section II.B). The NHP-genes of these triggers together with their control elements, should play the role of "master genes", interacting by their NHPs and controlling by the same NHPs, the activity of the "slave genes"; coding for the other proteins required by the cell machinery, but without acting upon the activation degrees of other proteins (Figure 18). Enzyme synthesis rates and concentrations will also be controlled by various post-transcriptional regulation processes and by lytic enzymes. The corresponding genes will also have a role within the hierarchical model.

The triggers will behave as ternary elements (instead of binary, Boolean elements) in a network of the type studied by Kauffman[175] (Section IV.D). The inactive (O), low activity (I), and high activity (II), states of each gene will be step functions of the concentration of one or more activating NHPs. The fact that the cells of some tissues are responsive toward hormone action inducing specific protein synthesis and differentiation while others are not, suggests that the active state of a gene may require the presence of more than a single protein. The *c-jun* gene seems to require, for its activation its own protein[139] (Section III.G).

Switches in the activity states of the triggers, and implicitly of the genes in the network, are induced by hormones and/or mitogens which should combine with certain NHPs and modulate their affinities toward the control elements of the trigger gene.

Post-transcriptional regulation processes and activation of lytic enzymes will modulate synthesis and decay rates of NHPs and may also produce switches in trigger states. Transpositions of genes or enhancers may also modify some links within the genetic network. Accordingly, while the state of the cellular automaton could be described by a set of ternary

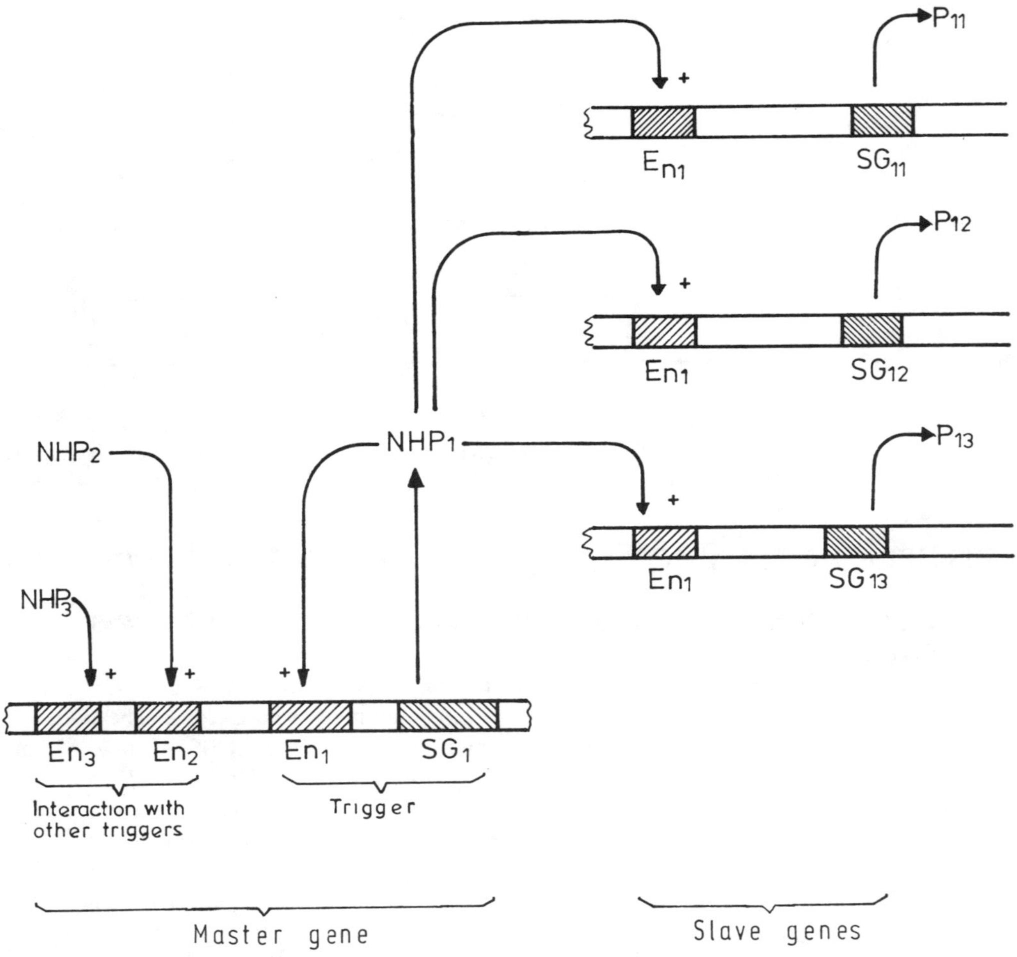

FIGURE 18.   Integration of the trigger in the hierarchical model[13] for cell regulation of gene activity. En_1, En_2, . . . En_6 — different types of activator sequences (enhancers); NHP_1, . . . different types of activator protein; P_{11}, P_{12}, P_{13} proteins with other functions; SG_1, SG_{11} . . . synthesis genes.

variables for gene activation degrees, the activity of some genes coding for transposition factors will produce changes within the network.

B. CELL PROLIFERATION AND DIFFERENTIATION

The control of these processes appears to be the key to carcinogenesis. Activation of some "mitotic" genes is certainly a basic element of carcinogenesis, but no realistic and sufficiently detailed model is available until now. Cell regulation is certainly more intricate than the simple and elegant model of Bullough[14,15] (see Section II.B). The irreversible activation of an oncogene can be the primary cause of carcinogenesis and there are several mechanisms which could achieve this, at least in principle (see Sections III.E and III.G). One such mechanism may involve a mutation (or two, in both alleles) producing a defect in the informational chain which transmits the growth stimulating or inhibiting chemical messengers to the trigger controlling an oncogene. The effect of a mutation, which makes activating NHP insensible to the action of an effector, which decreases the affinity of the NHP for an enhancer (in order to produce a deactivating switch), was discussed in Section V.E. The fact that our positive control trigger requires mutations in both alleles (allele coding for a given link of the transmitting chain for the deactivating switch) makes the gene control system of diploid cells more resistant against the effect of mutations (see also Section II.D).[178,184]

Nevertheless, one mutation of this type makes the deactivating switch more difficult (see Section V.E) and even mutation in both alleles may only decrease, and not annihilate, the action of the deactivating effector. This gives hope for, at least, a temporary cure for cancer by reversors which mimic the action of the defective link in the control transmitting chain. Reversors could be substances with the same action as the natural switch-effector, but which can be introduced in higher concentrations or have a higher affinity for the NHP and can be able to produce the switch deactivating the oncogene. The same would hold true for activating switches inducing differentiation.[178] Leukemia cells could be induced to differentiate in macrophages when cultured in media containing a high concentration of a differentiation factor.[200]

C. RETINOIC ACID — MECHANISM OF ACTION

Although the role of retinoids in malignancy is still not elucidated, they are tested as reversors in chemotherapy for some forms of cancer. They have been shown to have the property to block the phenotypic expression of transformed or even neoplastic cells, inhibiting the growth and inducing differentiation.[201] The differentiation-producing doses are in the concentration range 10^{-9} to 10^{-12} M.

The most frequently investigated reversor, retinoic acid, promotes differentiation of various neoplastic cell types, such as HL-60 cells, F9 murine embryocarcinoma cells (the most widely employed systems both for screening purposes and for investigating the mechanism of retinoic action), but affects differentiation and proliferation of many types of cells such as: ectodermal, endodermal and mesodermal, epithelial, fibroblastic and mesenchymal. Retinoic acid was identified as the first natural morphogen.[203] The retinoic acid receptors belong to the same family as the receptors for steroid and thyroid hormones and the *v-erbA* oncogene product.[202] The bicoid gene protein also has the role of a morphogene in the *Drosophila* embryo;[204] it acts as a concentration-dependent transcriptional activator.[205]

The differentiation promoting activity is usually associated with effects upon cell growth, but the accumulated evidence suggests the existence of different mechanisms of action for retinoids including regulation of:[201] (1) synthesis of several enzymes; (2) modulation of membrane functions; (3) modulation of the effects of many mutagens and transforming growth factors; (4) binding proteins; (5) modulation of transcriptional or post-transcriptional expression; (6) extracellular effects; (7) immunological activity and (8) protein kinase C cascade system.[206]

Such a pleiotropic mechanism of action suggests that there are several different receptors for retinoic acid. Actually, the manifold of differentiation and cell regulation processes is controlled by a rather limited number of natural chemical messengers, probably in various combinations. The idea that a receptor site for such a messenger is coupled (by exon transpositions during evolution) to intracellular proteins with different regulatory functions does not seem obsolete.

The existing evidence for the mechanism of action of retinoids is in favor of regulation of gene activity, as the main process.[201] Significant changes in the spectrum of cellular mRNA are produced by retinoids within 1 to 2 h. The abundance of transcripts of a repeated interspersed DNA sequence from a human teratocarcinoma line varies upon differentiation induced by retinoic acid.[202] The induction of differentiation of HL-60 and embryocarcinoma cells is associated with the suppression of *myc* oncogene transcription. Most of these cells contain receptor proteins for retinoids, the cytoplasmic retinol binding and the retinoic acid binding protein (CRBP and CRABP), respectively. Probably the transformed or tumoral cells express higher numbers of binding proteins, which can increase their sensitivity to the inhibition of growth or induction of differentiation by retinoids. Like the steroid hormone, retinoids were supposed to order gene expression, but work undertaken in the past years has not discovered similar mechanisms. The binding is to nuclear membrane receptors (estimated up to 10,000 to 300,000 binding sites) and not to DNA.[206] In spite of the fact that no CRABP could be detected in HL-60 cells or in U937 cells, they differentiate in the presence of retinoic acid. In addition, some melanoma cell lines resistant to the effect of retinoids have a concentration of binding proteins equal to, or higher than, the one detected in responsive cell lines. This could mean that receptor proteins for retinoids alone may not be sufficient for the growth inhibition and differentiation inducing properties.

In the framework of our positive trigger model,[207] retinoic acid should be an effector which by combination with an activating NHP (or with several NHPs) modulates its affinity toward the corresponding promoter or enhancer, inducing a switch in the state of the trigger and in the activation degrees of the controlled genes. The action of retinoids upon cells without detectable receptors (CRABP) could be also explained hereby. The CRABP should be an activating NHP and the corresponding trigger in the inactive "O"-state. Only a few NHP molecules per cell are available, resulting in accidental transcription of the trigger gene. By combination with the retinoid, the affinity of the NHP toward the enhancer and/or its lifetime are increased (K_1 and λ_P are decreased) so that these few NHP-RA complexes become able to activate the trigger gene and induce the O $\rightarrow$ I switch.

In certain cases, retinoids stimulate growth and inhibit differentiation, enhancing the expression of the transformed phenotypes. The complex mechanism controlling these processes and the variety of regulating factors which modulate the transformed phenotype make it difficult to explain what determines different cells to respond divergently to retinoids.[201]

VII. CONCLUSIONS

Carcinogenesis is a consequence of various genetic and epigenetic mechanisms, among which defects in regulation of gene activity play a major role. Activation of proto-oncogenes to oncogenes by point mutations, translocations and chromosomal disorders were proved as major mechanisms in several cases. In the last years, considerable progress has been made in the study of gene control in eukaryotes, for both normal and malignant cells. This control is predominantly positive, although the recently discovered tumor suppressor genes imply a negative control also. The differential, histospecific gene activity is produced by various mechanisms, such as gene amplification, DNA methylation or loss of a nucleotidic sequence which renders the transcribed mRNA stable toward degradation (activation of the *c-fos* proto-oncogene). Autoregulation of genes, activation of a gene by its own encoded, activating protein was recently discovered and this seems a most promising mechanism for stable and histospecific on and off switches of gene transcription.

Mathematical models for gene regulation in normal and malignant cells and tissues, including the simulation of genetic networks, were set up in the 1960s and early 1970s but based upon the negative repressor-operator control.

A trigger for autoregulation of genes is studied here by qualitative analysis of the corresponding system of differential equations and by computer simulations. This study rationalizes several experimental facts, such as the requirement for cooperative action of at least two protein molecules upon the gene activating sequences and the discontinuous ranges for the possible transcriptional activation degrees (the three cellular mRNA abundance classes). Computer simulations prove the stability of the two or three steady-states of this trigger and the possibility of switches between states by external effectors which temporarily modulate the affinity of activator proteins for the activating gene sequences. The simulation for the autoregulation of a gene encoding a steroid receptor protein yields reasonable results for time lags of activating and deactivating switches and for the per cell number of mRNA and receptor protein molecules in a stable (moderate transcriptional activity) state.

In the frame of this model, certain proto-oncogenes could encode proteins controlling the transcription of genes implied in cell growth and differentiation. A transformation to the active, oncogenic state could take place following mutations which render the encoded protein unresponsive to effectors which transmit growth inhibiting signals or following a (very rare) mutation increasing the affinity of the protein for activating sequences of the controlled gene. Some aspects of the differentiation promoting activity of retinoids are rationalized by this model.

VIII. MATHEMATICAL APPENDIX

A. APPENDIX 1 — STEADY-STATE SOLUTIONS FOR THE JACOB-MONOD TRIGGER OF INTERRELATED OPERONS

Consider Equations 5a,b, Section IV.B. If y_2 is expressed as a function of y_1 for the steady-state ($y_1 = 0$, $y_2 = 0$), using Equation 5b and introducing in Equation 5a, one obtains the second order equation:

$$y_1^2 + \left[K_2 + \frac{kK_2}{\lambda_2 K_1} - \frac{k}{\lambda_1} \right] y_1 - \frac{kK_2}{\lambda_1} = 0$$

whose solutions are:

$$y_1 = \frac{1}{2}\left[\frac{k}{\lambda_1} - \frac{kK_2}{\lambda_2 K_1} - K_2 \right] \pm \left(\frac{1}{4}\left[\frac{k}{\lambda_1} - \frac{kK_2}{\lambda_2 K_1} - K_2 \right]^2 + \frac{kK_2}{\lambda_1} \right)^{1/2}$$

As all constants are positive, the square root term is larger (in absolute value) than the first term and a single positive solution is possible for the second order equation. The negative solution (negative steady-state concentration) has no physical sense.

For the Equations 7a,b, corresponding to a cooperative repressor-operator interaction, also for the steady-state,

$$dy_1/dt = 0, \; dy_2/dt = 0: \; y_1 = \frac{kK_1}{\lambda_1(K_1 + y_2^n)}; \; y_2 = \frac{kK_2}{\lambda_2(K_2 + y^n)}; \; n \geqslant 2$$

and the steady-state solutions are obtained, in the y_1, y_2-plane, at the intersection of the two curves, $y_1(y_2)$ and $y_2(y_1)$. Figures 19a and 19b illustrate the situation for $n = 1$ and $n \geqslant 2$. The difference exists because for $n = 1$ one obtains:

$$\left(\frac{dy_1}{dy_2} \right)_{y_2=0} = \frac{k}{k_1\lambda_1}; \qquad \left(\frac{dy_2}{dy_1} \right)_{y_1=0} = \frac{k}{k_2\lambda_2}$$

while for $n \geqslant 2$;

$$\left(\frac{dy_1}{dy_2} \right)_{y_2=0} = 0; \qquad \left(\frac{dy_2}{dy_1} \right)_{y_1=0} = 0$$

For the noncooperative case, $n = 1$, the two curves intersect in a single point (Figure 19a), while for $n \geqslant 2$ there are 3 intersection points, A, B, C (Figure 19b), the middle one, B corresponding to an unstable solution.

B. APPENDIX 2 — STEADY-STATE SOLUTIONS FOR THE TRIGGER WITH POSITIVE FEEDBACK

Considering Equations 9a to c, with the steady-state assumption for mRNA concentration, $dx/dt = 0$, and eliminating x between Equations 9a and 9b one obtains:

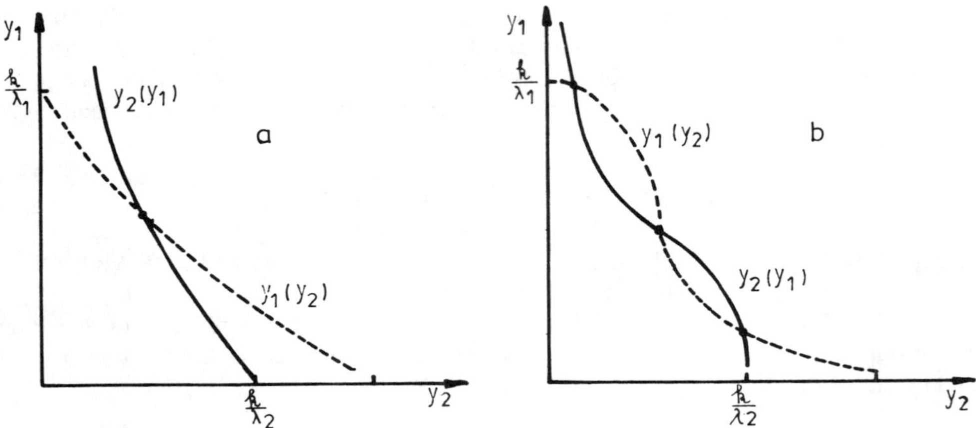

FIGURE 19.   Intersection of curves of repressor concentrations. $y_1(y_2)$ and $y_2(y_1)$, in reciprocal dependence, for the Monod-Jacob trigger; (a) noncooperative behavior — single steady-state; (b) cooperative behavior, two stable steady-states.

$$\frac{dy}{dt} = \frac{\Psi}{V\lambda_N} \left[\frac{\varphi_1 y_1^n}{K_1 + y_1^n} + \frac{\varphi_2 y_1^n}{K_2 + y_2^n} \right] - \lambda_P y = SR(y) - \lambda_P y$$

with $K_1 \ll K_2$ and $\varphi_1 \ll \varphi_2$. The positive term, SR, on the right hand represents NHP-synthesis rate, while the negative term, $-\lambda_P y$ stands for NHP decay. The steady-state solutions correspond to the intersections of $SR(y)$, with $\lambda_P y$. In the vicinity of stable steady-state solutions, y_s, the derivative dy/dt and the deviation Δy from y_s must be of opposite sign, such that y should tend from $y_s + \Delta y$ towards y_s.

For $n = 1$, the derivatives of the synthesis rate, SR is:

$$\frac{d}{dy}(SR) = \frac{\Psi}{V\lambda_N} \left[\frac{K_1\varphi_1}{(K_1 + y)^2} + \frac{K_2\varphi_2}{(K_2 + y)^2} \right]$$

$$\left(\frac{d}{dy}(SR) \right)_{y=0} = (\dot{SR})_0 = \frac{\Psi}{V\lambda_N} \left[\frac{\varphi_1}{K_1} + \frac{\varphi_2}{K_2} \right]$$

It decreases with increasing y (for $y \geq 0$). The decay rate $\lambda_P y$ will intersect SR only for $y = 0$ if $\lambda_p > (\dot{SR})_0$. The solution $y = 0$ is stable as for $y = \Delta y \ll K_1$, $\lambda_P y > SR$ and $dy/dt < 0$. For $\lambda_p < (\dot{SR})_0$, there are two intersections between SR and $\lambda_P y$; for the intersection (solution) $y = 0$, $dy/dt > 0$ and this solution is unstable.

For high cooperativity, $n \gg 1$, the synthesis rate, SR, will be a quasi-step function (see Figure 20), and if conditions (Equation 13) Section V.B are satisfied, there are five intersections (A, B, C, D, E) between SR and $\lambda_P y$.

Intersection A corresponds to $y = 0$; B to $y \cong K_1^{1/n}$; C to $y \cong \varphi_1 \Psi/V \lambda_N \lambda_P$; D to $y \cong K_2^{1/n}$ and E to $y \cong \varphi_2 \Psi/V \lambda_N \lambda_P$. The first, third and fifth solutions are stable, the second and fourth unstable. For example, in the vicinity of C, with $y = y_c + \Delta y$ for $\Delta y > 0$, we have $\lambda_P y < SR$ and $dy/dt < 0$, tending to bring back y to y_c. Also for $\Delta y < 0$, one has $\lambda_P y < SR$ and $dy/dt > 0$, tending to increase y towards y_c. In the vicinity of D, with $y = y_D + \Delta y$, for $\Delta y > 0$ one has $SR > \lambda_P y$ and y continues to increase toward y_E; for $\Delta y < 0$ one has $SR < \lambda_P y$, y decreases towards y_c. By the same type of reasoning, y_A and y_E are stable and y_B is unstable.

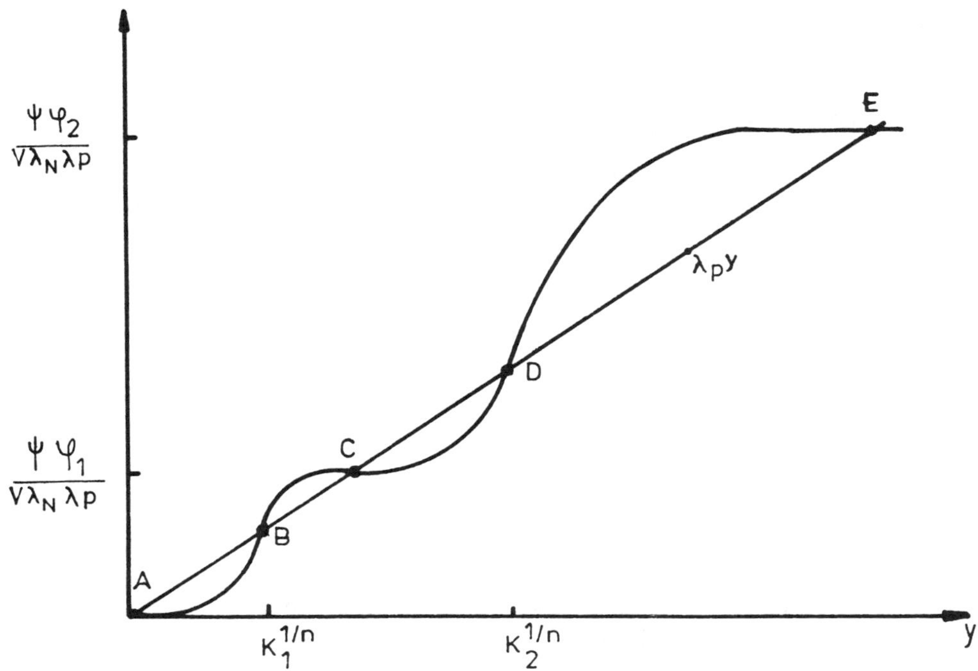

FIGURE 20. Intersection of synthesis rate curve, (SR) and decay rates, $\lambda_P y$, for the activator (NHP) concentration y. A, C, E correspond to the three stable steady-states, B, D — to intermediate steady-states.

C. APPENDIX 3 — COMPUTER PROGRAM FOR SIMULATIONS OF TRIGGER FUNCTION (G. I. MIHALAŞ)

A second order Runge-Kutta method (improved Euler method or Heun method) was used for the computer program, written in Fortran IV.[209] A set of options defines the total number of iteration, the step T1 (time interval) and the transition switch IT (0 for no transition, 1 for transition). Input parameters were read from a file (NFIS) as a vector P(II); φ_1, φ_2, K_1, $K_2\Psi$, λ_1, λ_2, x_o, y_o, K_2, y_4^o (or entered from the console; $V = 1$ is considered for all simulations). The values K_{2N} and y_4^o are not used for IT $= 0$, while for IT $= 1$, $K_2 = P(4)$ (i.e., K_{2N}) for $y \geqslant y_4^o$, and $K_2' = P(10)$ (i.e., the modified K_{2N}' value) for $y < y_4^o$.

The program was implemented on a Felix M-18 computer (56 kbytes RAM memory, 2 floppy 8-inch disks, line printer, MTU, graphic display with hard copy).

Since the error of a Runge-Kutta method of order 1 is Kh^{P+1} (in our case h $= T1$ and p $= 2$), it may be strongly reduced by lowering the step T1. Thus, low values (0.01) were used especially for studying transitions while higher values (0.1) were good enough for the other cases.

In our study concerning stability towards mutation (see also Section V.E) the x,y-concentration vs. time plots are printed directly in a semi-logarithmic scale (log x — straight line, log y — broken line, vs. t). A number of 40 time units and a 0.1 unit time step are used in each run. For each run one starts from the steady-state x_o, y_o values, for an interval of five time units and changes hereafter K_2 to K_{2P} (wild type) or to $2K_2K_{2P}/(K_2 + K_{2P})$ (mutant). The dissociation constant is changed back to K_2 when the condition $y \leqslant y_P$ is fulfilled. For the simulation of the I $\rightarrow$ O switch, the same type of changes are performed for K_1. The t values for the two switches in K_2 and K_1 are marked by arrows ($\uparrow$) in the legend of Figure 20.

D. APPENDIX 4 — STEADY-STATE SOLUTIONS FOR THE STEROID HORMONE CONTROLLED TRIGGER

For the system of Equations 22a to f, Section V.F, the steady-state values for the inactive "O" state should correspond to $v = 0$ for the gene activation degree, the state "I" values to an activation degree, $v = 1$. For $v = 0$, and $v = 1$, Equations 22a and 22b yield the approximate solutions (Equation 24). With the resulting $y_I = 10^{-10}\,M$ and $K_2 = 10^{-8}\,M$ for the dissociation constant, most of the NHP protein will be in the monomer state, for this situation ($v = 1$).

For the unstable intermediate solution, which is on the separating curve between the active "I", and the inactive "O" state, the activation degree should be about $v = {}^1/_2$. From Equations 22c, d, e one has $u = K_4$, $z = K_3K_4$ and the approximate conditions (Equation 25) result.

ACKNOWLEDGMENTS

Computer programs and simulations were performed by Dr. G. I. Mihalaş (Institute of Medicine Timişoara). The permission to use the M-18 computer of the Laboratory of Medical Informatics of the Institute of Medicine Timişoara is hereby gratefully acknowledged, as well as the technical assistance of Mrs. Elisabeta Baranyi. The authors acknowledge the support of the Library of the Institute for Cellular Biology and Pathology (Bucharest) and of Dr. A. Vlad (Timiş District Hospital, Endocrinology Section) in providing the necessary scientific literature.

REFERENCES

1. **Freifelder, D.,** *Molecular Biology,* Jones and Bartlett Publishing, Boston, 1986.
2. **Lewin, B.,** *Genes,* John Wiley & Sons, New York, 1987.
3. **Antohi, S. and Gavrilă, L.,** *Progrese în Genetica Moleculară,* Edit. Didactică şi Enciclopedică, Bucureşti, 1981.
4. **Barrett, J. C.,** Genetic and epigenetic mechanism in carcinogenesis, in *Mechanisms of Environmental Carcinogenesis,* Vol. 1, Barrett, J. C., Ed., CRC Press, Boca Raton, FL, 1987, chap. 1.
5. **Ptashne, M. P., Bachman, K., Humarjan, M. A., Jeffrey, A., Maurer, R., Meyer, B., and Sauer, R. T.,** Autoregulation and function of a repressor in the lambda bacteriophage, *Science,* 194, 156, 1976.
6. **Monod, J. and Jacob, F.,** Teleonomic mechanisms in cellular metabolism, growth and differentiation, *Cold Spring Harbor Symp. Quant. Biol.,* 26, 389, 1961.
7. **Clemens, M.,** Development in development, *Nature,* 330, 699, 1987.
8. **Hunter, T.,** A thousand and one protein kinases, *Cell,* 50, 823, 1987.
9. **Draetta, G., Pivnica-Worms, H., Morrison, D., Drukker, B., Roberts, T., and Beach, D.,** Human adc2 protein kinase is a major cell cycle regulated tyrosine kinase substrate, *Nature,* 336, 438, 1988.
10. **Popescu, N. C., Chahinian, A. P., and Di Paolo, J. A.,** Non random chromosomal alterations in human malignant mesothelioma, *Cancer Res.,* 48, 142, 1988.
11. **Hershkovits, J. and Hagen, D.,** The lysis-lysogeny decision of λ phage, *Annu. Rev. Genet.,* 14, 399, 1980.
12. **Ptashne, M., Jeffrey, A., Johnson, A. D., Maurer, R., Meyer, B. J., Pabo, C. G., and Roberts, T. M.,** How the λ repressor and cro work, *Cell,* 19, 1, 1980.
13. **Davidson, E. H. and Britten, R. J.,** Organisation, transcription and regulation of the animal genome, *Q. Rev. Biol.,* 48, 565, 1973.
14. **Bullough, W. S.,** *The Evolution of Differentiation,* Academic Press, London, 1967.
15. **Bullough, W. S.,** Chalones, in *Growth Kinetics and Biochemical Regulation of Normal and Malignant Cells,* Drevinko, B. and Humphrey, R. M., Eds., University Park Press, Baltimore, 1977, p. 77.
16. **Patt, L. M. and Houck, J. C.,** The incredible shrinking chalone, *FEBS Lett.,* 120, 163, 1980.
17. **Konyshev, V. A.,** Chemical nature and systematisation of substances regulating animal cell growth, *Int. Rev. Cytol.,* 47, 195, 1976.
18. **Sachs, L.,** The molecular control of blood cell development, *Science,* 238, 1374, 1987.

19. **Ruoslahti, E. and Pierschbacher, M. D.,** New perspectives in cell adhesion, RGD and integrins, *Science,* 238, 491, 1987.

20. **Cunningham, B. A., Humperley, J. J., Murray, B. A., Drediger, E. A., Brackenbury, R., and Edehman, G. M.,** Neural cell adhesion molecules: structure, immunoglobuline like domains and alternative RNA splicing, *Science,* 236, 799, 1987.

21. **Matsukawa, T. and Bertram, J. S.,** Augmentation of post confluence growth arrest of 10t1/2 fibroblasts by endogenous c-adenosine-3′,5′-monophosphate, *Cancer Res.,* 48, 1874, 1988.

22. **Beer, D. G., Neven, M. J., Paul, D. L., Rapp, U. R., and Pitot, H. C.,** Expression of the c-rat protooncogene, γ-glutamyl transpeptidase and gap junction protein in rat liver neoplasms, *Cancer Res.,* 48, 1610, 1988.

23. **Loewenstein, W. R. and Kanno, Y.,** Intercellular communications and tissue growth control: lack of communications between cancer cells, *Nature,* 209, 1248, 1966.

24. **Loewenstein, W. R.,** Intercellular communications by gap junctions, *Physiol. Rev.,* 61, 829, 1981.

25. **Kenyon, C. and Kamb, A.,** Cellular dialogs during development, *Cell,* 58, 607, 1989.

26. **Bishop, J. M.,** The molecular genetics of cancer, *Science,* 235, 305, 1987.

27. **Temin, H. M.,** Evolution of cancer genes as a mutation driven process, *Cancer Res.,* 48, 1697, 1988.

28. **Sandberg, A. A.,** Role of chromosome changes in carcinogenesis in *Mechanisms of Environmental Carcinogenesis,* Vol. I, Barrett, J. C., Ed., CRC Press, Boca Raton, FL, 1987, chap. 6.

29. **Sanderberg, A. A., Turc-Carel, C., and Gemmill, R. M.,** Chromosome in solid tumors and beyond, *Cancer Res.,* 48, 1049, 1988.

30. **Farber, E., Rotstein, J. B., and Erikson, L. C.,** Cancer development as multistep process experimental studies in animals, in *Mechanisms of Environmental Carcinogenesis,* Vol. II, Barrett, J. C., Ed., CRC Press, Boca Raton, FL, 1987, chap. 9.

31. **Barrett, J. C.,** A multistep model for neoplastic development: role of genetic and epigenetic changes, in *Mechanisms of Environmental Carcinogenesis,* Vol. II, Barrett, J. C., Ed., CRC Press, Boca Raton, FL, 1987, chap. 13.

32. **Warburg, O.,** *Stoffwechsel der Tumoren,* Springer, Berlin, 1926.

33. **Bullough, W. S.,** Chalones, *Biol. Rev.,* 50, 49, 1976.

34. **Duesberg, P. H.,** Activated protooncogenes: sufficient or necessary for cancer?, *Science,* 228, 669, 1985.

35. **Cooper, G. M. and Lanc, M. A.,** Cellular transforming genes and oncogenes, *Biochem. Biophys. Acta,* 738, 9, 1984.

36. **Rhim, S. J., Fujita, J., and Park, J. B.,** Activation of H-ras oncogene in 3-methylcholantrene-transformated human cell lines, *Carcinogenesis,* 8, 1165, 1987.

37. **Graffen, J., Stephenson, J. R., Heisterkamp, N., de Klein, A., Bertram, C., and Grosveld, C.,** Philadelphia chromosomal break-points are clustered within a limited region, *bcr,* in chromosome 22, *Cell,* 36, 93, 1984.

38. **Murphee, A. L. and Benedict, W. F.,** Retinoblastoma clues to human oncogenes, *Science,* 223, 1028, 1984.

39. **Knudson, A. G., Jr.,** Hereditary cancer, oncogenes and antioncogenes, *Cancer Res.,* 45, 1437, 1985.

40. **Weinberg, R. A.,** Finding the anti-oncogene, *Sci. Am.,* 259, 34, 1988.

41. **Maelicke, A.,** Kontrolle des Zellwachstums und Krebs, *Nachr. Chem. Technol. Lab.,* 36, 997, 1988.

42. **Xu, H.-J., Hu, S.-X., Hashimoto, T., Takahashi, R., and Benedict, W. F.,** The retinoblastoma susceptibility gene product: a characteristic pattern in normal cells and abnormal expression in malignant cells, *Oncogene,* 4, 807, 1989.

43. **Frearon, E. R., Hamilton, S. R., and Vogelstein, B.,** Clonal analysis of human colorectal tumors, *Science,* 238, 193, 1987.

44. **Angel, P., Allegretto, J., Okino, S. T., Hattori, K., Boyle, W. V., Hunter, T., and Karin, M.,** Oncogene *jun*-encodes sequence specific transactivator similar to AP-1, *Nature,* 332, 166, 1988.

45. **Gilman, A. G.,** Irreversible activation of the ras protein-cyclasic function by mutation, *Cell,* 36, 577, 1984.

46. **McCormick, F.,** rasGTPase activating protein (GAP): signal transmitter and signal terminator, *Cell,* 56, 5, 1989.

47. **Jakulski, D., Kim de Riel, J., Mercer, W. E., Calabretta, B., and Baserga, R.,** Inhibition of cellular proliferation by antisense oligonucleotide to PCNA-cyclin, *Science,* 240, 1544, 1988.

48. **Van der Walter, L., Aronson, D., and Braman, V.,** Alteration of fibronectin receptors (integrins) in phorbol ester treated human promonocytic leukemia cells, *Cancer Res.,* 48, 5730, 1988.

49. **Sachs, L.,** Control of normal differentiation and the phenotypic reversion of malignancy in myeloid leukemia, *Nature,* 274, 535, 1978.

50. **Kaldor, J. M. and Day, N. E.,** Interpretation of epidemiological studies in the context of multistage models of carcinogenesis, in *Mechanisms of Environmental Carcinogenesis,* Vol. II, Barrett, J. C., Ed., CRC Press, Boca Raton, FL, 1987, chap. 10.

51. **Barrett, J. C. and Fletcher, W. F.,** Cellular and molecular mechanisms of multistep carcinogenesis in cell culture models, in *Mechanisms of Environmental Carcinogenesis,* Vol. II, Barrett, J. C., Ed., CRC Press, Boca Raton, FL, 1987, chap. 12.

52. **Maelicke, A.,** Die Entstehung von Krebs ein Mehrstuffenprocess?, *Nachr. Chem. Technol. Lab.,* 31, 898, 1983.

53. **Knudson, A. G., Jr.,** Mutations and cancer: statistical study of retinoblastoma, *Proc. Natl. Acad. Sci. U.S.A.,* 68, 820, 1971.

54. **Farber, E.,** The multistep nature of cancer development, *Cancer Res.,* 44, 4217, 1984.

55. **Bohr, V. A.,** Differential DNA repair within the genome, *Cancer Res.,* 47, 28, 1987.

56. **Igo-Kelemes, T., Hörz, W., and Zacchau, A. G.,** Chromatin structure in eukaryotes, *Annu. Rev. Biochem.,* 51, 89, 1982.

57. **Moyne, G., Freeman, R., Sawayosti, S., and Yaniv, M.,** A high resolution EPR study of nucleosomes from SV-40 chromatin, *J. Mol. Biol.,* 149, 735, 1981.

58. **Thoma, F., Koller, T. H., and Klug, A.,** Involvement of H1 in the organisation of the nucleosome and in the salt dependent superstructures of chromatin, *J. Cell. Biol.,* 83, 403, 1980.

59. **Adolph, K. W., Cheng, S. M., Pauson, J. R., and Laemmli, I. I.,** Isolation of a protein scaffold from mitotic HeLa cell chromosomes, *Proc. Natl. Acad. Sci. U.S.A.,* 74, 4937, 1977.

60. **Muskavits, M. A. T. and Hogness, D. S.,** Hypersensitivity to DNAase I of transcribed DNA sequences, *Cell,* 29, 1941, 1982.

61. **Bishop, J. O., Morton, J. G., Rosbach, M., and Richardson, M.,** Three abundance classes in HeLa cell messenger RNA, *Nature,* 250, 149, 1974.

62. **Ordahl, A. I. and Ordahl, Ch. P.,** Irreversible gene repression model for control of development, *Science,* 201, 120, 1978.

63. **Davidson, E. H. and Britten, R. J.,** Regulation of gene expression: possible role of repetitive sequences, *Science,* 204, 1052, 1979.

64. **Simon, Z.,** Messenger RNA abundance and gene regulation in eukaryotes, *Nature,* 255, 171, 1975.

65. **Sarkar, C. and Sommer, S. S.,** Access to a messenger RNA sequence or its protein is not limited by tissue or species specificity, *Science,* 244, 331, 1989.

66. **Green, J., Goldberg, B., and Todaro, J. G.,** Types of differentiated cells and regulation of collagen synthesis, *Nature,* 212, 631, 1966.

67. **Lasch, B., Heins, J., Hilse, H., Bath, A., and Oehme, P.,** Die Aktivität der Dipeptidyl-Peptidase IV in verschiedenen Organen und Geweben der Ratte, *Die Pharmazie (DDR),* 36, 161, 1981.

68. **Pekkel, V. A.,** Adenylate deaminase in animal tissues, *Uspehi Sovrem. Biol. (Moscow),* 89, 377, 190.

69. **Dixon, M. and Webb, E. C.,** *Enzymes,* Longmans, London, 1958, p. 642.

70. **Maniatis, T., Goodburn, S., and Fischer, J. A.,** Regulation of inducible and tissue specific gene expression, *Science,* 236, 4837, 1987.

71. **Echols, H.,** Multiple DNA-protein interactions governing high precision DNA-transactions, *Science,* 233, 1050, 1986.

72. **Graydon, R. D., Costa, R. H., Xanthopoulos, K. G., and Darnell, J. E.,** One factor recognizes the liver specific enhancers in d_1-antitripsyn and transthyretin genes, *Science,* 239, 786, 1988.

73. **Müller, H. P., Sogo, J. M., and Schefner, W.,** An enhancer stimulates transcription in trans when attached to the promoter via a protein bridge, *Cell,* 58, 767, 1989.

74. **Guarante, L.,** The UASs and enhancers: common mechanism of transcriptional activation in yeast and mammals, *Cell,* 52, 303, 1988.

75. **Lichtsteiner, S., Wuarin, J., and Schibler, U.,** The interplay of DNA bindings proteins on the promoter of mouse albumin gene, *Cell,* 51, 983, 1987.

76. **Chereghin, S., Raymondjean, M., Carranca, A. G., Herbonnel, Ph., and Yaniv, M.,** Factors involved in control of tissue specific expression of albumine gene, *Cell,* 50, 627, 1987.

77. **Share, D. and Nasmyth, K.,** Purification and cloning of a DNA-binding protein from yeast that binds to both silencer and activator elements, *Cell,* 51, 721, 1987.

78. **Scholler, H., Haslinger, A., Heguy, A., Holtgrave, H., and Karin, M.,** In vivo competition between a metallothionein regulatory element and the SV40 enhancer, *Science,* 232, 76, 1986.

79. **Dynan, W. S.,** Modularity in promoters and enhancers, *Cell,* 58, 1, 1989.

80. **Wingender, E. and Seifart, K. H.,** Transkription in Eukaryoten-die Rolle von Transkriptionskomplexen und ihren Komponenten, *Angew. Chem.,* 99, 206, 1987.

81. **Muramatsu, M.,** U.S.-Japan seminar on oncogenes in relation to developmental and transcriptional control, *Jpn. J. Cancer Res. (Gann),* 78, 1287, 1987.

82. **Kagan, L., Gill, G., and Ptashne, M.,** Separation of DNA binding from the transcription activating function of a eukaryote regulatory protein, *Science,* 231, 699, 1986.

83. **Ma, J. and Ptashne, M.,** The carboxyl-terminal 30 amino acids of GAL 4 are recognised by GAL 80, *Cell,* 50, 137, 1987.

84. **Wu, C., Wilson, S., Walker, B., David, I., Paisley, T., Zimarino, V., and Ueda, H.,** Purification and properties of the *Drosophila* heatshock activator protein, *Science,* 238, 1247, 1987.

85. **Davidson, J., Xiao, J. H., Rosales, R., Staub, A., and Chambon, P.,** The HeLa cell protein TEF-1 binds specifically and cooperatively to two SV40 enhancer motifs of unrelated sequences, *Cell,* 54, 931, 1988.

86. **Tsai, S. Y., Duke, J. C., Weigel, N. L., Dahlman, K., Gustaffson, J. A., Tsai, M., and O'Malley, B. W.,** Molecular interactions of a steroid hormone receptor with his enhancer element: evidence for receptor dimer formation, *Cell,* 55, 361, 1988.

87. **Hlazonetis, T. D., Georgeopoulos, K., Greenberg, M. E., and Leder, Ph.,** c-jun dimerises with itself and with c-Fos, forming complexes of different DNA binding affinity, *Cell,* 55, 917, 1988.

88. **Kumar, V. and Chambon, P.,** The estrogen receptor binds tightly to its responsive element as a ligand induced homodimer, *Cell,* 55, 145, 1988.

89. **Ma, J. and Ptashne, M.,** Converting an eukaryotic transcriptional inhibitor into an activator, *Cell,* 55, 443, 1988.

90. **Picard, D., Salser, S. J., and Yamamoto, K. R.,** A movable and regulable inactivation function within the steroid binding domain of the glucocorticoid receptor, *Cell,* 54, 1073, 1988.

91. **Glass, C. K., Helloway, J. M., Devary, O. V., and Rosenfeld, M. G.,** The thyroid hormone receptor binds with opposite transcriptional effects to a common sequence motif in thyroid hormone and estrogen response elements, *Cell,* 54, 313, 1988.

92. **Jaynes, J. B. and O'Farrell, P. H.,** Activation and repression of transcription by homeodomain containing proteins that bind at a common site, *Nature,* 336, 744, 1988.

93. **Maelicke, A.,** Jahresüberblick Molekularbiologie 1988, Oncogene, *Nachr. Chem. Technol. Lab.,* 37, 166, 1989.

94. **Green, M. R.,** When products of genes and antioncogenes meet, *Cell,* 56, 1, 1989.

95. **Biggin, M. D. and Tjian, R.,** A purified *Drosophila* homeodomain protein represses transcription in vitro, *Cell,* 58, 433, 1989.

96. **Yu, H., Porton, B., Shan, L., and Eckhardt, L. A.,** Role of the octamer motif in hybrid cell extinction of immunoglobuline gene expression: extinction is dominant in a two enhancer system, *Cell,* 58, 441, 1989.

97. **Meyer, M.-E., Gronemeyer, H., Turcotte, B., Bocquel, M.-T., Tasset, D., and Chambon, P.,** Steroid hormone receptors compete for factors that mediate their enhancer function, *Cell,* 57, 432, 1989.

98. **Holzer, H. and Rubinstein, N.,** Quantal mitosis, in *Cell Differentiation in Microorganisms, Plants and Animals,* Nover, L. and Mothes, K., Eds., VEB Gustav Fischer, Berlin, 1977, p. 450.

99. **Cook, P. R.,** Hypothesis on differentiation and the inheritance of gene structure, *Nature,* 245, 23, 1973.

100. **Weintraub, H. H.,** Assembly and propagation of repressed and derepressed chromosomal states, *Cell,* 45, 705, 1985.

101. **Grosschedl, R. and Marx, M.,** Stable propagation of the active transcriptional state of an immunoglobuline gene requires continuous enhancer function, *Cell,* 55, 645, 1988.

102. **Marx, J. L.,** A parent's sex may affect gene expression, *Science,* 239, 352, 1988.

103. **Hodkin, J.,** *Drosophila* sex determination, a cascade of regulated splicing, *Cell,* 56, 905, 1989.

104. **Cohen, J. B., Broz, S. D., and Levinson, A. D.,** Expression of the H-ras oncogene is controlled by alternative splicing, *Cell,* 58, 481, 1989.

105. **Bender, T. P., Thompson, C. B., and Kuehl, W. M.,** Differential expression of a *c-myb* mRNA in murine B lymphomas by a block to transcription elongation, *Science,* 237, 1437, 1987.

106. **Gay, D. A., Yan, T. J., Lau, J. T. Y., and Cleveland, D. W.,** Sequences that confer B-tubulin autoregulation through modulated m-RNA stability reside within exon 1 of B-tubulin mRNA, *Cell,* 50, 671, 1987.

107. **Gillies, S. D., Morrison, S. L., Oi, V. T., and Tonegawa, S.,** A tissue specific enhancer is located in the major intron of a rearranged immunoglobulin heavy gene, *Cell,* 33, 717, 1983.

108. **Nasmyth, K. and Shore, D.,** Transcriptional regulation in the yeast life cycle, *Science,* 237, 1162, 1987.

109. **Benditt, J.,** Genetic skeleton, *Sci. Am.,* 259, 14, 1988.

110. **Pienta, K. J., Partin, A. W., and Coffey, D. S.,** Cancer as a disease of DNA organisation and dynamic cell structure, *Cancer Res.,* 49, 225, 1989.

111. **Cedar, H.,** DNA methylation and gene activity, *Cell,* 53, 3, 1988.

112. **Simon, Z.,** Recognition between biological macromolecules, *J. Theoret. Biol.,* 9, 414, 1965.

113. **Sadler, J. R. and Smith, T. F.,** Mapping the lac operon, *J. Mol. Biol.,* 62, 139, 1971.

114. **Simon, Z.,** Specific interactions. Intermolecular forces, steric requirements and molecular size, *Angew. Chem. (Int. Ed),* 13, 719, 1974.

115. **Heinemann, U.,** Molekulare Basis der Genkontrolle, *Nachr. Chem. Technol. Lab.,* 32, 712, 1984.

116. **Bohm, S. and Dracher, D.,** Protein structure and specific DNA sequence recognition, *Stud. Biophys. (Berlin),* 107, 237, 1985.

117. **Singer, P. B.,** Acid blobs and negative noodels, *Nature,* 333, 210, 1988.

118. **Evans, R. M. and Hollenberg, S. M.,** Zinc fingers; guilt by association, *Cell,* 52, 1, 1988.

119. **Freedman, L. P., Yamamoto, K. R., Luisi, B. F., and Sigler, Z.,** Zinc fingers in hand, *Cell,* 54, 444, 1988.
120. **Frankel, A. D. and Pabo, C. O.,** Fingering to many proteins, *Cell,* 53, 675, 1988.
121. **Berg, J. M.,** DNA binding specificity of steroid receptors, *Cell,* 57, 1065, 1989.
122. **Danielsen, M., Hinck, L., and Ringold, G. M.,** Two aminoacids within the knuckle of the first zinc finger specify DNA response element activation by the glucocorticoid receptor, *Cell,* 57, 1131, 1989.
123. **Umesono, K. and Evans, R. M.,** Determination of target gene specificity for steroid/thyroid hormone receptors, *Cell,* 57, 1139, 1989.
124. **Gehring, W. J.,** Homeoboxes in the study of development, *Science,* 236, 1245, 1987.
125. **Desplan, C.,** Autoregulatory function for the engrailed protein, *Nature,* 318, 630, 1985.
126. **Hocy, T. and Levine, M.,** Divergent homeobox proteins recognise similar DNA sequences in *Drosophila, Nature,* 332, 858, 1988.
127. **Kusiora, M. A. and McGinnis, W.,** Autoregulation of a *Drosophila* homeotic selective gene, *Cell,* 55, 477, 1988.
128. **Klein, G.,** The approaching era of the tumor suppressor genes, *Science,* 238, 1539, 1987.
129. **Marx, J. L.,** The *fos* gene as master switch, *Science,* 237, 854, 1987.
130. **Verna, I. M. and Sassone-Corsi, P.,** Proto-oncogene fos: complex but versatile regulation, *Cell,* 51, 513, 1987.
131. **Struhl, K.,** The jun oncoprotein a vertebrate transcription factor, activates transcription in yeast, *Nature,* 332, 649, 1988.
132. **Bohman, D., Bos, T. J., Adma, A., Nishimura, T., Vogt, P. K., and Tjian, R.,** Human proto-oncogene *c-jun* encodes a DNA binding protein with structural and functional properties of transcription factor AP-1, *Science,* 238, 1386, 1987.
133. **Short, N. J.,** Regulation of transcription. Fraudulent promotion, *Nature,* 331, 393, 1988.
134. **Turner, R. and Tjian, R.,** Leucine repeats and an adjacent DNA binding domain mediate the formation of functional c-Fos-c-Jun heterodimers, *Science,* 243, 1689, 1989.
135. **Curran, T. and Franza, B. R., Jr.,** Fos and Jun, the AP-1 connection, *Cell,* 55, 395, 1988.
136. **Sassone-Corsi, P., Ransone, L. J., Lamph, W. W., and Verna, I. M.,** Direct interaction between fos and jun nuclear oncoprotein: role of the leucine zipper domain, *Nature,* 336, 692, 1988.
137. **Kouzarides, T. and Ziff, E.,** The role of the leucine zipper in the fos-jun interaction, *Nature,* 336, 646, 1988.
138. **Gentz, R., Rauscher, F. J., Abate, C., and Curran, T.,** Parallel association of Fos and Jun leucine zippers juxtaposes DNA binding domains, *Science,* 243, 1695, 1989.
139. **Angel, P., Hattori, K., Smeal, T., and Karin, M.,** The jun proto-oncogene is positively autoregulated by the product jun/AP-1, *Cell,* 55, 875, 1988.
140. **Thayer, M. J., Tapscott, S. J., Davis, R. L., Wright, W. E., Lassar, A. B., and Weintraub, H.,** Positive autoregulation of the myogenic determination gene myo D_1, *Cell,* 58, 241, 1989.
141. **Horowits, D., Ish, D., Pinchin, S. M., Ingham, P. W., and Gyurkovits, H. G.,** Autocatalytic ftz activation and metameric instability induced by ectopic ftz expression, *Cell,* 58, 223, 1989.
142. **Jones, K. A., Kadonaja, J. T., Luciw, P. A., and Than, R.,** Activation of the AIDS virus promoter by the transcription factor Sp1, *Science,* 232, 755, 1986.
143. **Leung, K. and Nabel, G. J.,** HTLV-1-transactivator induces interleukin-2 receptor expression through an NF-K3-like factor, *Nature,* 333, 776, 1988.
144. **Hasseltine, W. A. and Wong-Stahl, F.,** The molecular biology of the AIDS virus, *Sci. Am.,* 259, 34, 1988.
145. **Cullen, B. R. and Greene, W. C.,** Regulatory pathways governing HIV-1 replication, *Cell,* 58, 423, 1989.
146. **Okamoto, T., Matsuyama, T., Mori, S., Hamamoto, Y., Kobayashi, N., Yamamoto, N., Josephs, S. F., Wong-Staaland, F., and Schimotohuo, K.,** Augmentation of human immunodeficiency virus type 1 gene expression by tumor necrosis factor, *AIDS Reso Hum. Retroviruses,* 5, 131, 1989.
147. **Reichel, R., Kovesdi, I., and Nevins, J. R.,** Developmental control of a promoter specific factor that is also regulated by the E1A gene product, *Cell,* 48, 501, 1987.
148. **Fromental, C., Kanno, M., Nomiyama, H., and Chambon, P.,** Cooperativity and hierarchical levels of functional organization in the SV40 enhancer, *Cell,* 57, 943, 1988.
149. **De Vos, A. M., Tong, L., Milburn, M. V., Matias, P. M., Jancarik, J., Noguchi, S., Nishimura, S., Miura, K., Ohtsuka, E., and Kim, S. H.,** Three dimensional structure of an oncogene protein catalytic domain of human c-H-ras-p21, *Science,* 239, 888, 1988.
150. **Dickson, R. L., Rosen, N., Gelman, E. P., and Lippman, M. E.,** Receptor and signaling transduction-related proto-oncogenes in breast cancer, *TIPS,* 8, 372, 1987.

151. **Guerassio, A., Avanai, G. C., Pegoraro, L., Estwille, X., Serra, A., Glubellino, M. G., Fierro, M. T., Novarino, A., Foa, R., and Saglio, G.,** Rearrangement of the c-myc oncogene with heavy chain immunoglobuline enhancer in tumor DNA from an acute lymphoblastic leukemia patient, *J. Natl. Cancer Inst.,* 78, 845, 1987.

152. **Akhurst, R. J., Fee, F., and Balmain, L.,** Localized production of TGF-mRNA in tumor promoter stimulated mouse epidermis, *Nature,* 331, 364, 1988.

153. **Carter, T. H.,** The regulation of gene expression by tumor promoters, in *Mechanisms of Environmental Carcinogenesis,* Vol. I, Barrett, J. C., Ed., CRC Press, Boca Raton, FL, 1987, chap. 4.

154. **Jones, P. A.,** Role of DNA methylation in regulating gene expression in *Mechanisms of Environmental Carcinogenesis,* Vol. I, Barrett, J. C., Ed., CRC Press, Boca Raton, FL, 1987, chap. 2.

155. **Reitz, R. H.,** Role of cytotoxicity in the carcinogenic process, *Bambury Rep.,* 25, 107, 1987.

156. **Heinmets, F.,** Elucidation of induction and repression mechanisms in enzyme synthesis by analysis of model systems with the analog computer, in *Electronic Aspects of Biochemistry,* Pullman, B., Ed., Academic Press, New York, 1964, p. 415.

157. **Simon, Z.,** Multi-steady state model for cell differentiation, *J. Theoret. Biol.,* 8, 258, 1965.

158. **Simon, Z. and Ruckenstein, E.,** Regulation and synthesis processes in the living cell. III. Triggers of interrelated operons as elements of the cellular automaton, *J. Theoret. Biol.,* 11, 314, 1966.

159. **Grigorov, L. N., Polyakova, M. S., and Chernavsky, D. S.,** Modelling studies for trigger sequences and the differentiation process, *Mol. Biol. (Moscow),* 1, 410, 1967.

160. **Babloyants, A. and Nicolis, G.,** Chemical instabilities and multiple steady state transitions in Monod-Jacob type models, *J. Theoret. Biol.,* 34, 185, 1972.

161. **Goodwin, B. C.,** *Temporal Organization in Cells,* Academic Press, London, 1963.

162. **Goodwin, B. C.,** Oscillatory behaviour in enzymatic control processes, *Adv. Enzyme Regul.,* 3, 425, 1965.

163. **Knorre, W. A.,** Analog-computer Simulation der Enzymsynthese in Bakterien, *Stud. Biophys. (Berlin),* 6, 1, 1968.

164. **Tivary, J., Fraser, A., and Beckman, R.,** Genetical feedback repression. I. Single locus model, *J. Theoret. Biol.,* 45, 311, 1974.

165. **Fraser, A. and Tivary, J.,** Genetical feedback repression. II. Cyclic genetic systems, *J. Theoret. Biol.,* 47, 397, 1974.

166. **Smith, H.,** Oscillations and multiple steady states in a cyclic gene model with repression, *J. Math. Biol.,* 25, 169, 1987.

167. **Cartianu, D.,** A study of the stability of realistic models of oscillating chemical reactions by using concepts derived from the rules of flow graphs, *Rev. Roum. Chim.,* 33, 489, 1988.

168. **Churaev, R. N. and Ratner, V. A.,** Modelling molecular-genetic control systems in the language of automaton-theory. I. Operons and operon systems, in *Issledovany Teoreticheskoy Genetiki,* Ratner, V. A., Ed., Academy of Science, Novosibirsk, USSR, 1972, 210.

169. **Tsanev, R. and Sendov, B.,** Model for a regulatory mechanism of cell multiplication, *J. Theoret. Biol.,* 12, 327, 1966.

170. **Sendov, B. and Tsanev, R.,** Computer simulation of the regenerative process in the liver, *J. Theoret. Biol.,* 18, 90, 1968.

171. **Tsanev, R. and Sendov, B.,** A cancer model studied by computer, *J. Theoret. Biol.,* 20, 124, 1969.

172. **Tsanev, R. and Sendov, B.,** Possible molecular model for cell differentiation in multicellular organisms, *J. Theoret. Biol.,* 30, 337, 1971.

173. **Kovarski, V. A. and Porfir, A. V.,** Trigger mechanism for the temperature activation of the TS-mutant of the src-oncogene in the model of Georgiev, *Biofizika (Moscow),* 34, 259, 1989.

174. **Sugita, M.,** Functional analysis of chemical in vivo systems by use of logic circuit equivalent. The molecular autonom idea, *J. Theoret. Biol.,* 4, 179, 1963.

175. **Kauffman, S. A.,** Metabolic stability and epigenesis in randomly constructed genetic nets, *J. Theoret. Biol.,* 22, 437, 1969.

176. **Bignone, F. A. and Bordo, D.,** Gene regulation: computer modelling with randomly connected boolean nets, *Cell Biol. Int. Rep.,* 10, 153, 1986.

177. **Simon, Z.,** Three steady state trigger with positive control for regulation of gene activity in eukaryotes, Preprint University of Timişoara, *Serie Chemie,* 4, 1984.

178. **Simon, Z. and Niculescu-Duvăz, I.,** Positive control, growth homeostasis, carcinogenesis. A hypothetical model, *Rev. Roum. Biochem.,* 23, 59, 1986.

179. **Mihalaş, G. I., Niculescu-Duvăz, I., and Simon, Z.,** Trigger with positive control for gene activity regulation. Computer simulation, *Stud. Biophys. (Berlin),* 107, 223, 1985.

180. **Besis, M.,** *The Cell,* Vol. V, Brachet, J. and Mirsky, R., Eds., Academic Press, New York, 1961, chap. 3.

181. **Paul, J.,** *Cells and Tissues in Culture,* Vol. I, Wilmer, E. N., Ed., Academic Press, New York, 1965, chap. 7.

182. **Starodub, N. F.,** Molecular basis of the differentiation of eritroid cells and regulation of the biosynthesis of different hemoglobin types, *Usp. Sovrem. Biol. (Moscow)*, 89, 124, 1980.

183. **Bachman, A.,** Turnover rates for mRNA and proteins in mammalian cells, *Science*, 234, 179, 1986.

184. **Simon, Z. and Mihalaş, G. I.,** Stability towards constitutive mutations in diploid cells with positive gene control. Computer simulation, *Stud. Biophys. (Berlin)*, 115, 113, 1986.

185. **Schrader, W. T. and O'Malley, B. W.,** Molecular structure and analysis of progesterone receptors, in *Receptors and Hormone Action*, Vol. II, O'Malley, B. W. and Birnbaumer, L., Eds., Academic Press, New York, 1978, 189.

186. **Baxter, J. D. and Ivarie, R. D.,** Regulation of gene expression by glucocorticoid hormones. Studies of receptors and responses in cultured cells, in *Receptors and Hormone Action*, Vol. II, O'Malley, B. W. and Birnbaumer, L., Eds., Academic Press, New York, 1978, p. 251.

187. **Clark, J. H., Pecker, E. J., Jr., Hardin, J. W., and Erickson, H.,** The biology and pharmacology of estrogen receptor binding. Relationship to uterine growth, in *Receptors and Hormone Action*, Vol. II, O'Malley, B. W. and Birnbaumer, L., Eds., Academic Press, New York, 1978, 1.

188. **Leavitt, W. W., Chen, T. J., Do, Y. S., Carlton, B. D., and Allen, T. C.,** Biology of progesterone receptors, in *Receptors and Hormone Action*, Vol. II, O'Malley, B. W. and Birnbaumer, L., Eds., Academic Press, New York, 1978, p. 157.

189. **Notides, A. C.,** Conformational forms of the estrogen receptor, in *Receptors and Hormone Action*, Vol. II, O'Malley, B. W. and Birnbaumer, L., Eds., Academic Press, New York, 1978, 33.

190. **Sluyter, M., Ed.,** *Interaction of Steroid Hormone Receptor with DNA*, VCH Publishers, Deerfield Beach, FL, 1985.

191. **Greene, G. F., Gilna, P., Watersfield, M., Baker Hirst, Y., and Shine, J.,** Sequence and expression of human estrogen receptor complementarity DNA, *Science*, 231, 1150, 1986.

192. **Kumar, V., Green, S., Stuck, G., Berry, M., Jin, J. R., and Chambon, P.,** Functional domains of the human estrogen receptor, *Cell*, 51, 941, 1987.

193. **Simon, Z., Vlad, A., and Mihalaş, G. I.,** Positive gene control and steroid hormone receptor protein interactions. A mathematical model, *Stud. Biophys. (Berlin)*, 125, 137, 1988.

194. **Emerson, B. M., Lewis, C. D., and Felsenfeld, S.,** Interaction of specific nuclear factors with the nuclease hypersensitive region of the chicken adult β-globulin gene, Nature of the binding domain, *Cell*, 41, 21, 1985.

195. **Steiberg, R. A., Lewinson, B. B., and Tompkins, G. M.,** Kinetics of steroid induction and deinduction of tyrosine amino-transferase in hepatoma cells, *Proc. Natl. Acad. Sci. U.S.A.*, 72, 2007, 1975.

196. **Guichon-Montel, A., Loosfelt, A., Lescop, P., Sar, S., Atger, M., Perrot-Appland, M., and Milgrom, E.,** Mechanism of nuclear localisation of the progesterone receptor: evidence for interaction between monomers, *Cell*, 57, 1147, 1989.

197. **Tsai, S. Y., Tsai, M. J., and O'Malley, B. W.,** Cooperative binding of steroid hormone receptors contributes to transcriptional synergism at target enhancer elements, *Cell*, 57, 443, 1989.

198. **Cormier, E. M., Jordan, W. C., and Gorski, J.,** Biochemical evidence for the exclusive nuclear localization of the estrogen receptor, in *Gene Regulation by Steroid Hormones III*, Roy, A. K. and Clark, J. H., Eds., Springer, New York, 1987.

199. **Tata, J. R., Ng, W. C., Perlman, A. J., and Wolfe, A. P.,** Activation and regulation of the vitellogenin gene family, in *Gene Regulation by Steroid Hormones, III*, Roy, A. K. and Clark, J. H., Eds., Springer, New York, 1987, 205.

200. **Jimenez, J. J. and Yunis, A. A.,** Tumor cell rejection through terminal cell differentiation, *Science*, 238, 1278, 1987.

201. **Sherman, M. I., Ed.,** How do retinoids promote differentiation, in *Retinoids and Cell Differentiation*, Dawson, P. and Nakamura, M., Eds., CRC Press, Boca Raton, FL, 1986, chap. 8.

202. **La Mantia, G., Pengue, G., Maglione, D., Pannuti, A., Pascucci, A., and Lania, L.,** Identification of new human repetitive sequences, characterization of the corresponding cDNAs and their expression in embryonal carcinoma cells, *Nucl. Acid. Res.*, 17, 5919, 1989.

203. **Thaller, I. and Eichele, G.,** Identification of a morphogen: retinoic acid, *Nature*, 327, 625, 1987.

204. **Petkovich, M., Brand, N. J., Krust, A., and Chambon, P.,** Closing of the morphogen-receptor gene, *Nature*, 330, 444, 1987.

205. **Driever, W. and Nusslein-Volhard, C.,** The bicoid gene product as morphogen in the *Drosophila* embryo, *Cell*, 54, 83, 1988.

206. **Struhl, G., Struhl, K., and MacDonald, P. M.,** The gradient morphogen bicoid is a concentration dependent transcriptional activator, *Cell*, 57, 1259, 1989.

207. **Lippman, S. M., Kesaler, J. F., and Meyskens, F. L., Jr.,** Retinoids as preventive and therapeutic anticancer agents (Part 1), *Cancer Treat. Rep.*, 71, 391, 1987.

208. **Simon, Z., Mihalaş, G. I., Rottenberg, F., Nagy, I. I., Vlad, A., and Poari, M.,** Positive gene control model. Computer simulations, *Timişoara Medicală*, Suppl. XXXII, 36, 1987.

209. **Dorn, W. S. and McCracken, D. D.,** *Numerical Methods with Fortran Case Studies*, John Wiley & Sons, New York, 1972.

Chapter 3

QUANTITATIVE PREDICTION OF CARCINOGENIC ACTIVITY

Ion Niculescu-Duvăz and Nicolae Voiculetz

TABLE OF CONTENTS

I. INTRODUCTION

The rationalization of connections between molecular structure and biological activity of chemical carcinogens was undertaken very soon after the discovery of the carcinogenic properties of polynuclear aromatic hydrocarbons. However, because this property belongs to compounds with largely different chemical structures, even today, when computer-assisted, structure-activity programs are available this aim remains a very difficult task.

No general structure-activity relationship that would account for all the experimental data and for all types of carcinogens can be formulated as yet. However, such tentatives on limited series of structurally related compounds were done and some of them were in surprisingly good agreement with the facts.

Before detailing this aspect, we have to emphasize the critical importance of a suitable evaluation for the carcinogenic potency of various chemicals. The accuracy and reproducibility of this experimental parameter will determine the general reliability of the computed relations and thus their predictive capability.

Carcinogenic potency varies with many factors (mode of administration, animal species employed, etc.) and its measurement raises extremely difficult technical problems. Nevertheless, some indices have been developed which (at least in a general manner) are able to distinguish the relative potencies of chemicals to induce tumors. One of the earliest known is the Iball index,[1] expressed by the ratio between the percentage of animals developing tumors and the average latent period (in days) × 100.

Because most human cancers are of epithelial origin, an estimation of the carcinogenic activity based on tumor induction in this tissue would be most relevant for human condition. An index based on the number of skin tumors induced in a mouse by a single administration of a chemical was recently developed, the carcinogenicity of a compound being expressed in units of tumors per micromole of applied compound.[2] Unfortunately, this index has been determined for a very limited number of substances.

Besides their inherent imprecision, such types of assay are afflicted by their long duration (1 to 2 years) and the large number of animals, the expenditure being evaluated at 30,000 to 500,000 dollars/compound.[3]

This problem was partially answered by the development of mutagenicity tests (especially the Salmonella-microsome test by Ames) which has gained widespread acceptance as the initial assay for the identification of potential mutagens and carcinogens. These bacteria tests are inexpensive and easy to perform, thus furnishing rapidly accurate and reproducible data for thousands of chemicals.[4,5] A positive correlation between Salmonella mutagenicity and rodent carcinogenicity (ranging from 78 to 95%) was reported for a large number of compounds.[6-8] This mutagenicity parameter is extremely useful in developing quantitative structure-activity relationships in chemical carcinogenesis. However, the proportion of carcinogens detected as mutagens depends heavily on the specific classes of chemicals (i.e., only 40% of the chlorinated carcinogens are mutagens) and on the rodent species used to assess the carcinogenicity. These findings restrict, to a certain extent, the predictive guiding character for the identification of carcinogens (but not for noncarcinogens).[9]

The aim of this chapter is to rationalize the various theoretical approaches (mathematical models, often computer assisted) undertaken in this area, in order to correlate physicochemical, structural or electronic parameters of chemicals with their carcinogenicity.

II. CLASSIFICATION OF THEORETICAL MODELS DEVELOPED FOR PREDICTION OF CARCINOGENIC ACTIVITY

The effectiveness of the theoretical models employed in carcinogenic activity prediction greatly improved both with our better understanding of the chemical carcinogenesis mechanisms and with the development of new computational procedures.

A better knowledge of the metabolism of various chemical carcinogens and the discovery of fundamental differences in their mechanism of action allowed Williams[10] to classify them in genotoxic and nongenotoxic carcinogens, more precisely in DNA-reactive carcinogens and carcinogens indirectly affecting the structure (or function) of the genetic material (see Scheme 1).

For the first class including the overwhelming majority of the "classical" carcinogens, nowadays there are arguments which strongly suggest that their interaction with DNA is the trigger of the cellular malignant transformation. These arguments are:

1. Recognition of a positive correlation between the carcinogenic activity and the extent of DNA binding (for PAH and some alkylating carcinogens)[11-13]
2. Experimental verification that the metabolic pathway responsible for DNA binding is that which produces the most carcinogenic metabolites[14]
3. Identification of proto-oncogenes which can be activated by chemical carcinogens[15-17]
4. Finding of carcinogenesis inhibitors which act by decreasing the concentration of DNA-carcinogen adducts[18]
5. Association of deficient DNA-repair mechanisms (in *Xeroderma pigmentosum*) with increased incidence of skin cancer[19]
6. The transformed phenotype can be conveyed to normal cells by transfection, etc.

On the basis of their requirement for an enzymatic or nonenzymatic activation, the chemical carcinogens were divided into direct and indirect acting carcinogens. The enzymatic systems involved in the activation process (e.g., cytochrome P-450 monooxygenases, prostaglandin synthetase, etc.), as well as the stereochemistry and kinetics of the reactions yielding the "ultimate carcinogens" are known in many cases (for review, see References 20 to 22). Equally important are the spontaneous or enzymatic reactions which limit or decrease the concentration of "ultimate carcinogens", leading to detoxication products (the enzymatic systems involved being glutathione-S-transferases, UDP-glucuronyl-transferases, etc.). The activation-detoxication equilibrium often plays a key role in determining the carcinogenic properties of the compounds.

The direct interaction between "ultimate carcinogens" and DNA has been also studied in detail in several cases, and the influence of steric and electronic parameters on the reaction pathway and mechanism has been established. The structure of the reaction products (usually known as adducts) has also been accurately determined for some carcinogens.[23]

Despite numerous unresolved problems, a general and coherent picture has emerged, partially represented in Scheme 1.

However, we must keep in mind that not every induced DNA adduct represents a trigger of the carcinogenic process, namely: there are specific positions, both on the purine/pyrimidine moieties and along the DNA molecule, that have to be affected by the carcinogen in order to produce a promutagenic event leading to further miscoding. Such a position is O^6G, O^4T, etc. for alkylating agents (alkylation at N^7 is not a promutagenic event per se). For PAH (at least in the cases of benzo(a)pyrene BaP and 7,12-dimethyl-benz(a) anthracene-DMBA), the reaction products formed at N^6A seem to be responsible for their carcinogenic activity.[24,25] Finally, it is necessary for such a promutagenic adduct — in order to trigger the cellular transformation — to be located in specific regions along the DNA molecule. For instance, a carcinogen affecting the codon 12 or 61 of the H-*ras* oncogene[26] leads to cellular transformation, whereas a similar lesion situated on a DNA region lacking special biological significance is probably ineffective. There are also efficient repair processes which decrease the concentration of the adducts. They proceed with different rates for different adduct structures[25] and intragenomic localizations.

Nowadays there are various models which allow a satisfactory (sometimes surprisingly accurate) prediction of the carcinogenic properties for a limited class of compound. From

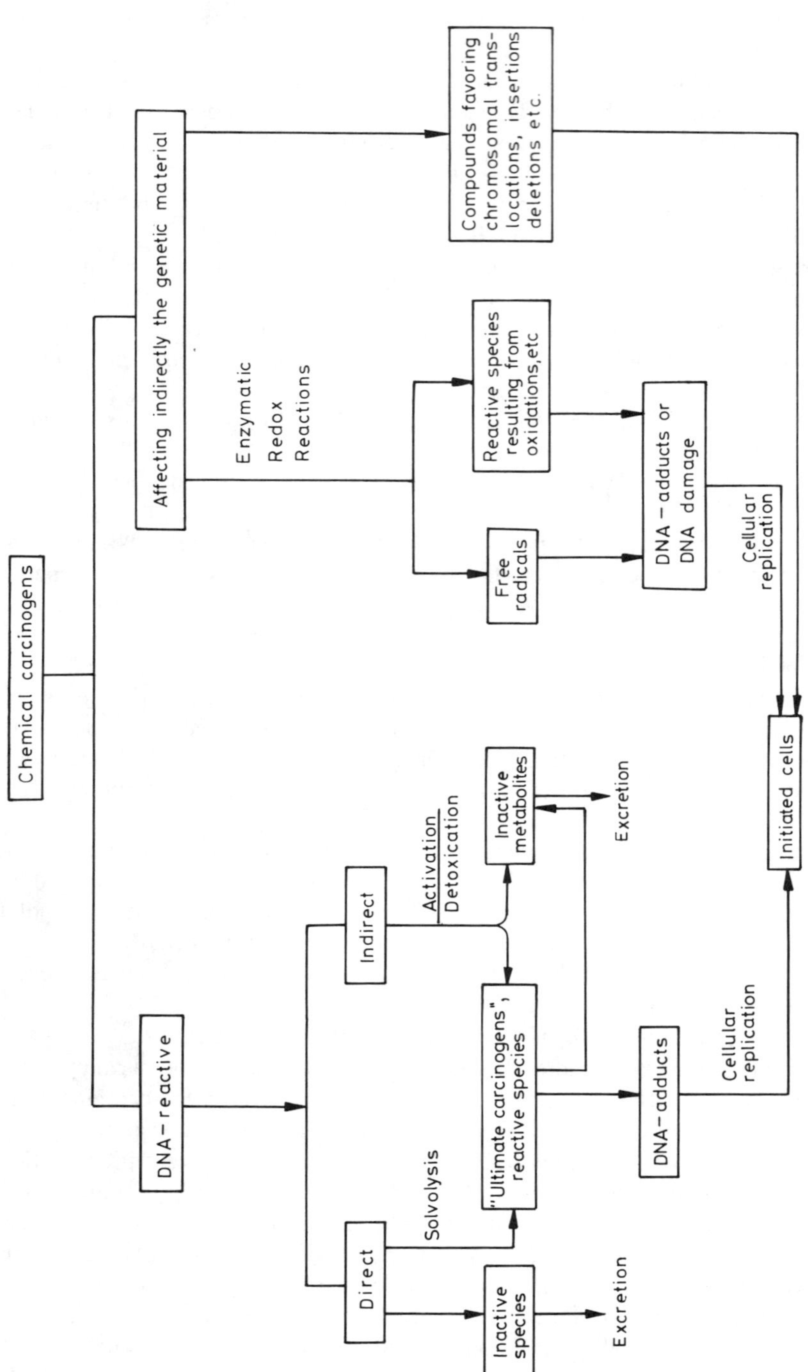

SCHEME 1.   Classification of carcinogens and of their mechanisms of action.

TABLE 1
Models Used for Carcinogenic Activity Prediction of DNA-Reactive Carcinogens

Type of carcinogen 1.	Determinant step taken into account for modeling[a] 2.	Predictive models[b] 3.	Parameters used in correlations with carcinogenic activity 4.
Direct-acting	Solvolysis (generation) of electrophilic species in aqueous media)	Reaction with water or other nucleophiles (NPB), etc. Electrophilicity and stereochemistry of the reactive intermediates Softness of alkylated species and alkylated sites Interaction with DNA *in vitro* and *in vivo*	Reaction rate constant Swain-Scott constants, competition factors, softness, quantum-mechanical parameters, electrostatic potential associated to nucleophilic centers in DNA, lipophilicity, etc.
	Electronic structure, size and shape of parent molecule	Quantitative description of electronic structure of parent molecule (K-, L-region theory, superdelocalizability indices, etc.) Reactions which involve a region of the parent molecule with particular electronic features, i.e., oxidation with OsO_4, etc.	Quantum-mechanical parameters, lipophilicity form indices, topological indices, Van der Waals volumes, reactive rate with OsO_4, free radicals, etc.
Indirect-acting	Enzymatic activation Spontaneous or enzymatic detoxication	Rate determining reactions involved in both carcinogens activation or detoxication	Reaction rates and equilibrium constants, quantum-mechanical parameters, steric or topological indices, etc.
	DNA interaction	Ultimate carcinogens reactivity (electrophilicity, stereochemistry, etc.) (Bay-region theory) Interaction with DNA *in vitro* and *in vivo*	Reaction rates and equilibrium constants nucleophilic substitution indices, quantum-mechanical parameters (computed by respect to ultimate carcinogens), topological indices, etc.

[a]   According to Scheme 1.
[b]   These models are developed for the computation of the parameters which correlated to the carcinogenic (or mutagenic) activity of DNA-reactive carcinogens.

this point of view, the polycyclic aromatic hydrocarbons are undoubtedly the most extensively studied class of carcinogens. There are many reasons for this choice. The first one regards the fact that carcinogenicity of PAH has been early discovered and measured for a relatively large number of structurally related compounds. The second reason consists in the particular electronic structure of aromatic systems which is very well suited for a quantitative description based on relatively easily performed theoretical, quantum-chemical calculations.

The alkylating carcinogens are also quite a large group of compounds for which the rational prediction of activity is possible. These are mainly direct carcinogens which by solvolysis release electrophilic species able to interact directly with DNA. The positive correlation found between the electrophilicity of these intermediates and the carcinogenic potency of the parent compounds appears to be an adequate basis for their activity prediction.

Such approaches were also noticed for other types of chemical carcinogens. An attempt to rationalize these prediction models for DNA-reactive carcinogens is given in Table 1.

For the "nonclassical" (epigenetic, nongenotoxic, etc.) carcinogens, which appear to

TABLE 2
Direct-Acting Carcinogens[a] with Alkylating Activity

No. 1.	Chemical class 2.	Typical carcinogens 3.
Alkyl halides		*n*-Propyl and isopropyl iodide; *sec-* and *tert*-butyl chloride, bromide and iodide; benzyl-chloride; 1,2-dibromoethane; 1,2-dichloroethane; 1,2-dibromo-3-chloropropene; 7-bromomethyl-benz(a)anthracene; 7-bromo-methyl-12-methylbenz(a)-anthracene
Alkyl phosphates		Dimethyl-2,2-chlorovinyl-phosphate; tris (2,3-dibromopropyl) phosphate
Alkyl sulfates		Dimethyl sulfate; diethyl sulfate; diisopropyl sulfate
Aziridines (mono- and difunctional)		Propyleneimine; triethylene-melamine; ethyleneimine; aziridine ethanol; *N*-caproyl-ethyleneimine; tris-(aziridinyl)-*p*-benzo-quinone; Thio-TEPA
Cyclic sulfides and sultones		1,3-propane sultone
Haloalkyl amines		Nitrogen mustard; Chlorambucil; Melphalan; Cyclophosphamide; naphthylamine mustard; uracil mustard, etc.
Haloalkyl ethers		Bis(chloromethyl) ether; 1,2,3-tris(chloro-methoxy)propane
Haloalkyl sulfides		Sulfur mustard
Lactones, oxetanes (4-membered rings), 5-membered rings and related compounds		β-propiolactone; β-butyrolactone; penicillinic acid; trimethyleneoxide; 3,3-dimethyl-2-oxethanone; β-dimethylmallic, maleic and succinic anhydride; vinylidene carbonate; sorbic acid, dehydroacetic acid
Methanesulfonates (mono- and difunctional)		Methyl methanesulfonate; ethyl methanesulfonate; alkyl methanesulfonates; Myleran; Mannitol Myleran
N-nitroso-guanidines		*N'*-methyl-*N'*-nitro-*N*-nitroso-guanidine
N-Nitrosourea		*N*-methyl-*N*-nitrosourea; *N*-ethyl-*N*-nitrosourea; 1(2-chloroethyl)-3-cyclohexyl-1-nitrosourea, etc.
Organo-metallic compounds		cis-Platin

[a]   Confirmed in animal tests.

be nonmutagenic and include hormones, peroxisomes proliferators, immunosuppressive carcinogens* etc., the complexity of the mechanisms involved precludes as yet any theoretical or quantitative approach with predictive capability.

Because we decided to review and to rationalize the theoretical models employed in the prediction of the carcinogenic activity for differernt types of compounds, our discussion is focused mainly on those models which allow a suitable description of the biological behavior of the various chemical carcinogens. The theoretical background of the correlational procedures used in the selection of the more appropriate parameters for such approaches is discussed in Chapter 5.

III. PREDICTIVE MODELS FOR THE CARCINOGENIC ACTIVITY OF ALKYLATING AGENTS (DIRECT-ACTING CARCINOGENS)

Biological alkylating agents, as defined by Ross,[27] are compounds which can replace a hydrogen atom by an alkyl group under physiological conditions (pH 7.0, 37°C, aqueous medium). Among them, there is a large number of chemical carcinogens with widely different structures.[28] They are summarized in Table 2.

---

*   In contrast to Weissburger and Williams' classification[10] we did not include promoters in this category; in the present author's opinions they represent a special group of agents involved in chemical carcinogenesis. A discussion of this aspect is, however, beyond the aim of this chapter.

Most of the biological alkylating agents also exhibit a pronounced cytotoxic effect against rapidly proliferating cells, being widely used as antitumor agents.[29]

The majority of the alkylating agents (direct-acting carcinogens) undergo *in vivo* a solvolytic decomposition to an electrophilic species which interacts directly with target cellular macromolecules (especially DNA). If this interaction is critical for the initiation step it is logical to assume a positive correlation between some properties of these electrophilic species and their carcinogenic activity. In order to substantiate this hypothesis, both *in vitro* and *in vivo* models were proposed.

The *in vitro* approach is mainly concerned with the finding of parameters which allow the quantitative description of the "ultimate carcinogens"-DNA interaction, under the most simple conditions. The employed models were focused on the direct reaction in aqueous media between: (1) pure "ultimate carcinogens" and nucleosides, nucleotides, or DNA and (2) carcinogens activated by microsomal, nuclear, or mitochondrial systems and DNA.

An alkylated DNA macromolecule is well characterized by two factors: the extent (i.e., the number of alkylated purine and pyrimidine units per DNA molecule) and the specificity (i.e., the reaction site on the purine or pyrimidine moieties) of the alkylation. Both factors may be rationalized in terms of stereochemistry and reactivity of the electrophilic species, reaction mechanism (S_N1 or S_N2), and nucleophilicity of the alkylated sites.

Usually, the relationships obtained between the DNA alkylation extent or specificity, and the aforementioned parameters are of linear or multilinear form. Unlike carcinogenicity, mutagenicity is much more dependent of the alkylation extent, as attested by several lines of evidence.[28]

The *in vivo* modeling of the same phenomenon is obviously more difficult by a series of supplementary factors leading to a picture which is much more difficult to express quantitatively. Among these factors we cite:

1. The necessity for the carcinogen to cross several barriers (i.e., cellular or nuclear membranes) and cytoplasmic compartments before reaching the desired target; the uptake and transport mechanisms in these systems are largely dependent on the chemical structure, as well as on the lipophilicity of the carcinogen. Moreover, this dependence often is no longer linear, becoming for instance, parabolic ($f(\pi,\pi^2)$).
2. Concurrent reactions with other nucleophiles (especially proteins, RNA, etc.) which diminish the number of carcinogen molecules reaching the target.
3. The existence of different repair processes, which decrease the overall concentration of the adducts induced by the carcinogen at the DNA level; mention must be made that these mechanisms are also selective, different adducts being repaired at different rates.

The development of the chemical dosimetry of carcinogenic and mutagenic agents, as well as of the quantitative expression of dose-effect relationships for the same type of compounds, furnished an improved background for the quantitative treatment of both mutagenesis and carcinogenesis. An excellent discussion of this topic belongs to Lawley.[28,30]

Two basic concepts have to be introduced before formulating any dose-response relationships in mutagenesis. The first is that DNA is the essential target for the mutagens. The second regards the contribution of the different repair processes.

Broad similarities exist between the action of chemical mutagens and radiation (e.g., both affect DNA, stimulate excision repair and postreplication repair, etc.) justifying the use for chemical mutagenesis quantification of the relationships developed for both radiation dosimetry and mutagenesis. Hence, Haynes[31] expressed the survival-fraction for UV inactivation of yeast, taking into account as repairing process the thymidine dimers excision from DNA. The following equation (of single hit and multitarget form) resulted, in which the repair system is inactivated by the mutagen according to a multitarget expression:

$$-\ln S = (1 - \tau_0)kD + \tau_0 kD(1 - \exp(-\beta D)^t) \tag{1}$$

where: S = survival fraction; τ_0 = fraction of potentially inactivating lesions repaired at zero dose; k = sensitivity of repairless line; D = dose; β = sensitivity of the enzymatic repair complex and t = multiplicity of hits necessary for the inactivation of the enzymatic repair complex.

Although this equation was derived with particular reference to the excision of pyrimidine dimers, it seems plausible that a similar treatment could also fit the chemical mutagenesis, because, as it was found in many cases, τ_0 is close to unity, which means a quasi-complete repair at zero dose) and linear term of Equation 1 disappears, as for instance in UV irradiation of yeast.[31] For chemical mutagenesis, no dose-response correlation containing the linear term of Equation 1 was ever obtained, all the curves being asymptotic to the abscissa. Therefore, the ratio of mutagenic hits to chemical hits affecting DNA (M/Z) should tend toward a constant value as the dose decreases. In contrast, the mutagenic efficiency (expressed as $M/-\ln S$) increases under the same conditions.

These considerations are in agreement with the survival curves obtained for the induction of mutations in V-79 hamster cells (resistant to 8-azaguanine) by two aralkylating agents: 7-bromomethyl-benzo(a)anthracene, 7-BrMBA (Equation 2) and BP-7.8-diol-epoxide, BPDE-*anti* (Equation 3).[32] The following expressions were obtained for the survival curves:

$$-\ln S = 1.09 \times 10^{-3}Z^2 + 0.156Z^3 \tag{2}$$

$$-\ln S = 6.5 \times 10^{-4}Z^2 + 1.56 \times 10^{-4}Z^3 \tag{3}$$

These curves are obviously nonlinear, being asymptotic to the abscissa, therefore giving for $\tau_0 = 1$.

Following a hypothesis which assumes that alkylating agents act by inactivating mutations, i.e., that an η-ploid cell dies if at least one important cistron is inactivated in all alleles, the probability of survival.

$$p_s = \left[(1 - (1 - \exp\left(-\frac{\alpha \cdot X}{\eta \cdot N}\right)^\eta \right]^{N\beta} \tag{4}$$

X = number of alkylations; η = ploidy; N = number of targets (nucleotide pairs per haploid chromosome sets; β = fraction of vital targets and α = probability of inactivation by one alkylation.

A diploid mammalian cell ($N = 2.5 \cdot 10^9$, $\eta = 2$, $\alpha = 1$, $\beta = 1$) should be killed by at least 2×10^3 alkylations in the cell DNA, which agrees with experimental values for cyclophosphamide and nitrogen mustard on hamster plasmacytoma (1×10^4 alkylations) but is much lower than the value for other alkylating cytostatics ($10^5 - 10^7$ alkylations).[33]

With regard to the relationship between mutational and chemical hits, a number of factors have to be taken into account. They are the specificity of the DNA alkylation, the nonrandom nature of this process, the existence of promutagenic lesions, the repair of the promutagenic bases before DNA replication, etc.

Not all the alkylated bases are equally effective in producing further miscoding.

If the alkylation of DNA occurs randomly, the following equation was proposed, containing a considerably larger number of variables,[34]

$$\frac{M}{Z} = n_M \times \sum_i \left(f_i \times P_{Mi} \frac{1 - r_{Mi}}{g_i} \right) \tag{5}$$

where: M = mutations induced per surviving cell; Z = extent of overall alkylation per nucleotide unit; n_M = number of nucleotidic sites at which a mutation can be induced; f_i = the fraction of total alkylations which affect the site supposed to cause miscoding (e.g., O^6G, O^4T, etc.); g_i = the proportion of a given i base in DNA to which the key mutation occurs (e.g., g_i = 0.21 for G in mammalian DNA); P_{Mi} = the probability that the alkylation of the considered site in the i base will produce miscoding and r_{Mi} = the proportion of the assumed miscoding base to be removed (by repair enzymes) before DNA replication.

Using this equation, Lawley and Martin[35] obtained a quantitative correlation between the extent of the T4rHAP72 bacteriophage alkylation and induced reverse mutation to wild-type T_4 with ethyl methanesulfonate. There are also other reports which support this expression.[28]

Concerning carcinogenesis, there is a very limited amount of data regarding its correlation with the extent of chemical alterations of target cells. Several dose-response relationships were empirically deduced. Thus, an expression correlating the administered dose and the medium time of induction was obtained for a series of carcinogens as for instance: 4-dimethylaminostilbene (n = 3), diethylnitrosoamine (n = 2.3) etc.[36]

$$Dt^n = k \tag{6}$$

where: D = daily dose of carcinogen administered; t = average duration of tumor induction and n = constant, depending on the carcinogen structure.

A critical factor in the attempts to correlate dose-response data for carcinogenesis with those for mutagenesis is the latent period for tumor induction. Except for this factor, the respective correlations are fairly good.

The interaction of alkylating (or aralkylating) carcinogens with DNA is a rapid reaction (i.e., 1 to 4 h with alkylating carcinogens such as nitrosourea, methyl methanesulfonate, etc., and 50 to 100 h with 7-BrMBA). The subsequent decrease of adduct concentration is due to the repair processes. But these reactions are typical for the initiation step. However, between this step and tumor formations a number of processes and selection steps occur, influencing at least the overall rate of the tumorigenesis process.

The analysis of a series of experimental data leads to the following expression of the incidence rate:

$$I_t = kD^m(t - t_o)^n \tag{7}$$

where: k = constant, depending on the animal type; D = administered dose; t = duration of exposure and t_o = apparent latent period.

The induction of malignant epithelial tumors in mice by continuous application of B(a)P to the skin is described by Equation 7, using the following parameters: t_o = 28 weeks, m = 2 and n = 3.

A model supporting the importance of specific alkylation reactions (promutagenic lesions) for carcinogenesis was also devised. Thus, a positive correlation was found between the O^6G alkylation and the number of induced thymoma in C57BL/cbi mice, following a single intraperitoneal injection of an alkylating carcinogen. The correlation (Equation 8) is of the same form as Equation 7

$$-\ln(1 - p_t) = (kD)^n(t - t_o) \tag{8}$$

where: p_t = probability of thymoma induction in C57BL/cbi mice; k = constant, depending on the alkylating agent and the animal line utilized; D = administered dose; t = time at which p_t is determined; t_o = minimal latency period, considered to be of approximately 70 days and n = the number of dose-dependent hits required for tumor induction (slope of the logarithmic curve). It was demonstrated that different values of n are obtained for structurally different alkylating carcinogens: n is 1 for *N*-ethyl-*N*-nitrosourea, 2 for ethyl methanesulfonate, and 3 for *N*-methyl-*N*-nitrosourea. In other words, this means that *N*-ethyl-*N*-nitrosourea is a more efficient carcinogen than *N*-methyl-*N*-nitrosourea, although the latter possesses a higher ability to alkylate DNA (i.e., the extent of O^6 — guanine alkylation in thymus DNA is 8 μmol/mol DNA-P at 2.1 mmol/kg b.w. dose for the former and 18 μmol/mol DNA-P at 0.8 mmol/kg b.w. for the latter).

A positive correlation between carcinogenicity and electrophilicity was also found for the alkyl- and aralkylbromides (e.g., 7-BrMBA) which produce sarcoma at the injection site, as well as for some alkyl halides which produce lung tumors in mice.[28]

Finally, all these processes, as well as some others (biodistribution, intercompartmental distribution, kinetics of the various cellular systems, etc.) make the answers of the *in vivo* models to be multilinear or nonlinear by respect to a part of the investigated parameters. For these parameters optimal values may be computed (for instance optimal lipophilicity, electrophilicity, etc.) by derivation of the deduced equations (with respect to the consideration parameter), the maximum or the minimum of the function being thus determined.

A large body of evidence is now available which suggests that the carcinogenic effectiveness of alkylating agents, expressed as tumor yield per unit of effective dose, depends on the reactivity of the carcinogen.

Both the alkylation extent of the biomolecules responsible for, or involved in the cell proliferation process and the specificity of this reaction depend on this parameter or on the factors affecting it. These factors, which can usually be quantitatively estimated, are

1. Mechanism of the reaction with the target molecules
2. Electrophilicity of the alkylating species
3. Softness of the alkylating moieties (according to Pearson's hard and soft acid-base theory)
4. Stereochemistry of the electrophilic species
5. Nature, reactivity and stereochemistry of the nucleophilic site

A. MECHANISM OF THE REACTION BETWEEN ALKYLATING AGENTS AND WATER OR NUCLEOPHILES

In nucleophilic substitutions, the breaking of an old bond and the formation of a new one occurs. The principal mechanistic variations are associated with the timing of these two events.

According to classical concepts, the nucleophilic substitutions can follow a unimolecular (S_N1) (Equations 9 and 10) or a bimolecular (S_N2) (Equations 11 and 12) pathway.

$$\text{Alk--X} \xrightarrow{k_1} \text{Alk}^+ + \text{X}^{-} \text{ (prior ionization)} \tag{9}$$

$$\text{Alk}^+ + \text{Nu}^{-} \xrightarrow{k_2} \text{Alk--Nu} \text{ for } k_1 \ll k_2 \tag{10}$$

$$\text{Alk--X} + \text{Nu}^{-} \xrightarrow{k_1} [\text{X}^{\delta-} \dots \text{Alk} \dots^{\delta-} \text{Nu}] \xrightarrow{k_2} \text{Alk--Nu} + \text{X}^{-} \tag{11}$$

$$d\,[\text{Alk--X}]/dt = -k_1[\text{Alk--X}] \cdot [\text{Nu}^{-}] \tag{12}$$

The $S_N 1$ mechanism proceeds through carbocations (Equations 8 and 9), X being the leaving group. For many alkylating agents the factors favoring one or the other of the two mechanisms have been determined.[27,37,38] In a different approach these mechanisms might be regarded as limiting cases of a common mechanism proceeding through ion pairs:

$$\text{Alkyl--X} \underset{k_{-1}}{\overset{k_1}{\rightleftharpoons}} \text{Alkyl}^+\text{X}\bar{:} \begin{cases} \overset{k_s}{\nearrow} \text{H}_2\text{O} \quad \longrightarrow \text{Alkyl-OH} \\ \underset{k_2}{\searrow} \text{Y}\bar{:} \quad \longrightarrow \text{Alkyl-Y} \end{cases}$$

$$k_{-1}/k_s \to 0 \to S_N 1$$

$$k_{-1}/k_s \to \infty \to S_N 2 \tag{13}$$

In the case of sulfur and nitrogen mustards, some mechanistic differences appear because of the "neighboring" group effect exerted by the sulfur and nitrogen atoms, respectively, on the reaction center.

Early concepts assumed that the alkylation of water molecules parallel (mechanistically and kinetically) that of nucleic acids, hence the hydrolysis (solvolysis) rate would be a suitable parameter for a quantitative correlation with the effectiveness of these alkylators. Thus, the hydrolysis rates for hundreds of alkylating agents were measured using a standard procedure ($Me_2CO{:}H_2O$ 1:1, 66°C, 30 min) developed by Ross.[27] The kinetics obtained for sulfur and nitrogen mustard hydrolysis under these conditions suggested that their mechanisms depend on the basicity of the heteroatom and that, from this point of view, aliphatic nitrogen mustards behave differently from aromatic ones.[27,38] Aliphatic nitrogen mustards cyclize rapidly to an ethyleneimmonium ion, which can be titrated (with thiosulfate) or detected by ^{1}H-NMR. This ion reacts further with nucleophiles in a rate-determining step:

$$\underset{\textbf{1}}{\text{RR}_1\text{NCH}_2\text{CH}_2\text{Cl}} \longrightarrow \underset{\textbf{2}}{\text{RR}_1\overset{+}{\text{N}}\!\!\bigtriangleup \; \text{Cl}^-} \overset{\text{Nu}\bar{:}}{\longrightarrow} \underset{\textbf{3}}{\text{RR}_1\text{NCH}_2\text{CH}_2\text{Nu}}$$

The less basic sulfur mustard shows a hydrolysis kinetics supporting ionization as the rate-controlling step, as required by a $S_N 1$ mechanism. There are no data supporting the accumulation of the cyclic sulfonium ion intermediate **5**, which further reacts with nucleophiles:

$$\underset{\textbf{4}}{\text{RS-CH}_2\text{CH}_2\text{Cl} + \text{H}_2\text{O}} \longrightarrow \underset{\textbf{5}}{\text{R}\overset{+}{\text{S}}\!\!\bigtriangleup \; \text{Cl}^- + \text{H}_2\text{O}} \longrightarrow \underset{\textbf{6}}{\text{RSCH}_2\text{CH}_2\text{OH}}$$

A similar behavior could be assigned to the aromatic nitrogen mustards, which are even less basic. The rate-determining step is the formation of the solvated carbocation, **8**, at equilibrium with the ethyleneimmonium ion, **9**.[39]

$$\text{Aryl}-\text{N}(\text{CH}_2\text{CH}_2\text{Cl}) \longrightarrow (\text{aryl}-\overset{+}{\underset{\underset{\text{CH}_2\text{CH}_2\text{Cl}}{|}}{\text{N}}}-\text{CH}_2)\,\text{Cl}^- \rightleftharpoons \text{aryl}-\overset{+}{\underset{\underset{\text{CH}_2\text{CH}_2\text{Cl}}{|}}{\text{N}}}\!\!\diagup\!\!\diagdown\ \text{Cl}^-$$

$$\qquad\qquad 7 \qquad\qquad\qquad\qquad\qquad 8 \qquad\qquad\qquad\qquad\qquad 9$$

Therefore the passage from the strongly basic nitrogen mustards to mustard gas and to the weakly basic (aromatic) ones does not alter the alkylation mechanism, which remains the nucleophilic attack of the cyclic intermediate. It also results that the basicities of the precursor amines are useful parameters in estimating the reactivity of the corresponding nitrogen mustards because they could be satisfactorily correlated to hydrolysis rates (log $k_{66°}$), in Ross's standard test. Thus, for a series of *m*-substituted nitrogen mustards Equation 14 was obtained:

$$\log k_{66°} = -6.60 + 0.580\ pK_a \tag{14}$$

Similar equations could also be derived for nitrogen mustard residues grafted on other aromatic systems.

However, we want to point out that the hydrolysis rate constants are of poor predictive value for their ability to alkylate DNA, because:

1. Solvolytic reactions are unsuitable for determining the reaction mechanisms, because the solvent effect leads to modified kinetics. The neighboring group effect also contributes to this situation.
2. The data thus obtained are useful only for comparing the reactivities of the derivatives belonging to the same homologous series of compounds.
3. Water, being a good solvent and also a hard Lewis base, does not represent a satisfactory model for the interaction between DNA and alkylating agents.

In order to avoid the previously mentioned disadvantages and also to find a parameter which could better define the reactivity of alkylating agents, the determination of the rate constant for the reaction with other nucleophiles than water was proposed, e.g., *p*-nitrobenzylpyridine (NBP),[10] 4-pyridine-aldehyde-2-benzothiazolylhydrazone (PBH),[40] etc. Among these reagents, the most widely used was NBP. According to this procedure, the reactivity of an alkylating agent is defined by the time-dependent alkylation of NBP in the presence of competing nucleophiles such as water or other solvent molecules.[37]

The concentration of alkylated NBP, determined under standard conditions, allows the calculation of the ''alkylating activity'' of the investigated derivative. This procedure could be applied to any chemical class of biological alkylating agents, excepting those requiring enzymatic activation. For the latter, the alkylating activity can be determined subsequent to their activation.

Usually, the reaction mechanism of NBP alkylation is of the S_N2 type.[37] However, first-order kinetics were also observed, but in such cases the observed NBP alkylation rate will only reflect the rate of the initial ionization step in forming the aziridinium intermediate.

NBP has also been used in determining the hydrolysis rates of the alkylating agents by measuring, in the absence of other nucleophilic partners than water, the decrease of alkylating activity in aqueous solutions. NBP competition is also a very useful procedure for determining Swain-Scott's constant (see also Section III.B).[41]

The alkylating activity offers a more accurate description for the reactivity of alkylating agents. Nevertheless, this parameter does not entirely reflect the behavior of alkylating agents against target macromolecules.

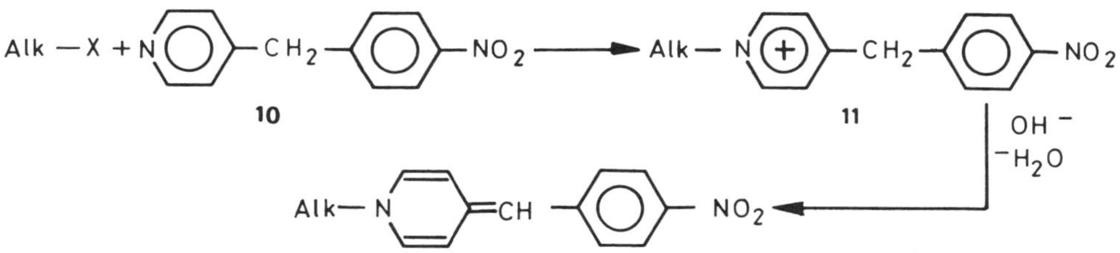

SCHEME 2. Alkylation of *p*-(nitrobenzyl) pyridine (NBP).

The electrophilic species generated during alkylation reactions are usually classical carbocations (carbonium ions), most often CH_3^+, $C_2H_5^+$, $C_6H_5CH_2^+$, etc., but also cyclic ions resulted from the solvolysis of the nitrogen mustards (i.e., aziridines, **13**), sulfur mustards, **14**, oxiranium ions, **15**, etc.

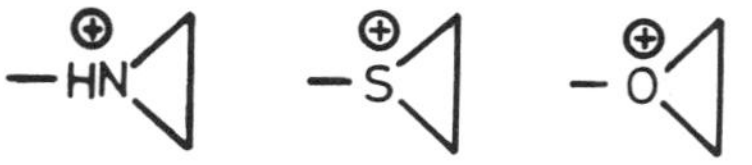

The reactivity of aliphatic carbocations, calculated from the dissociation energy of compounds RX to the corresponding carbenium ions, varies in the following order:

$$CH_3^+ > C_2H_5^+ > n\text{-}C_3H_7^+ > i\text{-}C_3H_7^+ \gg (CH_3)_3C^+ > CH_2 = CH\text{-}CH_2^+ >$$

$$C_6H_5CH_2^+ > (C_6H_5)_2CH^+ > (C_6H_5)_3C^+$$

The difference between the formation energy of the first and the last carbocation in this series is approximately 100 kcal/mol. However, this order of reactivity is valid for a S_N1 mechanism, where the appearance of the carbocation precedes their reaction with the nucleophile. In contrast, for the one-step (S_N2) alkylation reactions, an opposite order of reactivity was found, benzylic derivatives reacting faster than methylating agents.

The knowledge of the reaction mechanisms of the alkylating agents is necessary for the understanding of their behavior and the prediction of their biological properties. Thus, the alkylation efficiency of compounds reacting by the S_N1 mechanism (in contrast with those alkylating by S_N2) is independent of the concentration of the nucleophilic centers in the medium or in the target. On the other hand, agents reacting by the S_N1 mechanism would generally exhibit lower sensitivity to the nucleophilicity of the substrate, because of the high reactivity of the carbenium ion intermediates.

The reaction mechanism also determines, to a certain extent, the selectivity for the DNA nucleophilic sites. Thus, most of the agents alkylating by the S_N1 or S_N2 mechanism attack the nucleotides in the order of their increasing basicity: $G > A > C > T(U)$, whereas those alkylating by a radicalic mechanism exhibit a reverse order of attack.[38]

The category of alkylating agents reacting by an S_N1 mechanism includes several aromatic nitrogen mustards, clinically employed as antitumoral drugs. However, some of them, such as Melfalan, Chlorambucil and uracil-mustard exhibit high carcinogenic potentials in animals and probably also in humans.[28,42]

Their reaction mechanism with DNA is well known and has been extensively investigated *in vitro* and *in vivo* (Melfalan, uracil-mustard, etc.). The Swain-Scott factor, s (see Section III.B) parallels the stability increase of the generated carbocations, being for instance 1.39 for Chlorambucil, 1.18 for Melfalan,[41] 0.61 for triphenylmethyl and just 0.4 for *tert*-butyl.

According to similar kinetics but a slightly different mechanism (characterized as borderline S_N1/S_N2), *N*-methyl-*N*-nitrosourea and *N*-ethyl-*N*-nitrosourea ought to release, under physiological conditions, carbenium ions; however, because methyl and ethyl ions are too energy rich, they do not appear as such and instead pentacoordinated carbon atoms are involved in S_N2 transition states. A similar but much more complicated nonenzymatic activation occurs for 2-halomethyl-*N*-nitrosourea.[43]

Among the alkylating carcinogens reacting by an S_N2 mechanism one may cite aliphatic nitrogen mustards, sulfur mustards, β-propiolactone, methyl-methanesulfonates, primary and secondary alkyl halides, etc. (see also Table 2). In certain cases, discrimination between several possible mechanisms (S_N1, S_N2, borderline S_N1/S_N2) becomes quite difficult, because of the more complicated structure of ultimate carcinogens.

B. ELECTROPHILICITY OF ALKYLATING AGENTS

Usually, electrophilic species do not pre-exist in the reaction media, being formed *in situ* by reversible or irreversible reactions. A quantitative estimation of electrophilicity is a difficult task because it depends on several factors, such as: the magnitude of its electronic paucity; the facility of its formation; its stability in solution; etc. We mentioned previously that the alkylating activity (determined by the NBP procedure) parallels the reactivity of alkylating species satisfactorily, hence their electrophilicity.[44] However, besides the stereochemistry of the electrophilic species (which will be further discussed, see Section III.D) another aspect must be taken into account in order to accurately define this concept. This is the effect of the nucleophile on the reaction rate. The rate of the alkylation reaction depends on the nucleophilicity of the substrate. Swain and Scott (cited from References 27 and 28) expressed the nucleophilicity, n, of a reagent, by a linear-free energy relationship (Equation 15):

$$\log k/k_o = ns \tag{15}$$

where k is the second-order rate constant for the reaction between the considered nucleophile and the alkylating agent, k_o is the rate constant for the corresponding reaction with a standard nucleophile at 25°C (water), s is the Swain-Scott substrate constant, and n is the nucleophilic constant. The value of s = 1.00 for methyl bromide is the standard reference. Taking into account this reference standard, Swain and Scott computed a scale of nucleophilicities, assuming for water n_{H_2O} = 0.00. Using this scale they further calculated a series of substrate constants s. The preferential reaction of an alkylating agent with the stronger nucleophile relatively to a weaker one when both are present in excess will rise steeply with increasing values of the s constant. In other words, the nucleophilic selectivity increases in the same direction as the s parameter.[41]

Thus, if we consider *in vitro* alkylation of two nucleophilic sites A and B, with two electrophilic alkylators X and Y, the ratio of the relative extents of reaction at the two sites for the two reagents is given by the relationship:

$$\log \frac{\left(\dfrac{k_A}{k_B}\right)_X}{\left(\dfrac{k_A}{k_B}\right)_Y} = (s_x - s_y)(n_A - n_B) \tag{16}$$

where k_A, k_B = rate constants for the reactions between the electrophilic species X and Y and nucleophilic centers A and B; s_x, s_y = Swain-Scott constants for the two electrophilic alkylators and n_A, n_B = nucleophilicities of centers A and B (see also Section III.E).

These parameters are used in estimating the extent of alkylation at various nucleophilic centers in DNA by means of the competition factor F_y. This factor is related to s and n by Equation 17:

$$\log F_y = \log k/k_o - \log[H_2O] \tag{17}$$

where k and k_o have the same significance as for Equation 15. Replacing these values from Equation 15 we obtain:

$$\log F_y = sn - 1.74 \tag{18}$$

A series of n, s values for nucleophiles of biological interest may be found in References 27 and 28.

In fact, the Swain-Scott substrate constants afford a quantitative basis for the nucleophilic selectivity of alkylating agents. In particular it has been stressed that low nucleophilic selectivity may result in predominant alkylation of weaker nucleophilic sites.[41] Generally, the mutagenicity of the alkylating agents may be negatively correlated with their Swain-Scott constant, the more effective mutagens being those with low s values. Dose-response relationships for agents with s <0.55 have an exponential form.[28]

C. SOFTNESS OF THE ALKYLATING MOIETIES

An alternative way to express the selectivity of alkylating agents toward nucleophiles is the softness concept. An electrophilc A (electron acceptor) — nucleophile $\ddot{B}$ (electron donor) reaction could be regarded as a reaction between a Lewis acid and a Lewis base. The equilibrium constant K of such a reaction is determined not only by the strength factor s, but — according to Pearson's equation — by the introduction of the supplementary parameters σ_A, σ_B: which are called softness:

$$\log k = s_A \cdot s_{B:} + \sigma_A \cdot \sigma_{B:} \tag{19}$$

Some attempts to define softness were made by Pearson, Klopman,[46] etc. but a general consensus was not reached. Soft acids or bases are characterized by a large atomic radius, a small effective nuclear charge and a high polarizability, whereas hardness implies all the opposite properties.

In 1963 Pearson[45] expressed the Hard and Soft Acids and Bases (HSAB) principle, which claimed that hard acids (electrophiles) prefer to bind to hard bases and soft acids to soft bases. This statement is an extremely powerful qualitative rule, correlating the chemical behavior of alkylating agents toward cellular nucleophilic sites.

Although an exact softness scale is not available, an empirical systematization of various acids and bases was proposed. The alkylating agents (carbon Lewis acids) are relatively soft. The hardness sequence of several carbenium ions follows the order:

$$RCO^+ > CN^+ > C_6H_5^+ > \text{t-Bu}^+ > \text{i-Pr}^+ > (Et^+ > Me^+)$$

Replacement of the hydrogen atoms of CH_3^+ by electronegative groups would certainly harden the cation (i.e., $RCO^+ > RCOCH_2^+ > CH_3^+$; RCO^+ being borderline acid). Since H^- is one of the softer acids, CH_3^+ represents the extreme limit of the softness scale of the carbon Lewis acids bearing a positive charge. The corresponding carbene is even softer.

A correlation between softness and the s constant may be made. Generally, the soft alkylating agents are those with a higher s factor. An approximate scale of softness for Lewis acids and bases (or nucleophiles) is given in Table 3.[46]

TABLE 3

Classification of Hard and Soft Acids and Bases

Category	Acids	Bases
Hard	H^+, Li^+, Na^+, K^+, BF_3, $AlCl_3$, Al^{3+}, $Al(CH_3)_3$, CO_2, RCO^+, NC^+, N_3^+, RPO_2^+, $ROPO_2^+$, SO_3, Cl^{3+}, Cl^{7+}, HX (hydrogen bonding molecules), etc.	NH_3, RNH_2, N_2H_4 H_2O, OH^-, O^{2-}, ROH, RO^-, $CH_3CO_2^-$, CO_3^{2-}, NO_3^-, PO_4^{3-}, SO_4^{2-}, F^- (Cl^-)
Borderline	Fe^{2+}, Co^{2+}, Ni^{2+}, Zn^{2+}, R_3C^+, $C_6H_5^+$, $B(CH_3)_3$, NO^+, SO_2, etc.	$C_6H_5NH_2$, C_5H_5N, N_3^-, NO_2^-, SO_3^{2-}, BR^-
Soft	Cu^+, Ag^+, Au^+, Cd^{2+}, Pt^{2+}, BH_3, $Ca(CH_3)_2$, CH_2:, carbenes; acceptors such as chloranil, quinones, tetracyanoethylene, etc. HO^+, RO^+, RS^+, RSe^+, Br_2, Br^+, I_2, I^+, $RO^{\cdot}$, $RO_2^{\cdot}$, etc.	H^-, R^-, C_2H_4, C_6H_6, CN^-, RNC, CO SCN^-, R_3P, $(RO)_3P$, R_2S, RSH, RS^-, $S_2O_3^{2-}$, I^-

Note: R = alkyl.

D. STEREOSPECIFICITY OF ALKYLATING AGENTS

The stereochemistry, the van der Waals volume, and the hydration degree of the electrophilic species of alkylating agents represent important factors in determining the alkylation extent and specificity of the macromolecules, hence their biological properties. As the electrophilic reagents usually are carbocations of the R_3C^+ type (carbenium ions with sp^2 hybridization), their structure is mostly planar. Hence, the alkylation reactions of classical carbenium ions (as such or symmetrically solvated) are not stereospecific. However, the reactions of ions pairs or other ionic aggregates could occur stereospecifically, due to the chirality of these species. The nonclassical or bridged ions possessing a cyclopropane-like structure, admit geometric isomerism. The cyclic breakdown theoretically leads to disasterisomers, if the carbons are suitably substituted such reactions exhibit high stereospecificities.

E. REACTIVITY OF DNA MACROMOLECULES

Steric and electronic interactions between stacked bases and phosphate moieties in a DNA macromolecule lead to new qualitative effects which also affect the reactivity of the nucleophilic sites of the purine and pyrimidine bases.

The steric hindrance is one of the factors which drastically limit the access of exogenous electrophiles to nucleophilic sites. Thus, if the phosphodiesteric groups and the sugar hydroxy groups remain largely exposed to electrophilic attacks, some nucleophilic centers of the purine and pyrimidine bases are partially or totally hindered, either by: (1) their involvement in the DNA double helix or (2) the superposition of the electrostatic potential associated with the phosphate groups and the bases themselves. This fact greatly reduces their nucleophilic reactivity. Theoretically, only nucleophilic centers situated in DNA major or minor grooves or in their walls remain accessible to electrophilic attack.

The following nucleophilic centers contribute to hydrogen bonding: adenine, N^1 and 6-NH_2; guanine, N^1, 2-NH_2 and O^6; thymine, N^3 and O^4; cytosine, O^2, N^3, 4-NH_2. From these only N^3 and O^6 groups in guanine remain more or less easily accessible. Unexpectedly, in some cases (i.e., DNA alkylation with BCNU)* the alkylation of cytosine also appears to be an important reaction.

The role of the DNA macromolecule and its overall structure in the reactivity of its nucleophilic sites has become recently accessible to quantum mechanical exploration through the use of the concept of the electrostatic molecular potential.[47,48]

The electrostatic molecular potential (V) is defined by Pullman as the electrostatic

---

* BCNU — *N,N'*-bis(2-chloroethyl)-*N*-nitrosourea.

potential created in the neighboring space by the nuclear charges and the electronic distribution in the system. For a given wave function with the corresponding electron distribution $\rho(i)$ the value of such a potential V(P) at a point P in space is given by

$$V(P) = \sum_{\alpha} \frac{Z_{\alpha}}{|ap|} - \int \frac{\rho(i)}{|pi|} \, d\zeta i \tag{20}$$

where Z_{α} is the charge of the nucleus.[48]

This concept is particularly well suited for the study of the interaction of various electrophiles with DNA. The quantum mechanical treatment of this concept affords a unitary criterion for estimating the reactivity of the various nucleophilic centers in DNA.

In this concept the most prominent potential minima (calculated for each nonhydrogen atoms) are associated to high nucleophilic reactivity. The deepest minimum is generally associated to N^7 of guanine. One of the most striking results of these computations is the progressive increase of the absolute value of the potential minima in the series: single bases < nucleosides < nucleotides ≪ single helix < double helix. This phenomenon may be explained by the penetration and overlapping of the strong electrostatic potential of the phosphate groups with that of the purine and pyrimidine bases when these are arranged into a regular structure.

The involvement of ring nitrogen atoms (i.e., N^1A, N^3C, etc.) in hydrogen bonding in the double helix produces a very strong depletion of the molecular potential minima.[47] These facts have the following major practical consequences regarding the nucleophilic reactivity of DNA sites — the increase in the net nucleophilic reactivity of some centers (by respect to the reactivity of the same centers in bases, nucleosides, nucleotides). Thus, reagents such as N'-methyl-N'-nitro-N-nitrosoguanidine, N-methyl-N-nitrosourea, dimethyl sulfate, etc. cannot methylate guanosine. However, the same reagents do alkylate the guanine residues (at N^3 and N^7) in synthetic polynucleotides (i.e., poly G, poly GC, etc.) or in DNA.[49] Other examples can be cited[50] of the possible reversal in the relative ordering of nucleophilic centers when we go from single bases to double helix. Thus, the order of nucleophilicity of various centers in double helix DNA is the following: $N^7(G) > N^3(G) > N^3(A) > O^2(T) > O^6(A)$, etc., different from that of the monomeric bases: $N^7(G) > N^3(G) > O^2(C) > O^6(G) > N^1(A) > N^7(A)$, etc. These theoretical predictions are in surprisingly good agreement with experimental data.

The pH was also shown to influence the nucleophilicity of the bases (i.e., at pH 10.5 the nucleophilicity of guanosine and deoxyguanosine significantly increases).[51] Because of the cell homeostasis, such a pH is unlikely in the living tissue, the biological importance of this phenomenon being minimal. However, the behavior of 7-methyl-guanine at physiological pH resembles that of guanosine at high pH.

Another potential alkylation site in DNA macromolecule — often neglected — is the phosphate moiety. Because of the overlapping of the electrostatic effects, in DNA double helix, minima associated with the phosphate groups increase considerably.[52] Therefore, they become more nucleophilic, as it was shown experimentally. Thus, the DNA reaction with ethylsulfate or ethyl-N-nitrosoamine, affords a significant percentage (16 and 70%, respectively) of phosphate triester groups. A similar amount of phosphate moieties are alkylated using N-(2-chloroethyl)-N-nitrosourea.[53] Despite the great amount of work spent in this area there are relatively few well-established relationships (both *in vitro* and *in vivo*) between carcinogenic potency of alkylating agents and the previously discussed parameters.

Nevertheless, some quantitative attempts (QSAR analysis, see also Chapter 5) can be mentioned for nitrogen mustards,[54] oxiranes,[55,56] triazenes,[57] organo-metallic compounds,[58] N-nitrosoamines,[59,60] N-nitrosourea,[61] etc. Mention should be made that some of them require metabolic activation in order to alkylate DNA. These correlations showed a good predictive potential for structurally related compounds.

IV. MODELS PREDICTING CARCINOGENIC ACTIVITY OF INDIRECT-ACTING CARCINOGENS (FOREMOST POLYCYCLIC AROMATIC HYDROCARBONS, PAHs)

Most of the known carcinogens require metabolic activation in order to interact with target (macro)molecules. For this reason the development of valuable predictive models for indirectly acting carcinogens is obviously more complicated, because we have to take into account not only the direct interaction between the ultimate carcinogen and the target molecule (i.e., DNA), but also a series of factors determining the activation/detoxication processes.

As we mentioned previously (see Section II), such models were developed especially for PAH. However, some quantitative approaches may also be cited for other classes of indirectly acting carcinogens, i.e., N-nitrosoamines,[62] nitroarenes,[63] aromatic amines,[64] etc. A tentative rationalization of these models was presented in Table 2.

A. MODELS CORRELATING CARCINOGENICITY WITH THE PARAMETERS DETERMINED FOR PRECARCINOGENIC MOLECULES

These models were the first attempts of a theoretical approach to carcinogenicity; therefore they are of rather historical interest. Although they are old, they will be reviewed succinctly because some of the correlations thus obtained even for a large series of compounds were quite convincing.

Qualitative examination of structure-activity relationship in the PAH area generated a series of empirical observations regarding the carcinogenic properties of these compounds which depend on three parameters: the *dimensions of the hydrocarbon molecule,* involving both its size and its thickness when it is nonplanar or substituted, *geometric structure* and *electronic structure* and *reactivity of the molecule.*

The *dimensional criterion* is interesting for at least three reasons namely:

1. The interaction with cytochrome P-450 dependent monooxygenasic activation system; although this system has a low substrate specificity vs. xenobiotics, a steric hindrance is expected, related to increasing of substrate size over certain limits.
2. The interaction between the electrophilic species resulted during PAH activation and DNA occurs difficultly over certain size limits. Such a restriction was reported for PAH intercalation in the DNA helix[65] and it is logical to assume that such a criterion also works for adduct formation.
3. Carcinogenic activity is necessarily dependent on the ability of PAH (or PAH-derived ''ultimate carcinogen'') to reach the activation system, or the target molecule, respectively.

This last property depends on the hydrocarbon lipophilicity which ensures the compound partition between the polar-nonpolar barriers to be crossed. Rogers and Cammarata (1969)[66] proposed the following equation for calculating this parameter:

$$\ln P = 0.667 \sum_r S_r - 2.540 \sum_r |q_r| + 0.478 \tag{21}$$

where: S_r = electrophilic superdelocalization index[67] and q_r = absolute atomic charges.

According to this equation, q_r is the term reflecting the hydrophilicity of the molecule, which for instance, for a neutral PAH is 0. Thus a direct relationship between PAH dimensions and $\ln P$ was demonstrated.

Recently, a similar equation was reported, successfully correlating the electrophilic superdelocalizability, S_E (computed by the Modified Intermediate Neglect of Differential

Overlap — MINDO/3 — procedure) with the same lipophilicity parameter for a series of 8 PAH.[68]

$$\log P = 0.974\, S_E + 0.102 \quad (r = 0.993,\ F = 2147.9) \tag{22}$$

According to Smith[69] the correlations obtained between molecular dimensions or lipophilicity of PAHs and their carcinogenicity are not significant. However, this is not surprising, because only linear regressions between these parameters were calculated.

The dimension parameter is also used in more recent approaches to carcinogenicity (cf. References 55 and 70 and references cited therein). In the Hopfinger approach, the quantitative comparison of molecular shapes is based upon a formalism called molecular shape analysis (MSA). Using this procedure one of the most active compounds is chosen (i.e., benzo(a)pyrene) as a reference standard, and each other compound is superimposed and the overlap steric volume V_o is computed. V_o serves as a quantitative measure of shape similarity. A positive correlation was obtained between mutagenic potency of 30 PAHs and this parameter (see Chapter 5).

The *geometric structure,* later more precisely defined as the topology of the molecule (see this chapter and Chapter 4). Most carcinogens are derivatives of the phenanthrenic, but not anthracenic system. There are, however, some exceptions, i.e., fluoranthene, benzo(k)fluoranthene, **16**, 6,12-dimethylbenzo(b)thionaphtheno (3,2 f), thiophenanthrene **17**, etc., which are carcinogens although they do not contain a true phenanthrenic system.

CH$_3$

S — S

CH$_3$

16 **17**

Electronic structure and reactivity of the molecule: Schmidt[71] was the first to draw attention to the importance of the electronic features in determining the biological properties of PAHs by correlating the existence of high electronic density area in the hydrocarbons molecule with their typical carcinogenicity. Svartholm (1941) (cited after Reference 72) developed this concept by introducing the resonance energy.*

The first convincing correlation between the cancerogenicity of PAHs and their electronic structure was developed, however, by Pullman and Pullman[73,74] taking advantage of the advances made at that time in quantum mechanics.

An index describing the total charge of the K region (mesophenanthrenic region) was initially chosen as a predictor of PAH carcinogenicity. Essentially, the reactivity of the K region (possessing the higher electron density of the molecules) parallels the PAH carcinogenicity. This observation is also true for some polyaromatic heterocycles (i.e., for benzoacridines). A positive correlation was also observed between the rate of osmium tetraoxide

---

* It is well known that benzene molecule is currently represented by a Kekulé structure (possessing alternately three simple and three double bonds in conjugation). In fact, simple molecular orbital (Hückel) treatment of its electronic structure affords quite a different picture showing the delocalization of the π electrons of the carbon atoms. This particular distribution corresponding to a minimum of energy explains the aromatic properties of this compound. The difference between the real energy of the benzene molecules and that calculated according to a Kekulé structure represents the resonance energy ($\sim$30 kcal/mol) and reflects the additional stability of the molecule acquired by π electrons delocalization.

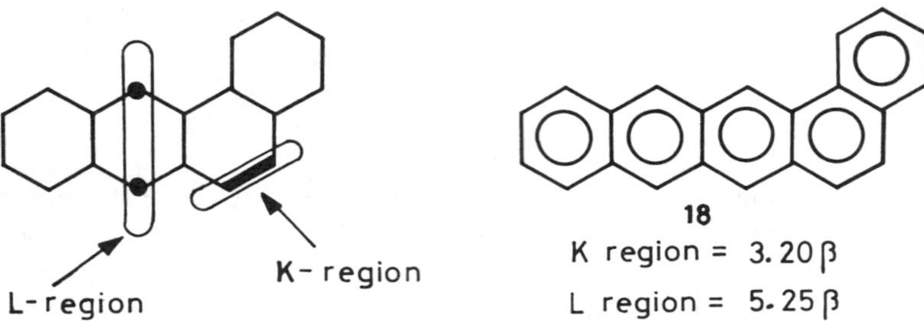

FIGURE 1.   K- and L-regions in PAH molecules.

addition to the K region of PAHs and their carcinogenicity. This experimental parameter is in fact a valuable predictor of PAH chemical reactivity and therefore has been proposed as an experimental predictor of PAH carcinogenicity. However, the numerous exceptions observed subsequently led to the modification of the theory, taking into account an additional region of the PAH molecule, namely the L-region (mesoanthracenic region, containing two *p*-ara carbon atoms). This one could inactivate the compound even though the activity of the K-region is adequate for carcinogenicity. A second index was introduced to express the reactivity of this region (the K- and L-region theory). In other words, a reactive L-region in a PAH precludes the expression of its carcinogenicity. Essentially, for a PAH to exhibit carcinogenic properties it has to have: a reactive K-region defined by a complex index OPE + CPE_{min} ≤3.31β and an unreactive L-zone, characterized by a complex index PPE + CPE_{min} ≥5.66β where: OPE = *ortho*-polarization energy; PPE = *para*-polarization energy and CPE_{min} = minimal carbon polarization energy. All indices are expressed in β units; (approximately 20 kcal/mol). They can be calculated by Hückel's molecular orbitals method.

According to this theory, for instance the 1,2-benzonaphthacene **18** is not carcinogenic, because, although the K-zone fits the required reactivity (OPE + CPE_{min} = 3.20β), the L-zone is too active (PPE + CPE_{min} = 5.25β).

This theory is of predictive value for a large number of unsubstituted PAHs and even of some heterocyclic systems. Similar calculations, performed for the series of monomethyl-benz(a)anthracene isomers (12 compounds), showed a significant correlation of carcinogenicity with the following indices:

1.   Free valence of the carbon to which the methyl group is bound
2.   Nucleophilicity of the compounds for the Ag^+ ion
3.   The bathochromic shift of the 287 nm band of benz(a)anthracene spectrum as a result of methylation
4.   Excitation energies calculated for an electron transition from HOMO to LUMO (see Appendix)
5.   The stability of aryl-methyl-cations derived from these compounds

Pullman's theory was improved by Mainster and Memery[75] by using the simpler I index (which is the sum of the superdelocalizabilities*, of the two atoms constituting the given

---

*   The π electron — superdelocalizability at the position r is defined as

$$S_r = 2 \sum_j \frac{c_{j,r}^2}{m_j} \tag{23}$$

where $c_{j,r}$ are carbon atom molecular orbital coefficients for molecular orbital j, the energy E_j of the occupied j orbital being

$$\epsilon_j = \alpha + m_j \beta$$

region), more easy to compute. They stated the carcinogenicity conditions as $I_K \geq 2.05$ and $I_L \leq 2.30$. The correlations with carcinogenicity are as good as for the latter indices, especially with unsubstituted PAHs and some types of heterocyclic systems.

Inconclusive correlation attempts were obtained with other parameters such as: electron donor — or electron-acceptor property of PAHs, photodynamic activity, hydrocarbon solubilization by DNA, etc.

However, the validity of these correlations has been made questionable by the finding that hydrocarbons lacking K-regions such as dibenz(a,c)anthracene, dibenz(a,c)naphthacene, etc. which ought to be inactive are in fact carcinogenic. Inadequacies also appear for methyl or halogen substituted PAHs and some heterocyclic systems.

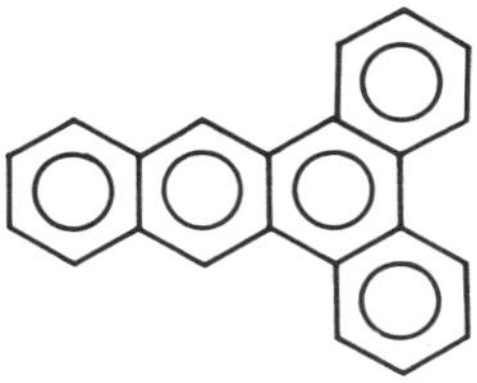

19 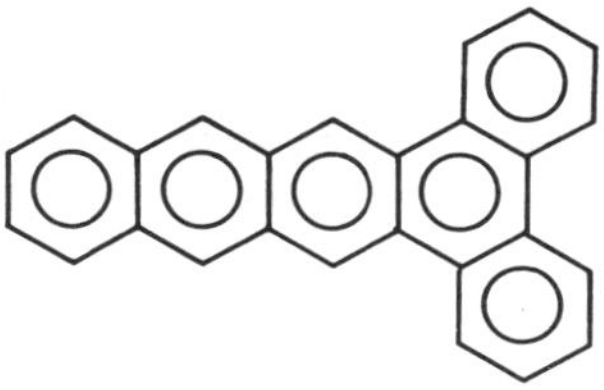   **20**

Similar more or less successful approaches were also reported for urethanes, fluoranthene-like hydrocarbons, heteroanalogs of the PAHs, benzo-derivatives of pyrrole, azo-compounds, etc.[76]

The parameters calculated for intact PAH molecules were actually based on the erroneous hypothesis of PAH molecules being carcinogenic per se. Moreover, because of the convincing correlations obtained, especially by Pullman's K- and L-region theory, the wrong conclusion was reached that the K-region was responsible for the carcinogenic properties of the PAH. This region was assumed to be involved in the interaction between the carcinogen and the biological target in a process representing the trigger of the malignant cellular transformation.

The most powerful objective to all these approaches was the finding that PAHs require activation in order to exert their carcinogenic potential, yielding an ultimate carcinogen directly interacting with DNA to give the promutagenic lesion. This active metabolite is usually a dihydrodiol epoxide (DE) structurally different by respect to the parent hydrocarbon. Because of the complexity of activation-detoxication mechanisms involved in the ultimate carcinogen generation, the simple correlation of the carcinogenic activity with indices computed on parent structures appears to be inadequate.

This criticism applies to all the aforementioned correlational approaches and also to more recent ones[77] suggesting the lack of predictive value of such parameters calculated on the parent molecule.

Moreover, such a criticism is also valid for the recently developed pattern recognition analysis of indirect-acting carcinogenes which use (shape or structure) descriptors of the parent molecules.

The quantum-mechanical indices calculated on the parent molecule may, however, be helpful for predicting other physicochemical or biological properties of PAHs. Thus for instance, highly significant correlations were obtained between quantum-mechanical calculated indices and the protein-binding constant to human serum albumin, the inhibition of dimethylnitrosamine demethylase, the rate of formation of 3-hydroxy-BaP, and mutagenic potency on *S. typhimurium* TA 100.[68]

However, most surprisingly, a number of predictions of the K- and L-region theory fit strikingly well with those of Jerina and Daly's bay-region theory (there are some exceptions which could not be explained by either theory; see also Section C.1).

An explanation of this situation emerged from a deeper analysis of both theories. Thus,

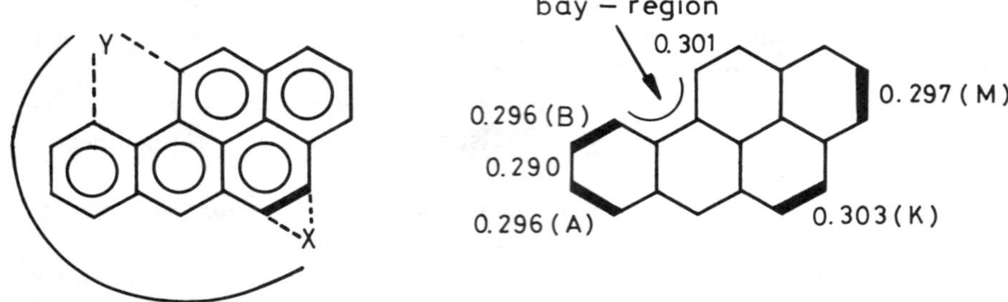

FIGURE 2.   Values of the superdelocalizability indices (S_{ab}^r) in the benzo(a)pyrene molecule.

a K-(mesophenanthrenic) region which implies an angular arrangement of benzenoid rings, is topologically equivalent to a bay-region provided that this "kink" is flanked by only one benzenoid ring (as in phenanthrene, benzo(a)pyrene, etc.). Second, the K-region seems to be required for the hydrocarbon interaction with the enzyme catalyzing bay-region or distal bay-region epoxidation. This last statement is based on the very plausible assumption that the initial interaction between the K-region and the enzyme alters the electronic distribution in the PAHs, and subsequently the reactivity of their bonds.[78] In order to substantiate this hypothesis a theoretical model was developed assuming two electron-accepting groups (X and Y) in the enzyme molecule interacting with K-(X) and bay-region (Y), respectively. Because this model is based on π-electron computation, the structure of the X and Y moieties of the enzyme cannot be defined.

Assuming the formation of a weak bond (of around 0.4 β_{C-C}) between the X group and the two carbons of the K-region of BaP the initial order of bond reactivity (4-5 > 11-12 > 2-3 > 9-10 $\cong$ 7-8 > 8-9, etc.) becomes 7-8 > 8-9 > 2-3 > . . . being in agreement with the primary epoxidation site. Similar results were obtained also for BA. It follows that an active K-region is a prerequisite condition for an adequate metabolization of the bay-region by the cytochrome P-450 dependent monooxygenases.

Some of the disagreements could be due to steric requirements as suggested by rather successful correlations for PAHs and alkylated derivatives in which the steric factor is accounted for by topological indices and the MTD-method.[79]

A conceptually similar mechanistic study was done in the case of a restricted set of carcinogenic *N*-nitrosourea[61] with the general structure:

$$R_1 R_2 \ N_{(6)} \!\!-\!\! \underset{\underset{O_{(5)}}{\|}}{C_{(4)}} \!\!-\!\! \underset{\underset{\underset{\overset{\|}{O_{(1)}}}{N_{(2)}}}{|}}{N_{(3)}} \!\!-\!\! \underset{\underset{H_{(\alpha)}}{|}}{\overset{\overset{H}{|}}{C_{(2)}}} \!\!-\!\! R_3$$

21

$$R_1, R_2 = H, CH_3 \ ; \ R_3 = H, CH_3, C_2H_5$$

The structure and reactivity of these compounds was studied using the semi-empirical MINDO/3 method,[80] with an original parametrization. The following parameters were calculated: net atomic charges (q_i), orbital energies (ϵ_{HOMO}, ϵ_{LUMO}), atomic electrophilic and nucleophilic superdelocalizabilities (S_i^E, S_i^N). The calculations of reaction enthalpies confirmed that *N*-nitrosoureas acted as S_N1 reagents. The most significant correlations showed that the indices involved in these equations are related (at least indirectly) to the centers of the initial step of the OH^- catalyzed biodegradation pathway (C_4 and N_2) or to the electronic structures of the α-carbon and α-hydrogen involved in the released alkyl carbocation.[61]

Finally, we mention the attempt to find a unified reactivity index which could be of predictive value for carcinogens belonging to structurally unrelated classes of compounds. In this approach, a 1,2-4-*trans* region (butadiene-like) was defined which is seemingly involved in the carcinogenic activity of different types of carcinogens. The sum of the LUMO coefficients (calculated by the simple Hückel method for the planar compounds and by the extended Hückel or CNDO/2 procedure for the nonplanar ones) increases in the order: precarcinogens < proximate < ultimate carcinogens.[81] However, no quantitative correlations were reported for a large series of structurally unrelated carcinogens in order to judge the efficiency of the proposed index.

B. MODELS CORRELATING CARCINOGENICITY WITH PARAMETERS OF ACTIVATION AND DETOXIFICATION REACTIONS

During the 1960s the situation dramatically changed because of the gradual realization that many carcinogens were not directly responsible for the triggering of carcinogenesis. They serve instead as a source of reactive metabolites (termed "ultimate carcinogens") which are responsible for the initiation step.[82] The complete sequence of intermediates between the parent carcinogen and DNA adduct is actually known for many compounds, and the structure of the ultimate carcinogens involved in these pathways was firmly established.

Based on the subsequent studies on BaP and other PAHs, the concept of bay-region* diol epoxides as ultimate carcinogens was proposed.[83,84] During these approaches two new elements emerged which may be of critical importance in developing a quantitative model of carcinogenesis process, namely:

1. The facility of ultimate carcinogen formation; this is based on (a) the activation-detoxication competition (representing the ratio between the rates of the main activation and detoxication reactions), and on (b) establishing the efficiency determining process in the series of concurrent reactions which led to the ultimate carcinogen.
2. The reactivity of ultimate carcinogens.

In this chapter we shall discuss the first aspect, focused on the well-known BaP metabolism. BaP activation involves a series of three enzymatic reactions: (1) a first epoxidation of BaP by cytochrome P-450 dependent monooxygenases at the bond adjacent to the bay-region yielding the 7,8-epoxide, **23**; (2) the enzymatic hydration (catalyzed by epoxide-hydrase) of the 7,8-epoxide leading to the corresponding *trans*-dihydrodiol, **27** and (3) a second epoxidation (mediated by the same cytochrome P-450) which affords the stereoisomeric bay-region 7,8,9,10-tetrahydrodiol-epoxides, **28** and **29**, whose *anti*-isomer, **29**, is the ultimate carcinogen.[85]

The primary epoxidation occurs on the distal bay-region bond termed A region.** The secondary epoxidation leading to diol-epoxide (DE) occurs at a double bond belonging to the bay-region, the B-region.

In order to determine the relative extent of activation and detoxication metabolism for each PAH, the reactivity of these regions in parent molecules and the corresponding dihydrodiols was calculated by quantum-mechanical procedures. This approach was founded on the assumption that, as long as the metabolism degree and specificity depends on the electronic properties of the substrate molecule, their tendency toward detoxication and ac-

---

* The notion of bay-region is of topological nature and represents a region of a PAH molecule with angularly condensed rings (see Figure 3 and Chapter 4).

** This region corresponds to the so-called, in early papers, M-region.

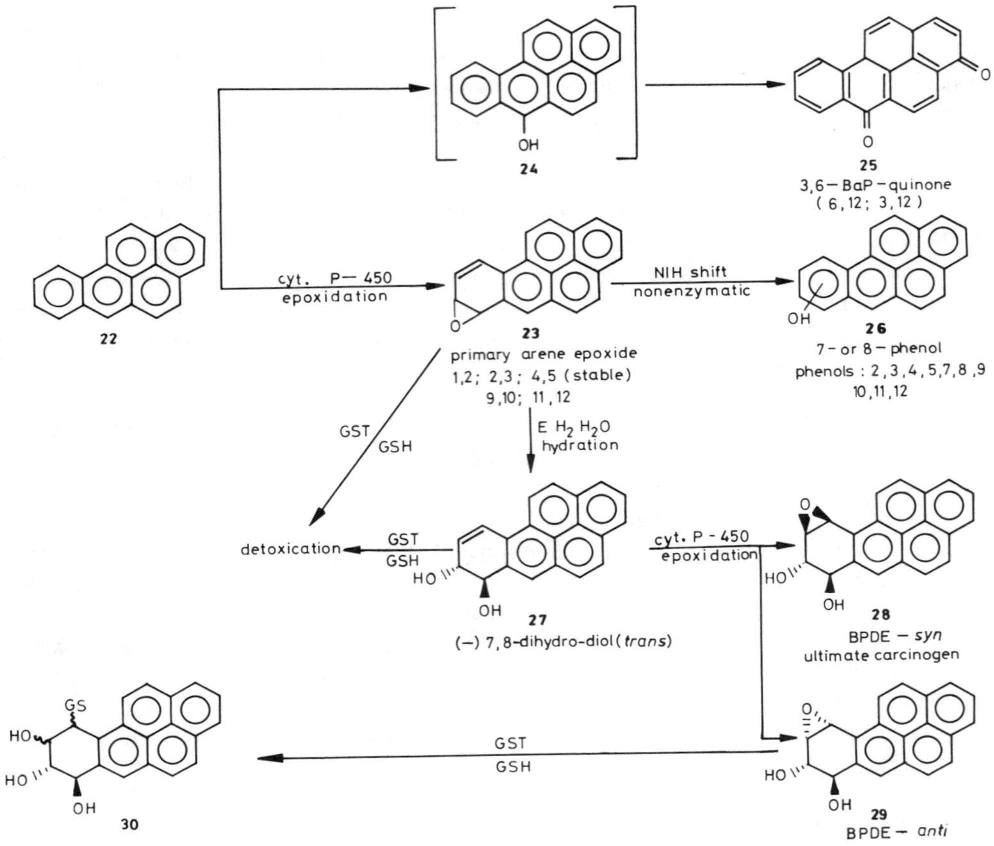

SCHEME 3.　Benzo(a)pyrene activation and detoxication.

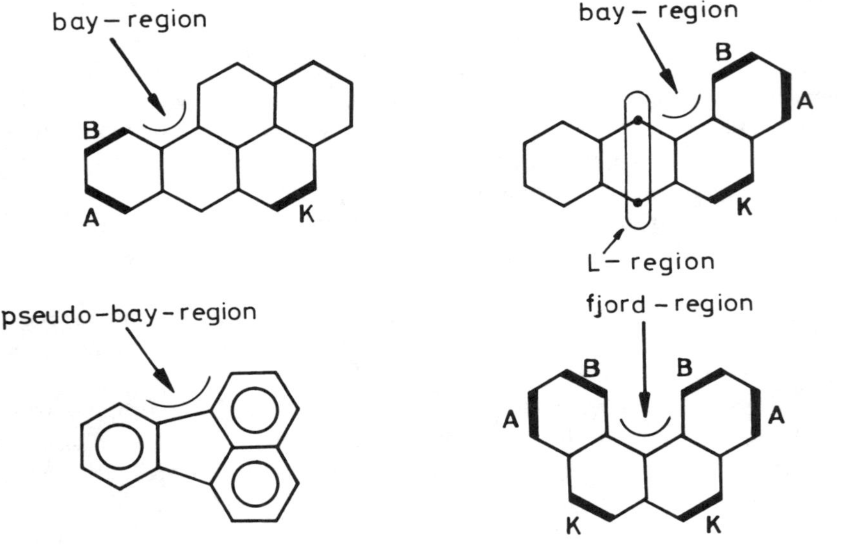

FIGURE 3.　A-, B-, bay-, pseudobay- and fjord-regions.

tivation could be quantitatively estimated. In order to evaluate the electronic structures and the reactivity parameters of the precursor PAH (primary epoxidation substrate), as well as for the bay-region distal dihydrodiols (secondary epoxidation substrate) extended Hückel theory and all-valence electron methods were used.[86,87,88]

The reactivity toward the epoxidation reaction R_{AB} in terms of π bond reactivity is expressed as:[89]

$$R_{AB}(\pi) = \sum_j \frac{\rho_{AB}(\pi)}{\epsilon_j} \qquad (24)$$

where $\rho_{AB}(\pi)$ is the density of the π electrons contributing to the bond between atom A and atom B in the j molecular orbital, and ϵ_j is the orbital energy.

Thus were calculated:

1. The superdelocalizability indices I_A, I_B, I_K of the intact hydrocarbons A-, B- and K-regions
2. The superdelocalization indices $1'_B$, $1'_K$ of the dihydrodiols resulted subsequently in the primary epoxidation
3. ΔE, i.e., π-electron energy difference between the parent molecule and the corresponding dihydrodiol, or between the latter and the corresponding DE
4. The reactivity toward oxidation centered at certain atoms

We recall the critical importance of the computation methodology employed in order to obtain suitable quantum-mechanical indices. For instance, whereas the simple Hückel molecular orbital method can be successfully applied to planar aromatic molecules (i.e., for computation of I_A, I_B, I_K indices), it leads to misleading results for the nonplanar ones (e.g., unsaturated diols, diol-epoxides, etc.). In these compounds only indices obtained with extended Hückel, iterative extended Hückel, or more sophisticated procedures would be appropriate for correlational purposes.

Because of the inadequate choice of the computational procedures some literature data appear to be conflicting.

Arene-oxide formation is the first step in PAH activation (see Scheme 3). The positive correlation found between the I_A indices and the carcinogenicity of the corresponding PAH was reported by several authors.[86-88] According to Smith et al.[69] the most potent carcinogens lack an L-region and have high I_A values >1.90. New data confirm the statistical significance of the correlation between I_A and Iball index (p <0.0008) for a sample of 24 unsubstituted PAHs, although the correlation index is rather low (r = 0.735).[90,91]

The reactivity of the K-zones toward primary epoxidation (expressed as I_K indices) does not correlate with the carcinogenicity of the corresponding PAH, independently of the method (simple or iterative extended Hückel) used for the computation of these indices.[86,87] These data support the important conclusion that the arene oxide formation could be the rate-determining step in the generation of diol-epoxides.

Hydration of arene oxides to afford dihydrodiols competes with their isomerization in aqueous solution (see Scheme 4).

The isomerization of the asymmetric arene oxides (i.e., via **31**) can afford two isomeric phenols, arising through ring opening in either direction (via zwitterions or via carbocations). Generally, one of the two possible phenols is formed preferentially.

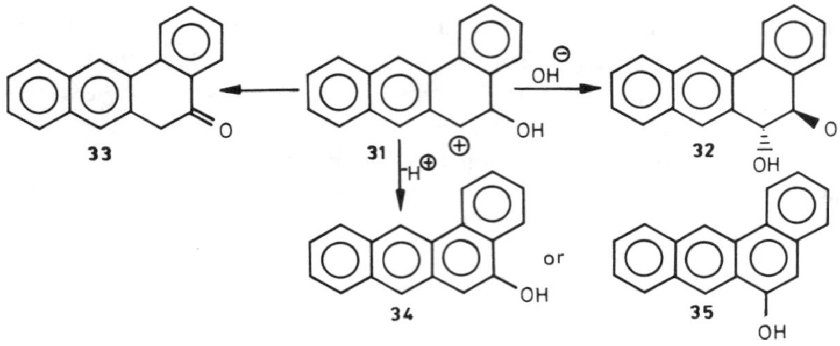

33   **31**   **32**

34   or   **35**

SCHEME 4.   Arene oxides isomerization and hydration.

The tendency toward phenol formation was expressed in terms of Dewar reactivity numbers*[92] or π-electron superdelocalizability (Equation 23).[88]

The products formed during arene-oxide hydration in aqueous media are known for a number of a cases, i.e., benzene oxide and phenanthrene-1,2- and 3,4-oxides undergo exclusive isomerization to corresponding phenols while K-region oxides of phenanthrene, BA, dibenz(a,h)anthracene and 3-methyl-cholanthrene yield important amounts (20 to 30%) of the corresponding dihydrodiols. These results are in good agreement with the theoretical predictions.[92] In contrast with this situation, enzymatic hydration of arene oxides affords mostly corresponding *trans*-dihydrodiols. The agreement between the theoretical prediction of the arene-oxide, enzymatic hydration and the experimental data is rather ambiguous.

The theoretical data obtained for the arene-oxide formation and hydration led also to the following additional conclusions:

1.   Saturation of a double bond (in a marginal ring) increases the reactivity toward oxidation of the adjacent double bond. The reactivity order of double bonds in various polyatomic systems is found in Figure 4.
2.   The reactivity of monoatomic centers to oxidation varies in Figure 5 (the L-region centers being the most reactive).

These calculations fully agree with the experimental data on the metabolite distribution for dibenz(a,c)anthracene, dibenz(a,h)anthracene, etc.[87,88]

Unexpectedly, a positive correlation was reported between carcinogenic potency and

---

* N_t = Dewar's reactivity number may be expressed by the equation:

$$N_t = 2(a_{or,1} + a_{or,2}) \tag{25}$$

where $a_{or,1}$ and $a_{or,2}$ are the NBMO coefficients for the adjacent positions to C (tetrahedral) atom-bearing oxygen. The following relation exists between N_t and the delocalization energy $\Delta E_{deloc}/\beta$

$$N_t = (2 - \Delta E_{deloc}/\beta) \tag{26}$$

For definition of NBMO coefficients see Appendix 1.

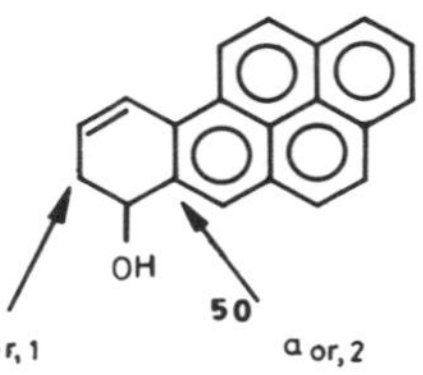

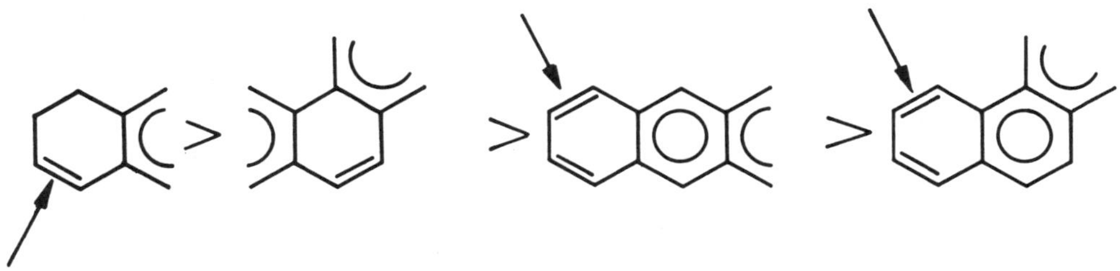

FIGURE 4. Reactivity of the different types of arene bonds in PAH.

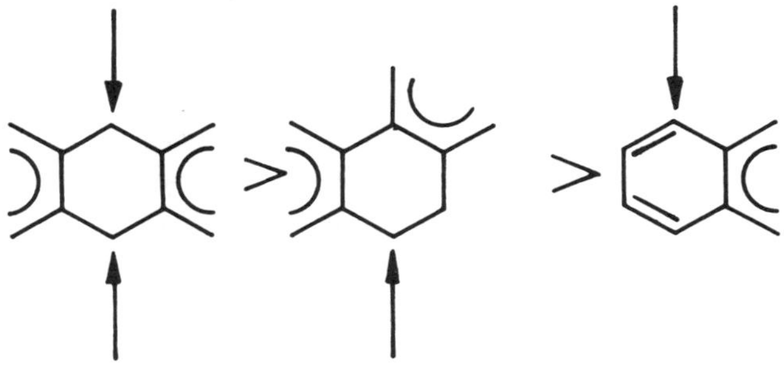

FIGURE 5. Reactivity of the different atomic centers in PAH.

parent compound reactivities toward atom-centered oxidation.[88] This is an entirely surprising observation which substantiates the possibility of PAH activation by one-electron oxidations occurring through radical-cations. This oxidation involves the 6-position in BaP and BA, the 7-position in dibenzo(a,h)pyrene and dibenzo(a,i)pyrene, and 8-position in dibenzo(a,e)pyrene, etc. Some experimental data[93] and the fact that 6-hydroxy-BaP is not itself a carcinogen[72] seem to rule out this possibility. However, no explanation could be advanced for this conflicting situation.

The secondary epoxidation of the dihydrodiol B-region is the following step and affords bay-region tetrahydrodiol-epoxides (see Scheme 2) representing the ultimate carcinogens.

The saturation of the distal bay-region double bond interrupts the aromaticity and therefore the bay-region styrenic double bond should be even more reactive toward epoxidation ($I_B' > I_B$) than the former. However, no correlation was found between these indices and the carcinogenicity of the corresponding PAH.[88] Mention should be made that the primary and the secondary epoxidation could occur by different mechanisms,[94] although some authors support the contrary opinion.[95]

Quantum-chemical calculations were also undertaken in order to determine the reactivity of some intermediates appearing in the decay process of some N-nitrosoderivatives,[60,96,97] in an attempt to correlate their reactivity with the carcinogenic potential of their parent compounds. For instance, candidate molecular descriptors of the metabolism and carcinogenic potency for a series of dialkylnitrosoamines were computed using the semi-empirical molecular method MINDO/3 and also the geometry optimization. Of all the properties examined, the initial enzymatic hydroxylation at C_α and C_β appear to be the major modulators of carcinogenic activity in the parent compounds. The electrophilicity of the diazonium ion $[(RN = N)^+]$ or of the alkyl cation (R^+) seems of little importance for differentiating their carcinogenic activity. Because of the high reactivity of these ionic species this conclusion is not surprising.[98]

C. MODELS CORRELATING CARCINOGENICITY WITH THE REACTIVITY AND STEREOCHEMISTRY OF ULTIMATE CARCINOGENS

If the reaction of the ultimate carcinogen with DNA is considered a prerequisite condition of malignant cellular transformation, then such an approach is fully justified. Therefore, after the evaluation of the rate-determining step (in the enzymatic activation of precarcinogens) to the overall expression of their carcinogenic properties, the importance of the ultimate carcinogen reactivity remained to be stressed. As we emphasized previously for the alkylating agents, the reactivity and the stereochemistry of the dihydro-diol intermediates, as well as that of the tetrahydro-diol-epoxides (ultimate carcinogens) may be positively correlated to their carcinogenicity.

1. Reactivity of the Electrophilic Species Generated by PAHs and Its Parametrization

The electrophilicity of epoxides and diol-epoxides (DE) results from their propensity to undergo specific ring opening affording carbocations during rate-determining reactions.

If we consider that among the PAH metabolites, only DEs are ultimate carcinogens, then an explanation of this property might be found in the difference of reactivity occurring between PAH simple epoxides and the diol-epoxides. However, this assumption is not entirely valid since there are also tetrahydro-epoxides derived from PAHs which behave as strong mutagens.

In order to substantiate this concept, the reaction of PAH epoxides or DE with water, nucleophiles, and DNA was studied both *in vitro* and *in vivo* in different conditions. Because the reaction between the ultimate carcinogens and DNA occurs in intracellular medium containing a large amount of nucleophilic species (including water), concurrent reactions must be considered (i.e., hydrolysis, reaction with other nucleophiles, intramolecular rearrangements*, etc.) all generally affording detoxication products.

The efficiency of the reaction between DE and DNA was evaluated by determining both the major reaction pathway (i.e., inferred on a thermodynamic basis), and the rates of the various concurrent reactions leading to the decrease of the DE concentration. For BaP and BA, it was shown that the formation rates of tetrols by nonenzymatic hydrolysis of precursor DE positively correlate with their mutagenic capacity.[99,100] This suggests that the reaction affording the DE-DNA adducts parallels mechanistically the DE reaction with water molecules. The elucidation of the DE-DNA reaction mechanism is of prime importance for estimating both the stereochemistry of the reaction products, and the factors controlling this reaction. Determination of these features could be of practical value for predicting carcinogenic potential.

A number of studies undertaken on the solvolysis of benzene-oxide, naphthalene-oxides and phenanthrene-oxides[101] showed that from a mechanistical point of view the ring opening in simple arene oxides and DE are similar. The reactions take place according to Scheme 5.

An important factor controlling the reaction extent of the ultimate carcinogen with DNA is the balance between the propensity of the arene oxides to undergo hydration or isomerization to corresponding phenols (NIH shift). The isomerization of simple arene oxides affords phenols, whereas that of DEs leads to the corresponding diol-ketone.[42] Both processes occur via zwitterionic intermediates or carbocations. Both phenols and diol-ketones are detoxication products. For the simple arene-oxide, the isomerization to phenols is distinctly favored thermodynamically with respect to the hydration pathway ($\Delta H = -17$ kcal/mol for hydration, vs. -29 kcal/mol for isomerization). In contrast, for DE none of the two routes are distinctly favored because the energetic difference between the two paths is small

---

* PAH phenols are formed during the solvolysis of the corresponding arene oxides by an intramolecular Wagner-Meerwein-Whitmore 1,2-shift called NIH shift or NIH rearrangement.

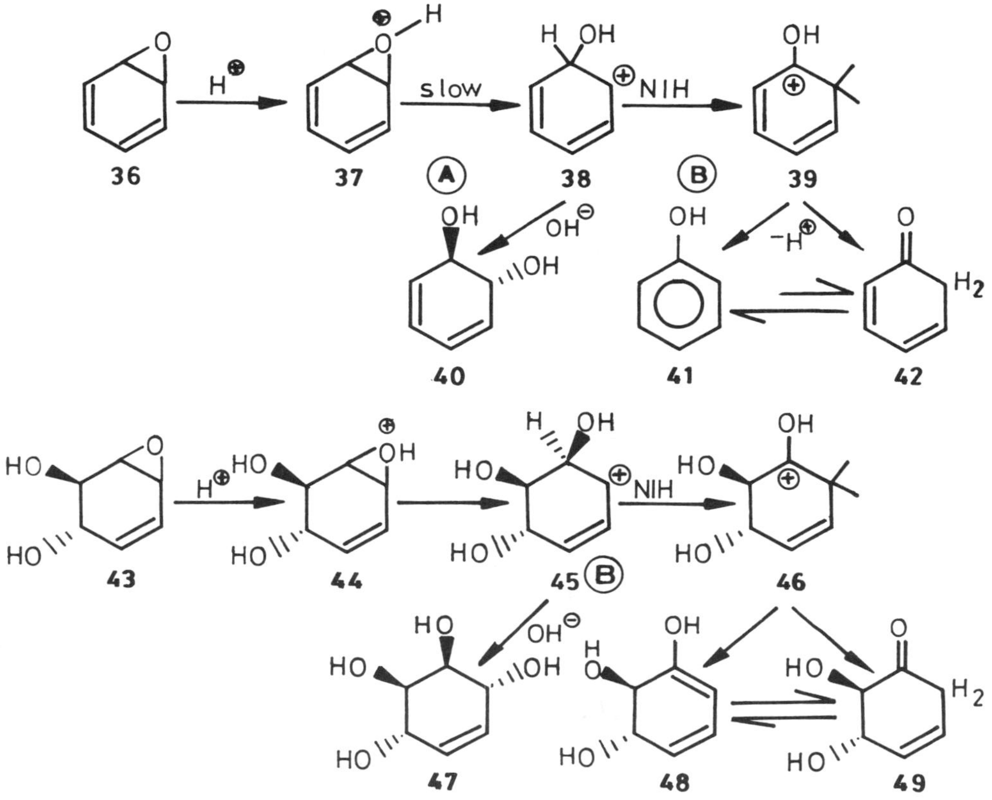

SCHEME 5.   Benzene-oxide and benzen-diol-epoxide solvolysis according. (From Ferrel, J. E. and Loew, G., *J. Am. Chem. Soc.*, 101, 1385, 1979. With permission.)

(approximately 1.5 kcal/mol); a slight advantage could be assigned to the hydration path. As the hydration of simple arene oxides is more exothermal than that of DEs, it follows that the former are better alkylating agents than the corresponding DEs (if both DNA attack and hydration occur by similar mechanisms) so that they would be more suitable candidates to ultimate carcinogens. However, because the propensity of simple arene oxides to undergo NIH shift is lower than that of the DEs, the latter react more extensively with DNA.

The formation of ketones **42** and **49**[102-104] during hydrolysis supports an S_N1 mechanism for hydration which occurs via the carbocations **38** and **45**, respectively (Scheme 5).

The quantum-mechanical calculation of formation energies for the C–O bonds in arene oxides showed that on protonation at oxygen these bonds are weakened (by approximately 70 kcal/mol), in agreement with the fact that acids are good catalysts for C–O bond breaking. This result also explains why the *syn*-isomers of PAH bay-region DEs (having a conformation which allows the formation of a hydrogen bond between the hydroxylic proton located in the benzylic position and the oxiranic ring oxygen, anchymeric assistance reacts with water or other nucleophiles more rapidly than the *anti*-isomers especially at neutral pH.[105]

A convenient prediction of the phenolic products resulting from the simple arene-oxide isomerization, of the stereochemistry of their hydration and dehydration products, as well as of the ratio of the hydration vs. isomerization products formed in these reactions could be performed by using Dewar's reactivity number N_t[92,106] calculated by simple MO methods (irrespectively, if these arene oxides do or do not belong to the K-region).

For ultimate carcinogens (DEs), similar calculations show that the reactions occur preferentially at the benzylic position (especially when this is located in the bay-region), the

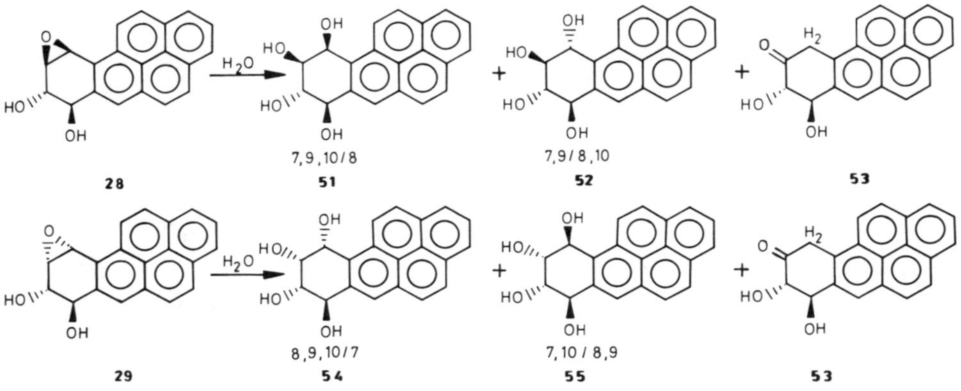

7,9,10/8
51

7,9/8,10
52

53

28

8,9,10/7
54

7,10/8,9
55

53

29

SCHEME 6.   Hydrolysis products of BPDE-*syn* and -*anti*.

ring opening being favored by the stabilization of the carbocation thus formed, by conjugation with the aromatic system of the PAH. This concept is supported by the data obtained for the reaction of styrene-oxide or PAH-DE with DNA or other nucleophiles.[107,108]

The regioselectivity of the enzymatic hydration of arene oxides (catalyzed by epoxy-hydrase) does not fulfill the theoretical predictions except for a few cases. The steric factors have a significantly larger contribution in this more complex reaction than in nonenzymatic ones.[92]

DE hydrolysis (nonenzymatic hydration) has been thoroughly investigated for a number of PAHs.[109-113] The following aspects have to be emphasized:

1. DE hydrolysis occurs via water addition to the epoxide moiety and affords vicinal *cis* or *trans* diols* depending on the structure of the arene oxide, pH, etc. For BPDE-*syn* (at pH 4 to 12), significant amounts (around 30 to 40%) of ketodiol **53** are formed (along with the tetrols).[103,114] The amount of ketone formed decreases with increasing reaction time; its presence has not been detected in the hydrolysis of BPDE *syn* at acidic pH.

   Regardless of pH, the major hydration route of the anti-diastereoisomer of BaP is the *trans* arene-oxide ring opening** the corresponding 7,10/8,9 tetrol **55** being formed in 60 to 95% yield, according to the experimental conditions (pH, ratio between organic solvent and water, buffer, ionic strength, etc.).[103,114] The greatest amount of 7,10/8,9 tetrol is formed during spontaneous hydrolysis (92 to 95%). Under these conditions and at short reaction times, traces of ketone are also noticed.[114] For the BPDE-*syn* diastereoisomer, the hydrolysis at pH 5 to 12 leads, via *cis* opening, to the corresponding 7,9,10/8 tetrol, its amount being approximately 60 to 80%, and increasing to 87% at pH lower than 5. The predominantly *cis* hydration of BPDE-*syn* could be explained by the neighboring group effect of 7-OH group on the oxiranic ring.

   A similar behavior was observed for the chrysene-DE or 5-methyl-chrysene-DE.[113,115] The *cis* opening is, however, more distinctly favored in the 5-methylchrysene-DE-*syn* (by respect to the unsubstituted hydrocarbon) which contains both the epoxidic ring and the methyl group in the same bay-region (the relative proportion between the two tetrols is 82% product of *cis*-opening to 18% product of the *trans*-one). It was shown for a DE series that the ratio between the amounts of *cis/trans* tetrols formed during hydrolysis increases proportionally with the facility of benzylic carbocation formation.[115]

---

*   The examples given concern BaPDE-*syn* and -*anti*.

** The *trans*- or *cis*-opening term refers to the reciprocal positions of C_9 and C_{10} substituents.

The data concerning the hydrolysis mechanism are conflicting. Some of them suggest carbocation formation both in spontaneous and in acid-catalyzed oxiranic ring opening.[101,116-118] Ketone formation during DE-*syn* solvolysis also suggests an S_N1 mechanism. However, the contribution of a S_N2 mechanism (at least partially) cannot be excluded (this being the major hydrolysis mechanism for simple arene oxides), since carbocations could not be trapped.[101]

2. Hydrolysis (in water or aqueous dioxane) follows kinetics expressed by the following equation:

$$k_{abs} = k_H \cdot a_H + k_o \qquad (27)$$

where k_o = constant of spontaneous neutral hydrolysis (s^{-1}), k_H = constant of acid hydrolysis ($M^{-1} \cdot s^{-1}$), and a_H = activity or concentration of the acidic catalyst.

The *syn*-diastereoisomers of DE are more reactive than the *anti*-ones at neutral pH (for instance, for BPDE, $k_{o,syn}$ is approximately three times higher than $k_{o,anti}$. In an S_N2 reaction with the *p*-nitrothiophenolate ion (in *t*-butanol), BPDE-*syn* is 150-fold more reactive than BPDE-*anti*;[119] k_H values are, on the contrary, approximately two times higher for the *anti*-isomer.

The reversal order of the hydrolysis rates of the two diastereoisomers in acid catalysis ($k_{H,anti} > k_{H,syn}$) is explained by the fact that the *anti*-diastereoisomer is much more sensitive to protonation than the *syn*-one which is already intramolecularly protonated.[120] The spontaneous hydrolysis rate also decreases with increasing proportions of organic solvent in the reaction medium.

3. In every studied case, tetrahydro-epoxides were more reactive under acid hydrolysis conditions than any of the corresponding DE-diastereoisomers. These differences in reactivity are too large to be attributed only to the inductive effects of the OH groups, therefore other stereoelectronic factors are probably involved.[103]

4. A positive correlation was obtained between the delocalization energy (ΔE_{deloc})* (computed by simple Hückel molecular orbital procedure, or other more sophisticated methods) and the hydrolysis rates (especially k_o) measured for the two diastereoisomeric DEs of a PAH series. This result supports the validity of the proposed hydrolysis mechanisms. It is of interest to mention that more sophisticated quantum chemical indices failed to significantly improve these correlations.[117]

The hydrolysis reaction of BPDE is catalyzed by: phosphate anions, acetate ions,[120] phenol,[121] nucleosides, nucleotides[110] and foremost DNA.[122-126] The results thus obtained suggest that physical binding of DE to DNA precedes both the hydrolysis (which is the major reaction) and adduct formation (namely 5 to 10% from BPDE at most is covalently linked to DNA).[127] This fact could be of critical importance for carcinogenesis prediction.

Among the nucleotides which catalyze this reaction, the most efficient are pdA and pdG (see Table 4).

---

* The delocalization energy (ΔE_{deloc}) is defined as the energy required for the formation of a carbocation during the ring opening of a PAH arene oxide. For instance:

29 → 56

For more details and its computation see Appendix 1.

TABLE 4
Catalytic Effect Exerted by
DNA, Nucleotides and
Nucleosides on BPDE
Hydrolysis Rate

Catalyst	$k_o(s^{-1}) \times 10^3$
Native DNA	45 ± 1
Denatured DNA	14 ± 1
pdA	5.8 ± 0.3
pdG	4.8 ± 0.3
pdT	1.8 ± 0.2
pdC	2.8 ± 0.2
dG, dT, dC	1.3 ± 0.1
dA	1.0 ± 0.1
Buffer	0.88 ± 0.05

SCHEME 7.   Hydrolysis of BPDE-syn, catalyzed by phosphate ions.

These data are in good agreement with an acid catalyzed ionic mechanism of DE hydrolysis under the influence of phosphate groups,[121] occurring probably according to Scheme 7.

This mechanism is probably also involved in alkylation of the DNA phosphate groups by BPDE, a reaction which leads to the breaking of the phosphodiesteric bonds.[128]

If this hydration mechanism is true, then DE detoxication in the cell occurs rather by hydrolysis processes involving acid catalysis than by scavengers of electrophiles (e.g., glutathione). This is in agreement with the low efficiency of SH-compounds for blocking *in vitro* DNA alkylation by BPDE, the scavenging process being effective only at $1:10^3$ *M/M* carcinogen:inhibitor ratios.[129]

During DE-DNA interaction, the hydrolysis rate increase is not exclusively the result of the large number of phosphate groups existing in the macromolecule. It was demonstrated that guanidine monophosphate anion (GMPH) exerts a 60- to 80-fold stronger catalytic effect than the inorganic phosphate ion on BPDE-*syn* and *anti*-hydrolysis, although the pK$_a$ values are very close.[110] This marked increase of the GMPH$^-$ catalytic power was attributed to its tendency to associate with BPDE-*syn* and *anti*. This concept is confirmed by the parallelism existing between the physical association strength (which actually decreases in the order:

TABLE 5
Hydrolysis Kinetic Data for Some HPA-DE

	Hydrocarbon 1.	$k_H(M^{-1}s^{-1})$[a] 2.	$k_o(s^{-1})$[b] 3.	Nucleophilic substitution index (NSI) 4.	$T_{0.5(min)}$ 5.
1.	Arene-oxide[c]	3.0.10	$1.2.10^{-3}$	2.10^{-2}	9.6[f]
2.	Naphthalene-1,2-oxide[e]	$1.4.10^2$	$2.9.10^{-3}$	9.10^{-3}	4.0[f]
3.	Phenanthrene-1,2-oxide[e]	$2.7.10^3$	$5.5\ 10^{-2}$	6.10^{-4}	0.2[f]
4.	Phenanthrene-3,4-oxide[e]	1.10^3	$3.1.10^{-2}$	8.10^{-4}	0.4[f]
5.	Phenanthrene-5,6-oxide[e]	1.10^2	$2.5.10^{-5}$	2.0	462[f]
6.	1,2-Epoxy-3,4-dihydroxy-tetrahydronaphthalene	6.0	$8.5.10^{-5}$	$1.1.10^{-1}$	136[f]
7.	Benzo(c) phenanthrene[d]	DE I 6.5.10	$6.0.10^{-6}$	—	920
		DE II $2.3.10^2$	$7.9.10^{-6}$	—	490
8.	Chrysene[d]	DE I $1.1.10^2$	$7.4.10^{-6}$	—	410
		DE II $1.1.10^2$	$7.4.10^{-6}$	—	610
			$1.1.10^{-4e}$		104[e]
9.	Benzo(a)anthracene[d]	DE I $1.3.10^2$	$3.1.10^{-4}$	—	37.3[f]
		DE II $2.8.10^2$	$2.8.10^{-5}$	—	413[f]
10.	Benzo(a)pyrene[d]	DE I $5.1.10^2$	$4.2.10^{-3}$	—	2.7
		DE II $1.4.10^3$	$1.3.10^{-4}$	—	43.0
11.	5-Methyl-chrysene[e]	DE I	$1.86.10^{-4}$	—	62
		DE II	$1.95.10^{-4}$	—	59
		DE I[g]	$2.14.10^{-3}$	—	5.4
		DE II[g]	$6.60.10^{-4}$	—	17.5
12.	Dibenzo(a,h)-pyrene[d]	DE II $8.5.10^2$	$3.2.10^{-4}$	—	29
13.	Dibenzo(a,i)-pyrene[d]	DE II $2.0.10^3$	$1.2.10^{-3}$	—	8.3

[a]   Acidic hydrolysis constant (DE I = *syn* diastereoisomer and DE II = *anti* one).
[b]   Constant of spontaneous hydrolysis reaction performed in 10% aqueous dioxane at 25°C and ionic strength of 0.1 *M*.
[c]   According to Reference 105.
[d]   According to Reference 118.
[e]   According to Reference 113; the measurements were made at 37°C.
[f]   Calculated from k_o.
[g]   Both methyl and oxiranic ring are in the same bay-region.

native DNA > denatured DNA > mononucleotides > mononucleotides > buffer) of these molecules and their catalytic ability.

The possibility of a benzylic carbocation (derived from PAH), to alkylate (or aralkylate) DNA depends not only on its reactivity and stereochemistry, but also of the accessibility of the nucleophilic centers in the nucleic acid macromolecule (see also Section III.E).

As a measure of DNA alkylation efficiency by ultimate carcinogens, a nucleophilic susceptibility index (NSI) was proposed. It expresses the relative rate of the nucleophilic addition of DE as compared to that of its hydration or its propensity to undergo intramolecular rearrangements.[105] NSI was defined for a given arene oxide as the ratio (A/B) of the second order rate constant between the considered arene oxide and the anion of 2-mercaptoethanol (A) and the first order rate constant for its aqueous solvolysis (B), in comparison with the same ratio (A_o/B_o) determined for ethylene oxide (standard molecule). Thus, for an NSI value of 1, the considered arene oxide has an electrophilicity identical to that of the standard molecule.

Some indices are summarized in Table 5, suggesting the following conclusions: (1) the K-region epoxides, followed by DE, are the least reactive in the solvolysis reaction and (2) only phenanthrene-9,10-oxide is more electrophilic than ethylene-oxide. DEs have an intermediate position, between K-region arene oxides and the standard molecule.

However, we have to mention that these indices concern the interaction with nucleophilic species moving freely in solution, in contrast with the nucleophilic centers spread along the DNA macromolecule and more or less sterically hindered.

A qualitative index of ultimate carcinogen reactivity (easier to handle than SNI) is the half-life determined for DE hydrolysis under standard conditions (pH 7.0 to 7.1, 25°C). This parameter has obviously only an orientative character regarding the tendency of a DE to interact with DNA; however, it provides useful indications concerning the effective life-times of ultimate carcinogens in aqueous media. Some of these life-times are summarized in Table 5. Obviously, a highly reactive DE has little chance in reaching the nuclear DNA target, while one that is too unreactive, once arrived would not be electrophilic enough to interact with this macromolecule. Therefore the cancerogenicity expression could be associated with an optimum lifetime of the ultimate carcinogens, or in other words with an optimum reactivity. There is a reactivity domain corresponding to the most favorable situation of ultimate carcinogens interaction with DNA. Just as for alkylating agents there are some specific features for aralkylating compounds. First regards the specificity of aralkylating agents for the exocyclic amino groups of the bases and especially of guanine. It was demonstrated for alkylating carcinogens that the selectivity toward the O^6 site is associated with the increase of the S_N1 character in the reactions (see Section III.B). However, although the aralkylating (e.g., benzylating) agents react predominantly via the S_N1 mechanism, they predominantly alkylate the N^2 amino group of guanine. A careful study of the factors influencing the product distribution over the N^7, O^6 and N^2 sites of guanosine during its alkylation with benzylating agents led to the following conclusions:[130] (1) the benzylating agents reacted at N^7, O^6 or N^2 guanine residues and (2) the increase of aqueous solvent concentration led to decreasing yield of N^7 alkylated products and increasing yield of N^2 or O^6 substituted bases; (3) changes from softer to harder leaving groups (in aralkylating agents) led to a substantial increase of solvolysis products and a decrease of the alkylated products and[131-137] (4) *para*-substitution of aralkylating agents favored reaction at the O^6 and N^2 sites.[134,135]

In an attempt to rationalize these findings, Dipple[130] suggested recently that two factors determine the site specificity of aralkylating agents, namely: (1) the ionic character of the reaction: the ultimate carcinogens, reacting through a more ionic intermediate (this means predominantly S_N1 mechanism), alkylate preferentially O^6 and/or N^2 sites and (2) the nature of the reactive intermediate; if the charge is well localized on the reaction center, then O^6 will be preferred and if the charge is delocalized (as in reactive intermediates resulting from PAH-DEs that are less than a full carbonium ion) reaction will occur at the N^2-site.

This concept could explain the relative extent of reactions observed in DNA-DE interactions, for instance the following amounts of DE bound to DNA under similar conditions: 6% for BaP, 32% for 5-methylchrysene and 65 to 70% for benzo(c)phenanthrene. Distortion from planarity for these PAHs parallels the sequence of increasing binding to DNA: BaP < 5-methyl-chrysene < benzo(c)phenanthrene. The distortion of the reaction centers from the plane of the aromatic ring retards the ionization and therefore decreases the hydrolysis rate. In these conditions the competition of amino groups in nucleotides for less than fully ionic intermediates (the more distorted structures) is favored.[130]

Another factor which has potential importance in PAH metabolism is the interaction of PAHs with specific proteic receptors. Such proteic receptors were found in several laboratories and their specificity and affinity for PAH were measured.[136,137] Via such PAH-receptor complexes, the carcinogen could be translocated into the cell nucleus inducing the enzyme systems (i.e., Ah gene) involved in their own activation and detoxication. On the other hand, such receptors could also be involved in the translocation of ultimate carcinogens — formed at microsomal level — into the nucleus. However, the contribution of these phenomena to the overall carcinogenicity of the PAH is unknown.

2. The Bay-Region Theory

If the carcinogenic properties of a PAH depend on the ability of the resulted DE to react with DNA, then it becomes obvious that a positive correlation ought to exist between the propensity of benzylic carbocation formation (from the corresponding DE) and the carcinogenicity of the parent molecule unless the metabolic activation to the ultimate carcinogenic DE is not hindered. In this respect, Jerina et al.[83,84,138] reported such a correlation between the experimentally determined carcinogenicity of a PAH and the ability of its corresponding DE to generate a trihydroxybenzylic carbocation (see the reaction **29 → 56**).

This propensity of PAH-DE to generate carbocations can be evaluated by using the delocalization energy (ΔE_{deloc}) which can be easily computed by a simple Hückel molecular orbital (HMO) procedure or by more sophisticated quantum-mechanical techniques.

The value of the delocalization energy is given by the expression:

$$\Delta E_{deloc} = 2(1 - a_{or})(\text{in } \beta \text{ units}) \tag{28}$$

where a_{or} = nonbonding molecular orbital coefficient (NBMO)* of the benzylic carbocation formed. The discovery of the BaP metabolic pathway, as well as the structure assignments for ultimate carcinogens[82] substantiate the bay-region theory of Jerina et al.[83,84,138] developed on the basis of the following theoretical and experimental observations:

1. Bay-region DEs exhibit significantly higher chemical reactivity and mutagenic potency than nonbay-region DEs; therefore the carcinogenicity of the PAH molecules may be related to a topological element defining their structures.
2. A substituent (methyl, halogen, etc.) which blocks the possibility of bay-region DE formation during the activation process usually cancels the carcinogenic properties (although some exceptions are known).
3. The results of the quantum-mechanical calculations (by the simple Hückel molecular orbitals method) predict an easier formation of benzyl carbocations for DEs whose oxiranic ring is located in the bay-, pseudo bay- or fjord-region. The ease of benzyl carbocation formation is expressed by the value of ΔE_{deloc} parameter. Its magnitude parallels the increase of carcinogenic potency for PAHs possessing bay-region(s), although some exceptions are known.[139,140] Some values for delocalization energies for a series of PAHs are given in Table 6.

The calculation is quite easy to perform, requiring an unsophisticated mathematical apparatus (some practical examples are given in the Appendix).

Jerina's bay-region theory was confirmed for at least 12 PAHs for which, according to theoretical predictions, bay-region DEs are demonstrated to be the ultimate carcinogens.[139]

The results discussed above were obtained by simple molecular orbital calculations which obviously give approximate values, but the general sense of correlations is not modified by the use of more sophisticated quantum-mechanical approaches which furnish much more accurate parameters. Mention should be made that Jerina's theory does not take into account the metabolic factors involved in DE formation, factors which could play an essential role in determining PAH carcinogenicity (for instance, the low carcinogenicity to BeP could not be explained by an inadequate ΔE_{deloc} value). However, it represents an accurate guide in the evaluation of PAH-generated ultimate carcinogen reactivity.

The quantum-mechanical procedure employed for delocalization energy computation plays an important role in the validity of the obtained correlation for other classes of

---

* The a_{or} (or NBMO) coefficients calculated by the simple HMO techniques are widely used in PAH carcinogenicity prediction. For the definition and computation of the NBMO indices, see Appendix 1.

TABLE 6
Delocalization Energies (ΔE_{deloc}) and Carcinogenic Potencies for Some PAHs

	Hydrocarbon	E_{deloc}[a]	Relative cancerogenicity[b]
1.	Naphthalene	0.488	−
2.	Anthracene	0.544	−
3.	Benzo(c)phenanthrene	0.600	+
4.	Chrysene	0.640	+
5.	Benzo(c)phenanthrene	0.647	+
6.	Phenanthrene	0.658	−
7.	Triphenylene	0.664	−
8.	Naphtho (2,3,b)pyrene	0.690	+ +
9.	Pentacene	0.710	−
10.	Benzo(e)pyrene	0.714	+
11.	Dibenzo(a,c)anthracene	0.722	+
12.	Dibenzo(a,j)anthracene	0.722	+
13.	Benzo(g)chrysene	0.728	+ +
14.	Dibenzo(a,h)anthracene	0.738	+ +
15.	Benzo(a)anthracene	0.766	+
16.	Dibenzo(a,e)pyrene	6.788	+ + +
17.	Benzo(a)pyrene	0.794	+ + + +
18.	Dibenzo(a,b)pyrene	0.808	+ + + +
19.	Tribenzo(a,e,i)pyrene	0.818	+ +
20.	Dibenzo(a,h)pyrene	0.845	+ + + +
21.	Dibenzo(a,i)pyrene	0.870	+ + + +

[a]   Computed for bay-region benzylic carbocation formation (β-units).
[b]   Relative indices for PAH carcinogenicity according to Reference 1.

compounds than unsubstituted PAHs. However, it cannot distinguish, for instance, between various methylated isomers.[83,84]

The Q_b (net π-electron charge) index was therefore developed:

$$Q_b = 1 - q_b \tag{29}$$

where q_b = the π-electron density at the benzylic carbon position of the tetrahydrotriol carbonium ion.

This index, which correlates with carcinogenicity, as well as ΔE_{deloc}, is more generally applicable than ΔE_{deloc}, being operational also for methylated isomers.[69] The free-valence index F*, as well as the atomic superdelocalizability at the bay-region carbocation position, S_b (see Equation 23), correlate also with carcinogenicity.[69]

As a matter of fact, as shown by Silverman,[141] in the estimation of the reactivity (or ease of oxiranic ring opening) of DEs the simple Hückel procedure and the Extended Hückel theory lead to totally different results, the former failing to give correct indices. This is due to the fact that the first method considers only ''through-bond'' interactions, whereas the second method also takes into account ''through-space'' interactions. According to this concept, the substituted (i.e., with CH_3, C_2H_5, halogens, etc.) carbons in PAH molecules

* The free valence index F, is given by the expression:

$$F = 1.732 - \sum_s \rho_{r,s} \tag{30}$$

where s refers to atoms bonded to the r atom and $\rho_{r,s}$ is the density of the π electrons contributing to the bond rs.

may be divided into "remote" and "nonremote" substitutional sites. The former ones are sites that are neither on the potentially activated benzene nucleus nor at the two positions that are adjacent to this ring.[142] The magnitude of the electronic effect resulted by methylation of these sites parallels the induced difference in the carcinogenicity for a number of PAHs.[143,144] For this situation ΔE_{deloc} can be calculated by the simple HMO procedure.

The methylation effect at the "nonremote positions" on carcinogenicity of PAHs could not be correlated with ΔE_{deloc} computed by the simple HMO procedure. The effect of intramolecular steric crowding on arene-oxide ring opening in DE and therefore on the ease of benzylic cation formation was recently investigated by Silverman.[141] A more sophisticated computational method based on Allinger's force field program[145] and molecular geometry optimization was chosen. The conclusions of this study indicate that methylation at "non-remote bay-region sites" of the PAH should be expected to induce changes in the relative conformations of DE diastereoisomers, thus influencing their stability and therefore their carcinogenicity.

Finally, we want to recall that a relationship between the bay-region theory and the K-region theory was observed and a possible explanation of this correlation was discussed (see also Section VI.1). A much better correlation was obtained between K-region indices and ΔE_{deloc}, if only primitive K-regions were considered (the primitive K-region is defined according to Loewe and Silverman[146] as "K-regions that are directly behind a bay-region, see **58**). In contrast the indices of nonprimitive K*-regions (more reactive than the former ones) correlate poorly with $\Delta E_{deloc}/\beta$.[146]

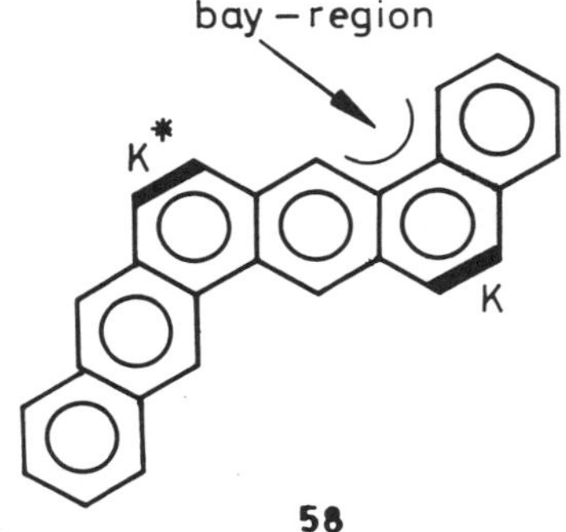

58

In a similar attempt at rationalizing PAH carcinogenicity, Fu et al.[92] calculated the Dewar reactivity indices, N_t, for benzylic carbocations derived from DE formed during PAH activation. As this index is defined also as a function of a_{or} by the relationship:

$$N_t = 2a_{or}/\beta \qquad (31)$$

(a_{or} having the same meaning as in ΔE_{deloc} expression, Equation 27), the results thus obtained are similar. This type of calculation was successfully applied for cancerogenicity estimation of cyclopenteno polycyclic aromatic hydrocarbons such as cholanthrenes.[147] The calculation showed that the five-membered ring has the following characteristics: its double bond has the highest bond order (or the highest olefinic character) and the carbocation resulted subsequent to oxiranic ring opening can be stabilized by the remaining aromatic system. ΔE_{deloc} having the same order of magnitude as that obtained for bay-region DE (see also Appendix) resulted in of ΔE_{deloc} of cyclopenteno-phenanthrene, CPP.[147]

Osborne[140] also found that the sum of the absolute values of all NBMO coefficients for a bay-region DE (for instance, $9 \times 11^{-1/2}$ for BaP) gives an even better correlation with the carcinogenicity of the respective molecules than their ΔE_{deloc} values.

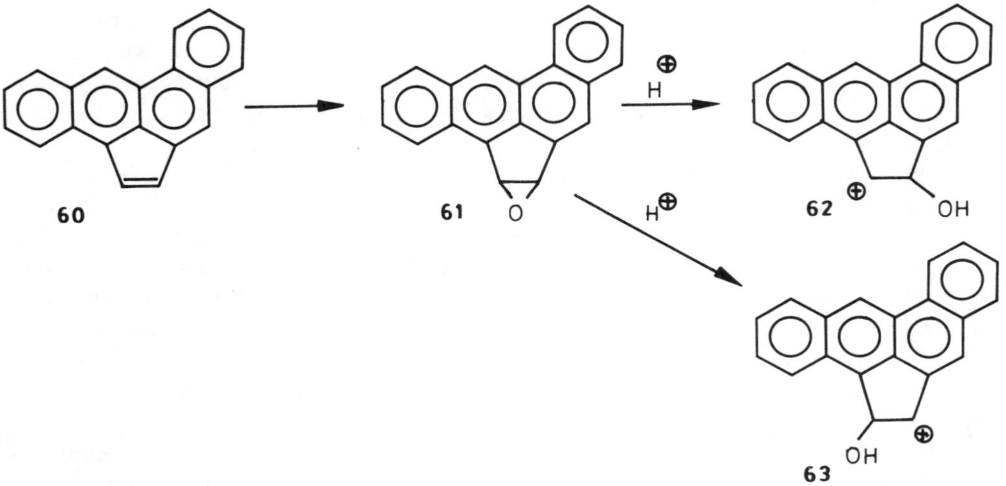

SCHEME 8.   Application of the $\alpha' > \alpha > \beta$ rule to cyclopenteno-benzo(a)anthracene. (From Loew, J. P. and Silverman, D. B., *Acc. Chem. Res.*, 17, 332, 1984. With permission.)

Summarizing these data, Loewe and Silverman[146] developed a simple rule for choosing the most stable carbocations, by substantiating the assumption that the stability of a benzylic carbocation depends on its location on the aromatic system, increasing in the order $\alpha' > \alpha > \beta$ by respect to the location of the CH_2^+ branch on the PAH fragment.

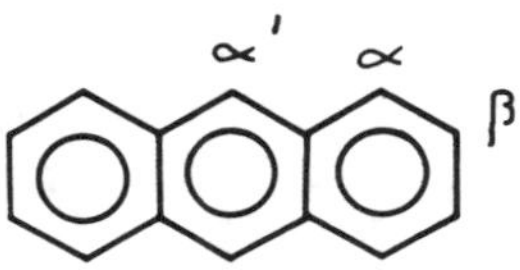

Positions α or β are those known in naphthalene (see **59**). The superiority of the α over β site for stabilizing a CH_2^+ side chain was recognized a long time ago[148] and was found to be true for many PAHs. The α' site is defined as the carbon atom between two fusion sites (as for instance a meso-anthracenic carbon, see **59**); this α' position is the best for stabilizing a CH_2^+ side chain. Although such sites do not appear in alternate carcinogenic bay-region PAHs, they can be of importance for the carcinogenicity of a nonalternate PAH (with odd-membered regions, as for instance in cyclopenteno-benzo(a)anthracene **60**, see Scheme 8).

This rule (known as the $\alpha' > \alpha > \beta$ rule), although not providing numerical values for the delocalization energy, is nevertheless useful for a rapid evaluation of carcinogenic potency of PAHs. This rule is also functioning for carcinogenic PAHs generating nonbay-region carbocations. For instance, if we have to decide which of the two benzylic carbocations formed by the activation of hydrocarbon **60** is the ultimate carcinogen, it follows immediately, according to the $\alpha' > \alpha > \beta$ rule, that carbocation **62** is more stable than **63**, being thus a more plausible candidate for the ultimate carcinogen than **63**.

The NBMO coefficients thus calculated might also serve for the carcinogenicity prediction of some substituted PAHs. For instance in the case of PAH methylation, the substituent when located in a ''remote position''* (i.e., 1, 2, 3, 4, 5, 12 for BaP) stabilizes the bay-region cation by hyperconjugation. Using quantum-mechanical calculations it is

* See also Section IV.C.2 for remote and nonremote positions.

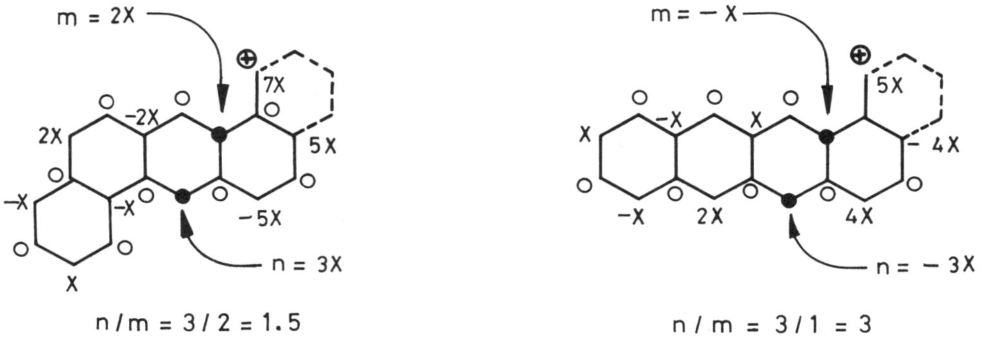

SCHEME 9. Computation of n/m ratio. (From Loew, J. P. and Silverman, D. B., *Acc. Chem. Res.*, 17, 332, 1984. With permission.)

possible to demonstrate that hyperconjugation is larger when the methyl group is attached to a site with larger absolute magnitude of the corresponding NBMO. Furthermore, for BaP benzylic (bay-region) carbocations a stabilizing of comparable magnitude results when methylation occurs at 1, 3, 4 and 12 positions $(11^{-1/2} = 0.302)$*. No stabilization should result from methylation at 2 and 5 positions (NBMO = O)*. This rule does not function for the "nonremote positions" because of the steric crowding appearing in these positions (see Section IV.C.2).

The effect produced on the carbocation stabilization energy by the rearrangement of the rings in the conjugated system may also be predicted by using NBMO coefficients of LEMO. The ion stability is directly proportional with the magnitude of the ratio of two NBMO coefficients namely n and m (see Scheme 9) calculated according to the method described in Appendix 1. For example, on this basis one can predict that the bay-region carbocation of benzo(a)tetracene would be more stable than that of dibenzo(a,h)anthracene. A generalization of this observation led to the rule that a kink in the aromatic system reduces the bay-region carbocation stability and is more destabilizing the closer it occurs to the bay-region.[146] This rule can be used to compare the carcinogenicity of nonbranched PAHs.

We briefly reviewed these aspects because they represent, in our opinion, an elegant and rapid procedure for estimating on the basis of simple but well-substantiated rules whether a PAH with a given structure can or cannot be carcinogenic.

A more difficult problem emerges in the carcinogenicity prediction of heteroatom-containing polycyclic aromatic hydrocarbons. Many such heterocycles (especially aza-PAHs) exhibit interesting carcinogenic properties. However, the extension of the previously discussed methods to the prediction of their carcinogenicity raises theoretical, as well as computational difficulties. First of all, they have to be activated according to the same general mechanism, affording bay-region DEs. This seems to be the case for a number of better known heterocyclic systems (i.e., the benzo(a)- and benzo(c)acridines or dibenz(c,h)acridines) which react with DNA via DE intermediates.[149,150] There are also other types of carcinogenic heterocyclic systems possessing other potential sites for metabolic attack (i.e., dibenzo(c)carbozole).[152]

Second, inclusion of an electronegative atom in the aromatic system will affect all types (σ, π) of electrons, thus the correct estimation of ΔE_{deloc} becomes more difficult. Simple quantum-chemical calculations performed on this type of heterocycles[153] showed that the position of the nitrogen atom in the cyclic system exerts a very important effect on benzylic carbocation formation (see Scheme 10).

The calculations by the simple Hückel method previously described using for $\alpha_N = \alpha$

---

* See Appendix.

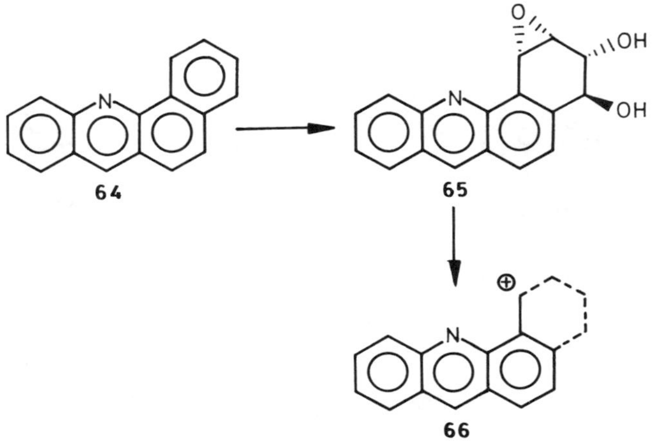

SCHEME 10.   Activation of benzo(c)acridine.

+ 0.5 β, as well as by the perturbational method, inferred that the tendency toward benzylic carbocation formation in the benzoacridinic system is lower than in the corresponding benzoanthracenic system.* These data correlate well with the mutagenic activity of several benzoacridine tetrahydroepoxides (**67-69**), which is lower than that of the corresponding benzoanthracene arene oxides. The data mentioned above are generally in agreement with the more sophisticated calculations (i.e., extended Hückel, INDO or Gaussian 70 *ab initio* SCF) performed by Loewe and Silverman[154] for similar systems.

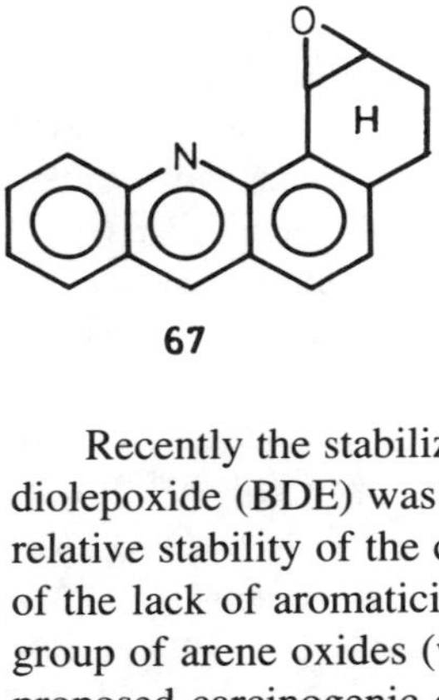

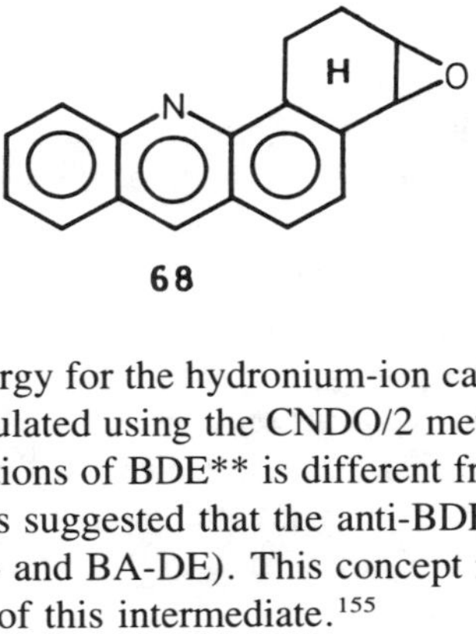

Recently the stabilization energy for the hydronium-ion catalyzed hydrolysis of benzene diolepoxide (BDE) was also calculated using the CNDO/2 method. Despite the fact that the relative stability of the conformations of BDE** is different from that of PAH-DE (because of the lack of aromaticity), it was suggested that the anti-BDE belongs to a highly reactive group of arene oxides (with BaP- and BA-DE). This concept is in good agreement with the proposed carcinogenic character of this intermediate.[155]

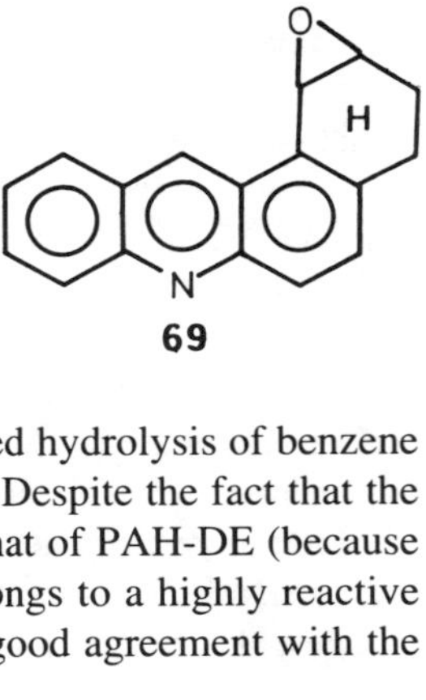

3. Stereochemistry of PAH-Reactive Intermediates

The stereochemistry of the PAH-reactive intermediates is of critical importance for their

---

* The $\Delta E_{deloc}/\beta$ for heterocyclic systems is expressed by the equation:

$$\Delta E_{deloc,N} = \Delta E_{deloc} - 0.5\, a_{or}^2 \tag{32}$$

where ΔE_{deloc} is the energy needed by the parent hydrocarbon to be converted into an arylmethyl carbocation and a_{or} is the NBMO coefficient of the same cation and at the position substituted by nitrogen.

** See also Section III.B.

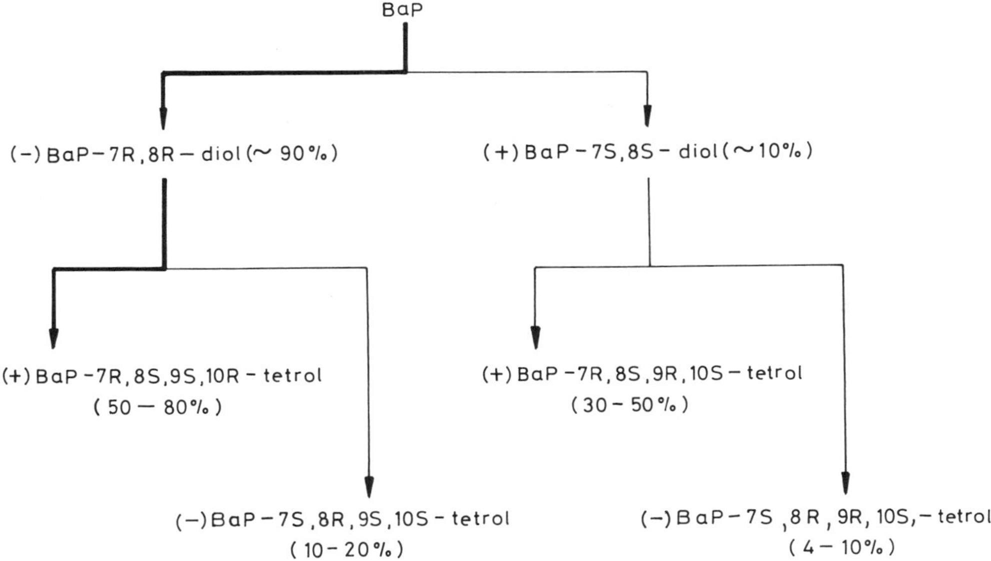

FIGURE 6.   Stereochemistry of BaP activation in mice cells.

carcinogenicity because it determines the effectiveness of both: their activation to ultimate carcinogen DE, and their interaction with DNA.

The concept of regioselectivity (or positional stereoselectivity) actually reflects the propensity of monooxygenasic systems for attacking preferentially certain regions or sites of the PAH molecules. For instance, the 4,5-,7,8- and 9,10-dihydrodiols formed subsequently to BaP activation by MC-stimulated microsomes are found in yields of 9, 12 and 20%, respectively.[156]

Considering the bay-region DE ultimate carcinogens, it is obvious that the amounts of the precursor diol, as well as the effectiveness of their further metabolization, are very important in determining the carcinogenic potential of PAHs. Thus, the conversion of BA into the corresponding 3,4-dihydrodiol (only 2%) accounts for its weak carcinogenicity, although the intrinsic carcinogenic activity of the ultimate carcinogen BA-DE is strong.[156] A remarkable stereoselectivity was observed during PAH activation. However, this factor is heavily dependent on the specific systems (i.e., origin of cells and microsomes, pretreatments, etc.) and the specific conditions under which it was determined.

It was thus demonstrated, for at least five PAHs that their MC-stimulated microsomal activation leads in an 80 to 90% proportion to dihydrodiols in (R,R) configurations. The stereochemistry of BaP activation is represented in Figure 6.

One of the key BaP metabolites, namely the 7,8-dihydrodiol is formed up to a 97% proportion as the (−)7R, BR enantiomer. This undergoes a further stereospecific oxidation, affording in up to 86% yield the (+)7R, 8S-diol-9S,10R-epoxy-7,8,9,10-tetrahydro-BaP ultimate carcinogen. The latter is formed with a total yield of approximately 82% with respect to the BaP-7R,8S-oxide. The metabolism of chrysene occurs similarly. The absolute configuration of these metabolites in the Cahn-Ingold-Prelog system, as well as their nomenclature, are presented in Table 7.

The monooxygenase epoxidation of PAHs is highly stereospecific, but the resulted DEs have a different configuration by respect to those in which epoxidation occurs under peroxyl radical oxidation.[157,158] The different stereochemistry of DEs formed by cytochrome P-450 and peroxylradicals is shown in Scheme 11.

A substantial carcinogenic activity is usually associated with only one enantiomeric DE, thus formed enzymatically as demonstrated for BaP where the (+)anti-7R,8S,9S,10R BPDE,

TABLE 7
Nomenclature and Stereochemistry of DE Resulted From BaP-Activation[a]

7,8-dihydroxy-9,10-epoxi-7,8,9,10-tetrahydro-benzo(a)pyrene

Diastereoisomer enantiomers	*anti* +[b]	*anti* −	*syn* +	*syn* −
α,β Nomenclature	(+)7β,8α,9α,10β	(−)7α,8β,9β,10β	(+)7α,8β,9α,10α	(−)7β,8α,9α,10β
CIP nomenclature	7R,8S,9S,10R	7S,8R,9R,10S	7S,8R,9S,10R	7R,8S,9R,10S
Common nomenclature	(+)diolepoxide 2	(−)diolepoxide 2	(+)diolepoxide 1	(−)diolepoxide 1

[a] This nomenclature could be applied to all PAHs, according to the numbering system used.
[b] The most carcinogenic enantiomer.

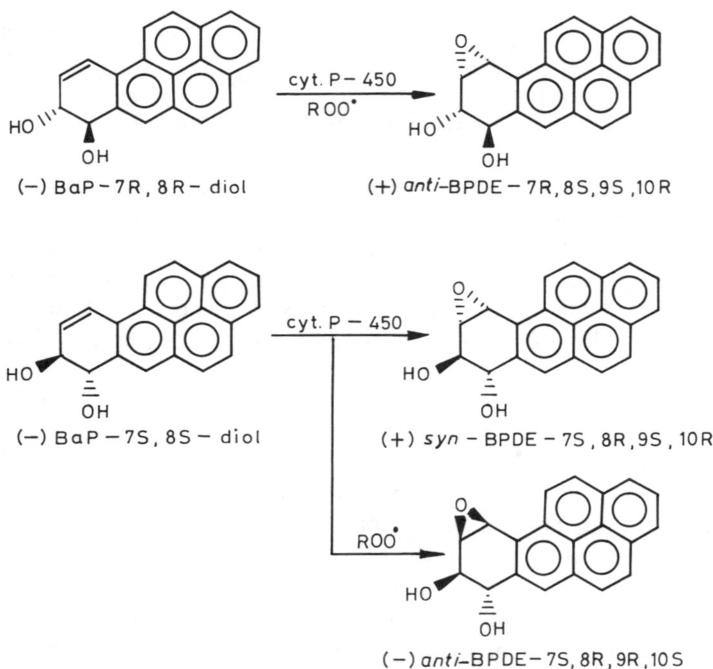

SCHEME 11.   Stereochemistry of diolepoxides formed under cytochrome P-450 dependent monooxygenase catalysis or under peroxyl-radicals attack.

is the most *carcinogenic*.[159] This observation is in agreement with the order of the *mutagenic* effects exerted by these four diastereoisomers on V-79 hamster cells, but not with the order of their mutagenic activities on *S. typhimurium* TA 98 and TA 100.[160]

Similar observations made for a number of PAHs suggest a possible correlation between the R,S,S,R (*anti*) configuration of the DE and their carcinogenic properties.

Both *conformation* and *configuration* of dihydrodiol intermediates and tetrahydro-DEs play an essential role in determining the carcinogenic properties of the parent PAHs.

Concerning the conformation of ultimate carcinogens, the *cis* and *trans* position of the oxiranic ring relative to the C-7 hydroxyl group, as well as the quasi-axial or equatorial character of both C-7 and C-8 hydroxyls are important in determining their: (1) reactivity;

(2) resistance against enzymatic hydration (by epoxy-hydrase) and (3) accessibility to nucleophilic centers in DNA.

Two physical methods are useful in accurately defining the configuration of these compounds: X-ray diffraction and nuclear magnetic resonance. The former gives a picture of the molecule (interatomic distances, angles, etc.) in solid (crystalline) state.

X-ray diffraction measurements demonstrate that the reciprocal position of hydroxylic groups in PAH-dihydrodiols is always *trans*.[161-163] If these hydroxylic groups of the precursor dihydrodiols are situated in a sterically crowded region (for instance, in a bay-region), then they have a diaxial conformation; if they are outside this region they adopt a diequatorial one.[164] These conformations are also maintained in solution. The ^{1}H-NMR procedure allows, by measuring the coupling constant J, of the adjacent C_7-C_8 protons to establish the equatorial or axial character of the hydroxy groups linked to the C-7 and C-8 atoms. Thus, a coupling constant $J_{7,8} = 12.7 \pm 0.2$ Hz corresponds to a diequatorial configuration, whereas $J_{7,8} = 2.0 \pm 3.1$ Hz corresponds to a diaxial configuration.[165]

The dihydrodiol conformations are important in determining the pathway and the yield of their subsequent metabolization. Generally, the diaxial conformation of the precursor dihydrodiols hinders DE formation whereas the diequatorial one favors this process. Thus, BaP-7,8-dihydroxy-7,8-diol possessing a pseudoequatorial orientation of the 7 and 8 hydroxylic groups ($J_{7,8} = 10.4$ Hz) is converted into their corresponding BPDE with high yields. BaP substitution can alter this situation. For instance, the 6-F-BaP dihydrodiol **70**, possessing a pseudoaxial conformation of the two 7,8 hydroxyls, ($J_{7,8} = 3.5$ Hz) because of the influence of the peri-fluorine, undergoes only a partial conversion into the corresponding bay-region 6-F-BPDE. This fact accounts for its weaker carcinogenic properties in comparison with BaP.[166] In 9F-BaP-7,8 diol ($J_{7,8} = 7.2$ Hz) the population of molecules with quasi-axial conformation of the hydroxylic groups equal that of molecules with a quasi-equatorial conformation, in contrast with 9-Me-BaP-7,8 diol **71** where the quasi-equatorial conformation is predominant.[165] The weak carcinogenicity of 7-Me-BaP, a compound which interacts with DNA via the 7-Me-BaP 7,8,9,10 tetrahydro-7,8-diol 9,10-epoxide, represents an interesting case. Because the hydrocarbon possesses a normal quasi-diequatorial conformation of the 7,8 hydroxyl groups[169] the very low amount of the corresponding ultimate carcinogen DE which results by metabolic activation could be related only to the unusual axial position of the 7-methyl group which hinders the monooxygenase attack.

The configuration of the intermediate dihydrodiols and of the DE formed during PAH activation is also extremely important for their carcinogenicity. The absolute configuration of DE ultimate carcinogens was determined for a number of cases, and an R,S,S,R configuration seems to be required for the carcinogenic DE.[160,168] This particular configuration is probably required for a specific interaction with the target DNA molecule.

We shall briefly examine the resulting stereochemistry of the DE during PAH activation, because it determines, together with the electronic factors, the mechanism and the kinetics of their reaction with DNA and furthermore, the structure of the resulted adducts. This step is obviously important for PAH carcinogenicity prediction. A second reason for this approach

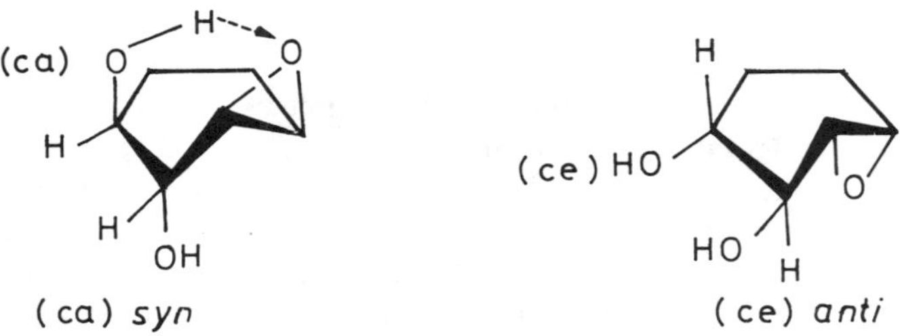

FIGURE 7.   Conformation of BPDE-*syn* and -*anti*.

is that the sterical features of the bay-region DE determine their resistance against enzymatic hydration (catalyzed by epoxi-hydrase), a unique property of these compounds which could also play an essential role for the carcinogenicity of PAHs.[139]

Depending on the location of the oxiranic ring with respect to the bay-region in PAH-DE, three distinct cases may be delineated. *The epoxidic ring is located in the bay-region and the two hydroxylic groups are outside this region.* As a general rule, the *trans*-dihydrodiols formed by enzymatic activation adopt a quasi-diequatorial conformation.[102] This favors the subsequent metabolism of dihydrodiols to the corresponding DE. However, generation of the oxiranic ring during bond oxidation by monooxygenases or peroxyl radicals leads to different ratios between the *syn* and *anti* diastereoisomers.

^{1}H-NMR spectra of the C_7- and C_8-protons in ($\pm$)BPDE-*syn* and -*anti* showed that the hydroxylic groups possess a quasi-diaxial conformation in *syn*- diastereoisomers and an *anti* quasi-diequatorial conformation.[169]

The mutagenesis and carcinogenesis data determined for these ultimate carcinogens suggest that the diequatorial conformation of the hydroxylic groups favors carcinogenic activity.[118,156] The significance of this fact is not yet fully elucidated. Data provided by X-ray analysis confirmed the proposed structures for BPDE-*syn* and -*anti* and also indicated that the epoxidic ring is folded at an angle of 103° related to the approximately planar polycyclic system of the hydrocarbon. Quantum-mechanical calculations indicate the possibility of the *syn*-isomer to adopt a conformation in which the hydroxy groups are fixed in a quasi-axial position, by establishing a hydrogen bond between the 7-OH axial group and the arene-oxide oxygen, the distance between them being 2.7 Å[170] (see Figure 7). This conformation strongly affects the reactivity of the ($\pm$)BPDE-*syn* diastereoisomers. The conformation of the *anti*-BPDE stereoisomer is much less favorable for stabilization through hydrogen bonding. Similar steric features were also determined for BA, DMBA, etc.[170a,171]

The DEs, where the epoxidic ring is located in a region which is sterically more crowded than a usual bay-region, possess some special biological properties which may be explained by this particular structure. Two distinct examples will be discussed. Benzo(c)phenanthrene, BcF, exhibits a so called "fjord-region". In the BcF-DE-*syn*-diastereoisomers the plane of the oxiranic ring is folded at an angle of 90° with respect to that of the aromatic system, whereas in the *anti*-isomer this angle is only 60°. Unlike the previously discussed case, both BcF-DE-*syn* and *anti*, **72** and **73**, exhibit a quasi-equatorial conformation of the hydroxy group linked with C-3 and C-4 atoms.[172-175]

This unusual conformation of both diastereoisomers accounts for their carcinogenic and mutagenic activities, which are among the strongest presently known for DEs and suggest the outstanding importance of the steric factor for carcinogenic activity.[130] *The hydrocarbons in which the bay-region is additionally crowded by a substituent (most often a methyl group).* Such a substitution usually leads to an exacerbation of the carcinogenic potency of the substituted hydrocarbon. Many examples could be cited: 7-methyl-benz(a)anthracene (7-MBA),7,12-dimethylbenz(a)anthracene (7,12-DMBA)[176,177] 5-methylchrysene,[178] 15,16-dihydro-11-methylcyclopenta(a)phenanthrene-17-one[179] 1,4-dimethylphenanthrene,[180] 11-methyl BaP,[181] all being more carcinogenic than the corresponding unsubstituted hydrocarbons. Overcrowding of the bay-region by fluorination can also produce a similar effect, as for 7-F-BA or 11-F-7,12-DMBA.[182] However, this rule is not always valid. The previously discussed facts suggest that when a substituent (methyl or fluorine) is located in a bay-region, either the epoxidation of the double bond adjacent to this region is favored, or the formed DE is intrisically more carcinogenic than the corresponding DE lacking this substituent.[126]

The former hypothesis seems not to be valid since the extent of 5-Me-chrysene-1,2-diol and 5-Me-chrysene-7,8-diol formation in the mouse epidermis was the same.[126] Therefore the strong tumorigenicity of 5-Me-chrysene is due to the unique reactivity and carcinogenicity of its DE possessing both the methyl group ($+B$ effect*) and epoxide ring located in the same bay-region (5-MeC-*anti*-DE-I). The fluorine substitution of 5-Me-chrysene provides strong supportive evidence for the hypothesis that 5-Me-C-*anti*-DE-I is a major ultimate carcinogen of 5-Me-chrysene (Amin, 1984).

X-ray crystallographic studies have shown that in 5-Me-chrysene, distortion from normal geometry occurs, in order to accommodate the methyl group in the bay-region. Out-of-plane distortions are greater in DMBA than in 5-Me-chrysene, probably paralleling the $+B$ effect. The stereochemistry of the corresponding DE has not yet been reported for all the discussed PAHs. However, the examination of precursor dihydrodiols derived from 7,12-DMBA and 7-hydroxymethyl-12-MBA,[171,183] with a coupling constant $J_{3,4} = 11.5$ Hz showed, as expected, a trans-diequatorial conformation of the hydroxy groups. The absolute configuration of the precursor bay-region dihydrodiols is R,R in the known cases (i.e., 7-F-BA).[184] However, PAH substitution could lead to configurational and conformational modifications of the diols obtained subsequent to metabolic activation. Examples such as 7-F-BaP,[166] or more recently 7-F-BA, were reported, in which the *trans*-7,8- and 8,9-dihydrodiols adopt a quasi-axial conformation under the effect of the fluorine atom.[184] Also, the P (peri) effect could be cited in this respect. When a methyl group (or a fluorine atom) occupies the peri-position adjacent to an angular ring (as in 6-Me-BaP, 6-F-BaP, 5,12-di-Me-chrysene, 12-F-5-Me-chrysene, etc.) the conformation of the angular ring *trans*-dihydrodiol will be diaxial because of the steric hindrance exerted by this group. Therefore this peri effect could inhibit carcinogenicity by altering the conformation of the precursor dihydrodiol.[185] An alternate explanation could be that the peri-methyl group may inhibit the formation of the dihydrodiol intermediate. This last assumption is substantiated by the inhibition of 6-Me-BaP-7,8-dihydrodiol formation during the activation of 6-Me-BaP.

Epoxy and two hydroxy groups located in the bay-region form another case. As the bay-region is a sterically crowded part of the PAH molecule, the precursor dihydrodiols located in this region possess an unfavorable quasi-diaxial conformation. This is the case of benzo(e)-pyrene (BeP), triphenylene, etc. These hydrocarbons possess two bay-regions, so that in their corresponding DE both the oxiranic ring and the two hydroxy groups occupy such regions.[1] H-NMR studies on both ($\pm$) BeP-9,10,11,12-tetrahydro-9,10-diol-11,12-epoxide,BeP *syn*, **74**, and *anti*, **75**, showed that all diastereoisomers have a quasi-diaxial

---

* $+B$ effect was defined as the key structural requirement for the enhanced tumorigenicity of methylated PAH.[126]

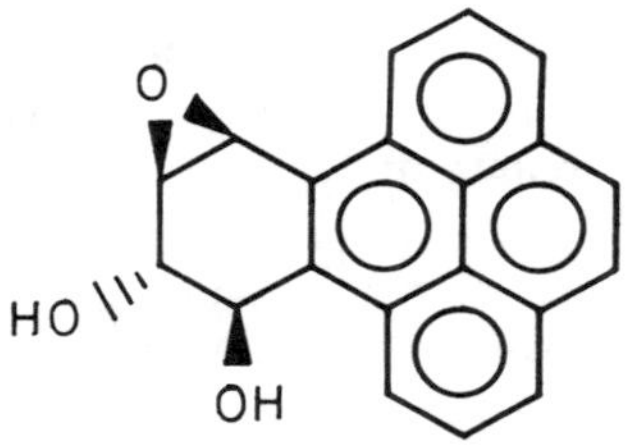

74 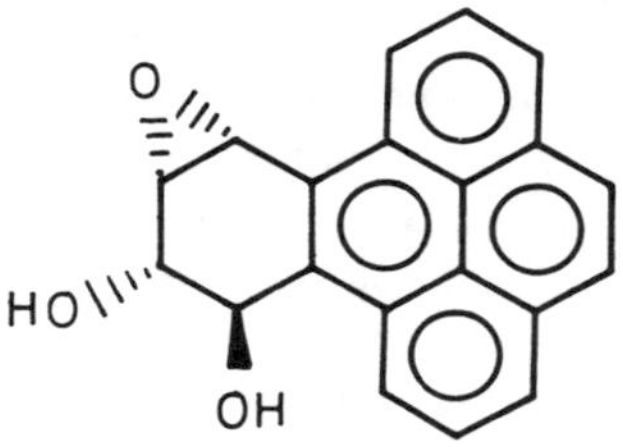   **75**

conformation of the hydroxy groups (coupling constants of the adjacent protons to the OH groups are $J_{9,10}$ = 1.7 to 3.5 Hz.[126]

In the BePDE *-anti*, **75**, the oxiranic ring is almost perpendicular to the plane of the aromatic system.[187]

BeP apparently does not fit the bay-region theory because of its weak carcinogenicity, despite the fact that this hydrocarbon possesses two bay-regions. Data concerning its metabolism demonstrate, however, that the precursor dihydrodiol, B(e)P-9,10-dihydro-9,10-diol, is formed in very small amounts,[139,188,189] and the diaxial conformation of their hydroxylic groups precludes its conversion to a DE ultimate carcinogen.[190] The unfavorable conformation of the corresponding DE could also account for the weak mutagenic and carcinogenic character of triphenylene-DE.[191]

The hydroxy groups are located in the bay-region, and the epoxidic ring outside it. This is the case of BaP-7,8,9,10-tetrahydro-7,8-epoxy,8,10-diol (reverse BPDE). The precursor BaP-9,10-dihydro-9,10-diol has a diaxial conformation of the hydroxylic group. We therefore expect for the corresponding reverse-BPDE diastereoisomers to have the same conformation. As we discussed previously, such a stereochemistry of the DE molecule is unfavorable for carcinogenicity expression and is in good agreement with the weak or nonexisting carcinogenic potency of this metabolite. Experimentally it was found that the adduct concentration obtained by reverse BPDE direct interaction with DNA is small in respect to BPDE *-anti*.[102]

Finally, the stereochemistry of K-region epoxides deserves some comments, because they are candidates of being ultimate carcinogens of some BaP phenols.[139,193] It was also shown, for methylated phenanthrenes, that the hindrance of 9,10-diols formation and the formation of 5,6-diols (K-region) is associated with increasing mutagenicity.[180]

The K-region is characterized by bonds shorter than usual aromatic ones (around 1.34—1.35 Å).[162,194] X-ray crystallographic studies of the K-region DMBA, BaP and phenanthrene epoxides showed that:

1.   Epoxidation reduces the planarity of the molecule (for instance, the angle between the marginal ring and the plane of the rest of the molecule increases from 23 to 35° in DMBA).
2.   In BaP and phenanthrene, the formed oxirane has the C–O bonds of practically equal length (1.48 and 1.46 Å, respectively).
3.   For DMBA (in which the K-region is sterically crowded by the 7-methyl group), the C-O bonds in the oxiranic ring are of inequal lengths, C^6–O being longer (1.457 Å) than C^5–O (1.445 Å). Therefore, the first to break during hydrolysis is C^6–O.[162]

Recent data demonstrate that the biosynthesis of BaP-5,6-oxide from the achiral BaP molecule is stereoselective and leads to almost exclusive formation of (+)BaP (4S,5R) oxide,[195] which by conjugation with glutathione further leads to the diastereoisomers corresponding to this configuration (see Scheme 12).

There are few compounds among PAH in which some tetrahydro-epoxides are more mutagenic than their corresponding DEs presumed to be the ultimate carcinogens. These are the tetrahydro-epoxides derived from phenanthrene, BeP, **79** and triphenylene, **80**.[196]

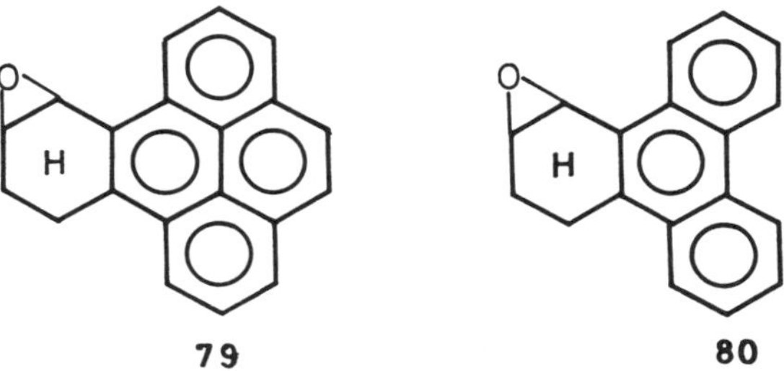

SCHEME 12. Stereochemistry of conjugation products resulted from BaP-4,5-oxide reaction with glutathione.

These intermediates seem to also have carcinogenic properties. It is not known whether one enantiomer is more carcinogenic than the other ones.

Stereochemistry of the active intermediates derived from PAH possess a pseudo-bay-region. There are known PAHs with intermediate or moderate carcinogenic potency which possess a so-called pseudo-bay-region; examples are the fluoranthenes.

Not much information is available regarding the activation of these hydrocarbons. However, the fact that the dihydrodiols **81** and **82** derived from benzo(k)fluoranthene and benzo(j)fluoranthene, respectively, are the most mutagenic intermediates known so far,[197,198] suggests that the corresponding DEs are the principal candidates for the ultimate carcinogens.

Their stereochemistry is unknown, but it is supposed to correspond generally to that of bay-region DEs. More recently it was demonstrated that indeed *syn-* and *anti*-fluoranthene-DE **83, 84**, are formed during rats' exposure to this hydrocarbon.[199]

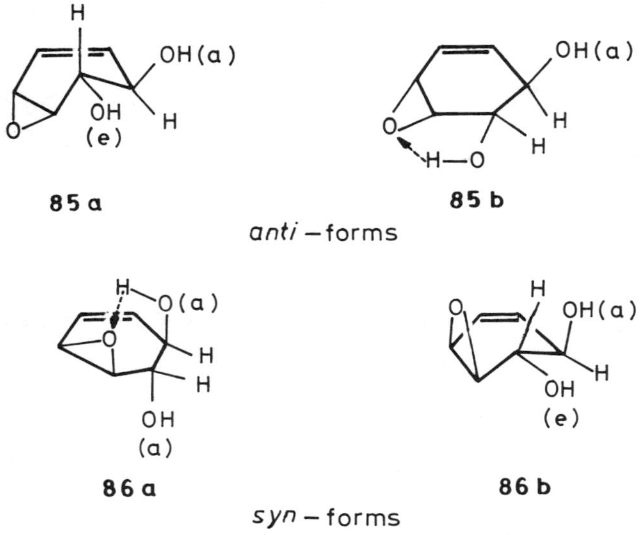

85 a

85 b

anti —forms

86 a

86 b

syn — forms

SCHEME 13.   Conformations of benzene diol-epoxides (BDE).

Stereochemistry of PAH-active intermediates sometimes *possess no bay-region*. Finally, we want to point out the existence of PAHs which, although not possessing a bay-region, are nevertheless carcinogenic. They are exceptions from Jerina's theory. The most simple and at the same time the one with the most obscure mechanism of action is benzene which exhibits leukemogenic activity to humans.[200,201] One metabolic route consists in its oxidation (in liver) to phenols (i.e., phenol, hydroquinone, pyrocatechol, 1,2,4,-benzenetriol) and even some higher oxidation products (i.e., quinones).[202,203] However, it seems that these intermediates fail to interact directly with DNA,[20] but some of them could induce (especially 1,2,4-benzenetriol) significant amounts of superoxide anions ($O_2^{\cdot-}$) which are able to denaturate DNA.

An alternate possible metabolic pathway is however possible via benzene-diolepoxides, BDE because it has been recently reported that 1,2-dihydroxy-3,4-epoxy-1,2,3,4-tetrahydrobenzene is a weak mutagen.[205] The semi-empirical molecular orbital CNDO/2 method was used to investigate theoretically the electronic structure and reactivity of BDE-*syn* and *anti*.[155] The results indicate that there are two possible conformations for BDPE-*anti* and *syn*, respectively (Scheme 13), the conformations **85a** and **86a** being the most stable. The *syn*-form is more stable than the *anti*-form.

Another example is cyclopenta(c,d)pyrene (CPP), a ubiquitous hydrocarbon with strong carcinogenic properties. CPP-3,7-oxide **87** was recognized to be the strongest mutagenic and carcinogenic intermediate among its metabolites, thus being a candidate for ultimate carcinogen.[206,207]

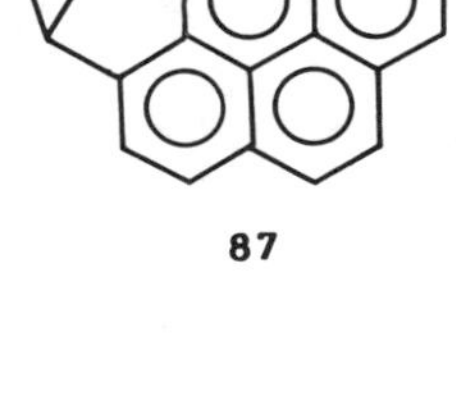

87

The stereochemistry of this intermediate is not known. By ring opening it affords reactive carbocations (for instance, a 1-pyrenyl or 7-pyrenyl carbocation) able to interact with DNA. Their ΔE_{deloc} are calculated in Appendix 1, and are high enough to account for the carcinogenic properties of this compound.

The structure and stereochemistry of the carbocations formed during the reaction of ultimate carcinogens with DNA could be inferred from the previously mentioned information. In every case, benzylic carbocations are formed, the positive carbon atom being located in a nonplanar ring.

The relatively sophisticated stereochemistry of these carbocations makes difficult the assignments of absolute configurations to the final products (adducts) formed during reaction with DNA.

The stereochemistry of the reactive intermediates resulted during PAH activation reveals extremely important aspects for the biological properties of these compounds, namely:

1. The diequatorial or diaxial conformations of the PAH *trans* dihydrodiols determines both the effectiveness of their metabolization to DEs and the stereochemistry of the latter. The diequatorial conformation favors the metabolic conversion to the corresponding DE.
2. The diequatorial or diaxial conformations of the hydroxy groups in the ultimate carcinogens DEs determines their carcinogenicity, the diequatorial structures favor the expression of this property. This conformation hinders the catalytic activity of epoxy-hydrase.
3. The configuration of the active intermediate and ultimate carcinogens also plays an important part in the specificity of their interaction with DNA, a single enantiomer being usually active (i.e., (+)BPDE-*anti*). Finally, it was recently reported that optical isomers of the same compounds, i.e., (+)-*syn*-BcP and (−)-*syn*-BcP can react with subtly different sequence selectivities in contrast with compounds with the same stereochemistry but with different hydrocarbon residue (i.e., (+)-*anti*-BaP and (−)-*anti*-BcP) which exhibit widely divergent sequence selectivities for c-H-*ras*-oncogene DNA.[208]

D. COMPLEX ELECTRONIC THEORIES OF CHEMICAL CARCINOGENESIS

The magnitude of delocalization energy satisfactorily correlates with the propensity of the ultimate carcinogens to react with DNA. However, it affords no information concerning the easiness of ultimate carcinogen formation (this problem was discussed in Section IV.B). Therefore, in order to improve the predictive potential of the correlations between PAH structure and their carcinogenic properties, the use of multilinear regression equations containing several indices describing different aspects of PAH behavior was proposed.

A three-term equation for a series of 21 PAHs using electronic energy indices combined with the superdelocalizability parameters for the atoms involved in the L-region, has been recently proposed for PAH activity prediction.[209]

$$S = 8.64\Delta E_{\pi} + 12.43\Delta E_{deloc} - 0.34I_L + 21.61$$

$$n = 21 \qquad s = 0.62 \qquad r = 0.91 \qquad F = 26.45 \qquad (33)$$

where: S = carcinogenicity expressed using an arbitrary value scale (0,1,2,3,4; 0 denoting inactivate PAH and 4 very active ones) ΔE_{deloc} = alteration of the PAH-DE molecule energy (β units) when being converted into a carbocation; I_L = sum of the atomic superdelocalizabilities involved in the L-region and ΔE_{π} = the energy change (β units) in forming the A-region dihydrodiol from the parent PAH.

A unification attempt was recently done by Szentpaly,[70,209] who proposed a three-

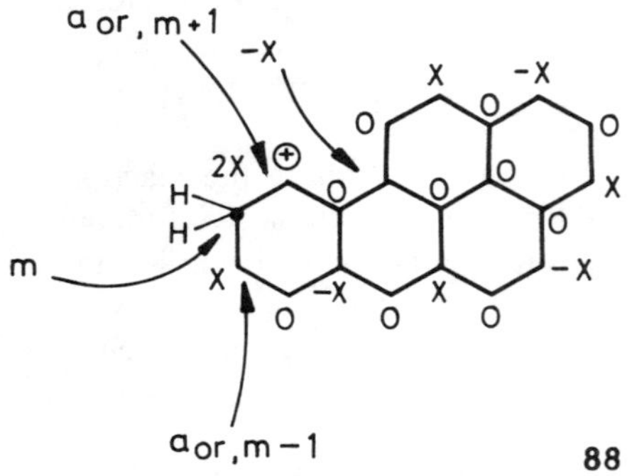

$$N_m = 2\left(\frac{1}{\sqrt{12}} + \frac{2}{\sqrt{12}}\right) = \frac{6}{\sqrt{12}} = 1.732$$

$$\sum_r a_{or,r}^{*4} = \frac{23}{11^2} = 0.190$$

a_{or}^{*} being the NBMO benzylic carbocation of BaP as in **88**

88

SCHEME 14.   Example for N_m and $\sum_r a_{or,r}$ calculation.

parameter model for PAH carcinogenicity prediction which correlates Iball carcinogenicity indices with three theoretical parameters.

A metabolic parameter, M (metabolic index A); was chosen based on the assumption that A-region primary epoxidation is the determinant reaction for the activation process because of the positive correlation found between A-region reactivity indices and carcinogenicity.[88] There exists evidence that epoxidation occurs by a nonconcerted addition of oxygen at the double bond beginning at the more reactive atom. Therefore, the ease of the epoxidation will be negatively correlated to the smaller of the Dewar numbers in this region, namely to the index N_m calculated as:

$$N_m = 2(a_{or'm-1} + a_{or,m+1}) \tag{34}$$

where: $a_{or,m-1}$ and $a_{or,m+1}$ are the NBMO coefficients calculated as mentioned above (see Appendix 1), at atoms $m-1$ and $m+1$ of the odd PAH which results if we interrupt the π-system at the m atom (for exemplification, see **88** epoxidation occurring at the m-m + 1 bond). An example of computation for index N is given in Scheme 14.

However, the centers or regions in which detoxication reactions occur must also be taken into account. The center with the lowest N_c Dewar index is chosen assuming that only the most rapid reaction is prevalent in detoxication. On the basis of these two Dewar numbers a metabolic index M is defined by the relation:

$$M = (N_m - N_c)^2 \tag{35}$$

It reflects both the sensitivity of PAH to primary epoxidation and the competition between the activation and the one-center detoxication reactions.

The second variable used describes the ease of active species formation from DE. Using a more sophisticated approach, the possibility of both a carbocation and a free radical formation is considered, the index used in the regression equation being the complex index E_R which is associated to the arylmethyl ion formation from DE, namely:

$$E_R = E_C + E_D \tag{36}$$

where: E_D represents the delocalization energy being equivalent to that calculated by HMO methodology (see also Section IV.C.1) for the benzylic carbocation:

$$E_D = (1.50 - 1.03a_{or,b})\beta \tag{37}$$

where: $a_{or,b}$ is the NBMO coefficient of benzylic carbocation. E_c is called the charge dispersal energy and was expressed as:

$$E_C = -41.71 + 56.64 \sum_r a_{or,r}^4 \tag{38}$$

Taking for β a value of -20 kcal/mol, E_C was obtained in kcal/mol with a correlation coefficient $r = 0.980$ for a number of 36 alternate hydrocarbons (for computation of $\sum_r a_{or,r}^4$ (see also Scheme 14).

Finally, a variable taking into account the size of the PAH molecule is introduced, according to the plausible idea that there is an optimal size of the PAH molecule which favors the carcinogenesis process. Considering the optimal size of a PAH molecule to correspond to a number of 20—24 carbon atoms, the following relation was employed:

$$\Delta = |n - 20|^3 \tag{39}$$

where: Δ is size parameter, and n is the number of carbon atoms of the PAH molecule.

Taking into account these three parameters, the following regression equation results, the Iball carcinogenicity index being the independent variable:

$$I_{calc} = -(80.47 \pm 9.46)M + (8.24 \pm 0.510)(E_D + E_C) - (0.074 \pm 0.010)\Delta - (331.7 \pm 21.6)$$

$$n = 36 \qquad r = 0.961 \qquad s = 6.8 \qquad F = 87.455 \tag{40}$$

The above correlation is obviously good. If the term E_C (responsible for free radical formation) is eliminated, the correlation value decreases significantly, r becoming 0.824. This method was recently extended with good results (r = 0.940) to heterocyclic and methylated PAHs.[210] A completely different approach, but with qualitatively similar results, is based on the topological study of PAH molecules[211] (see also Chapter 4).

The presently discussed aspects emphasize that it is relatively easy to perform MO procedures (pencil and paper calculations which are presently available allowing a reasonable prediction of PAH carcinogenicity. Generally, sophistication of calculations obviously leads to better results, eliminating and explaining a series of exceptions. However, these computational refinements are not always justified, partly because the observed tendency usually parallels the results inferred by simple MO methods, and partly due to the fact that the biological assays utilized for these correlations (i.e., Iball index, etc.) have far larger inaccuracies than the unsubstantial improvements in the precision of some electronic indices. However, one must take into account that for significant deviations from planarity — if they occur — or for the substitution at remote positions in PAHs the simple Hückel calculations fail. Considering these comments, the methods reviewed in this chapter represent a sufficient theoretical background for usual situations.

Unfortunately, all these theoretical developments have been applied almost exclusively to PAHs. Other classes of carcinogens have been more or less neglected, especially as their quantum-mechanical approach is much more difficult than that of aromatic systems. However, several of these classes were the object of QSAR studies. They will be discussed in Chapter 5.

APPENDIX

We do not intend to describe here the molecular orbital theories which were developed since 1930 and were extensively applied for a better understanding of the properties of many organic molecules. An outstanding presentation of this topic may be found in a number of reviews and some classical textbooks (Coulson[212]; Streitwieser[213]; Heilbronner[214]).

This appendix is concerned with the presentation of a minimum of data needed by a biochemist or an organic chemist (without a special background in quantum chemistry) to calculate without the use of a computer (with pencil and paper) a few simple quantum mechanical indices, for instance ΔE_{deloc} required for an *a priori* selection or discussion of the carcinogenic properties of PAHs.

It is well known that a covalent bond results from the overlap of two atomic orbitals. This concept may be quantitatively defined by the overlap integral S, in which Ψ_A and Ψ_B are normalized atomic orbitals wave functions:*

$$S = \int \Psi_A \cdot \Psi_B d\varphi \tag{41}$$

(The asterisk indicates the complex conjugate, and space element $d\varphi$ is integrated overall space); S depends on the distance between A and B. The principle of maximum overlap assumes a direct relationship between the magnitude of S and bond strength.

A diatomic molecule may be characterized by a two-center molecular orbital. This orbital can be constructed in different ways, but a simple approach is to define it as a linear combination of atomic orbitals (LCAO). The wave-function (Ψ_{mol}) of the orbital thus formed may be written:

$$\Psi_{mol} = c_A \Psi_A \pm c_B \Psi_B \tag{42}$$

where c_A, c_B are the coefficients indicating the contribution of each atomic orbital in the molecular orbital. The most elementary form of the molecular orbital theory is the Hückel approach which gives a successful account of the properties of many organic molecules. For conjugated multiple bonds or aromatic systems, the nonlocalized bonding molecular orbital theory was employed. This procedure separates the 6π- from the σ-orbitals (involved in σ-bonds) and we calculate only the first. Several simplifying assumptions were made for facilitating the computation, namely: coplanarity of the conjugated system; equality of all bond distances and neglect of all nonneighbor interactions.

Generally, from n atomic orbitals, n molecular orbitals are formed. Returning to our previous example of a diatomic molecule, containing a double bond A = B, by the LCAO procedure two molecular orbitals with different energies are obtained: a bonding orbital of lower energy with $\Psi_{mol} = c_A \Psi_A + c_B \Psi_B$, and an antibonding orbital of higher energy $\Psi_{mol} = c_A \Psi_A - c_B \Psi_B$.

In the fundamental state of the molecule, only the bonding orbital is occupied by two electrons (with opposite spins). The central problem of HMO is to find that set of coefficients which gives the best value for the energy of the molecular orbital. This may be easily done by computers.

Thus in benzene having six π-electrons, the six molecular orbitals $(\Psi_{mol})_i$ comprise the following linear combinations of carbon $2p_2$ atomic orbitals:

i	c_1	c_2	c_3	c_4	c_5	c_6
1.	0.408	0.500	0.289	0.289	0.500	0.408
2.	0.408	0	0.577	−0.577	0	−0.408
3.	0.408	0	−0.577	−0.577	0	0.408
4.	0.408	0.500	−0.289	0.289	−0.500	−0.408
5.	0.408	−0.500	−0.289	0.289	0.500	−0.408
6.	0.408	−0.500	0.289	0.289	−0.500	0.408

---

* The wave-function is defined for one electron by Schrödinger's equation

$$\mathcal{H}\Psi = E \cdot \Psi \tag{43}$$

where $\mathcal{H}$ is the Hamiltonian of the function Ψ and E is the energy of the electron.

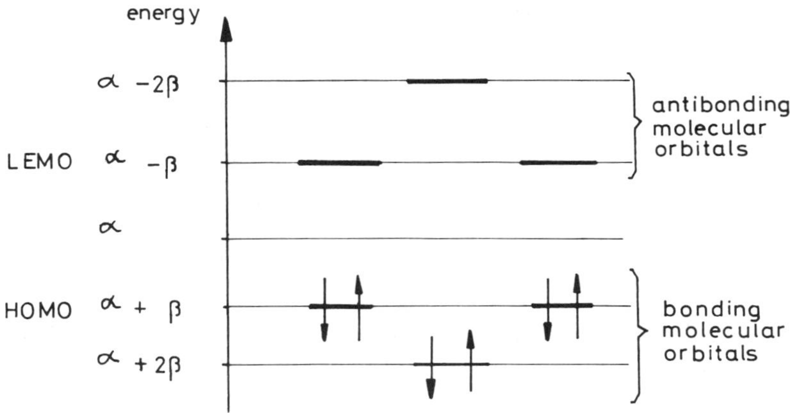

SCHEME 15.   Energy levels of the six benzene molecular orbitals.

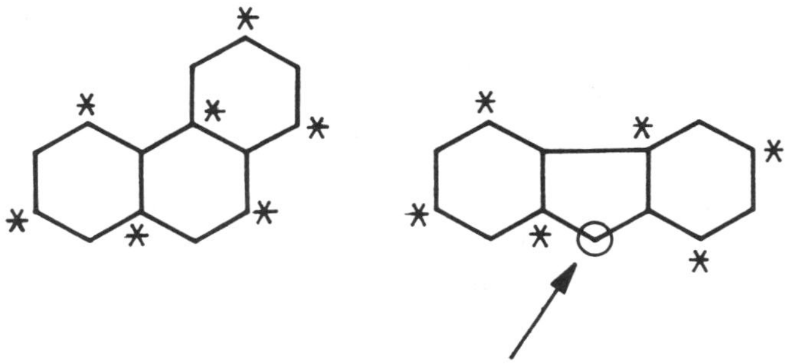

SCHEME 16.   Starring process for PAH with odd and even membered ring.

The energies of these orbitals calculated by a similar procedure are represented in Scheme 15.

From the six molecular orbitals, three are bonding and the other three are antibonding. In the ground state, only the three bonding orbitals are occupied by pairs of π-electrons. When the molecule is excited, an electron transition occurs from the highest occupied molecular orbital (HOMO, a bonding orbital) to the lowest empty orbital (antibonding one called lowest empty — or unoccupied — molecular orbital, LEMO or LUMO). The coefficients of Ψ_{LEMO} orbital (a_{or}) are of critical importance for the computation of several quantum mechanical indices employed for PAH carcinogenicity prediction.

The concept of alternate and nonalternate PAH must also be introduced.

If we look more carefully to the PAH class, then a very important distinction may be made between alternate and nonalternate hydrocarbons. Alternate hydrocarbons are planar conjugated hydrocarbons which have no odd-membered ring, and in which all carbon atoms can be divided into groups of starred (*) and unstarred carbons, such that no member of one group is adjacent to another atom of that group. For instance the, "starring process" may be successfully applied to phenanthrase, but not to fluorene (see Scheme 16).

The assignment of the first star is arbitrarily done. All alternate hydrocarbons have interesting properties, namely (Coulson-Rushbrooke theorems):

1.   In the energy diagram (see Scheme 15) the energy levels are symmetrically disposed about the zero or α level.

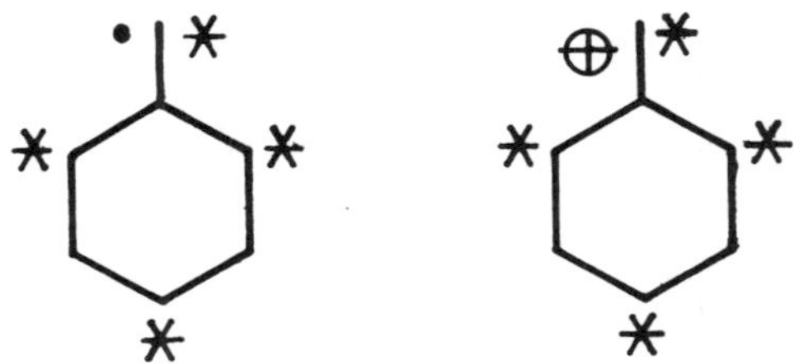

SCHEME 17.   Starring process for benzyl radical and carbocation.

2.   In the ground state of a neutral hydrocarbon (or hydrocarbon radical) atomic charges (q_i) on the various carbons, involved in the conjugation, are all equal to one.

These rules are also valid for odd-alternate conjugated hydrocarbons (alternate systems with an odd number of carbons) as for instance, the benzyl radical because in this case the starring process may also be successfully applied.

By removing one electron from the singly occupied nonbonding MO (NBMO) of an odd alternate hydrocarbon, the benzyl carbocation is formed. In this case the positive charge will be distributed among those carbon atoms for which the NBMO coefficients are not zero. As a general rule these coefficients are zero at the nonstarred position if the starred atoms are more numerous. The calculation of these NBMO coefficients (a_{or}) becomes very important.

A very elegant and simple procedure for the computation of the NBMO coefficients was developed by Dewar and Longuet-Higgins by studying the properties of the NBMO. This method represents a simple pathway for computing ΔE_{deloc} for different PAHs in which the interaction of ultimate carcinogens (DE) with DNA involves the formation of benzylic carbocation intermediates.

This type of computation may also be extended (however with a higher degree of imprecision) to heterocyclic aromatic hydrocarbons.

We present two models of calculating NBMO coefficients and the delocalization energy ΔE_{deloc}. The following operations have to be completed:[72,146]

1.   The aromatic system is drawn and a zero is placed where the branch representing the benzylic carbocation joins the aromatic system (in other words, where the CH_2^+ is linked to the aromatic ring). For instance, for the carbocation resulted by BPDE activation (which may be assimilated to a 3-methyl-pyrenyl carbocation, as the saturated cyclohexanic ring does not significantly influence the aromatic system), a zero is placed as in **88**.

2.   A zero is placed at every second carbon atom, throughout the aromatic system (as in **89**).

88	**89**	**90**

3. The first NBMO value, x, is placed at a nonzeroed carbon atom far from the branch (as in **90**).

4. The NBMO values of the other nonzeroed carbons are calculated according to the following rule: the sum of coefficients around a zero-noted carbon atom must always vanish (see **91**).

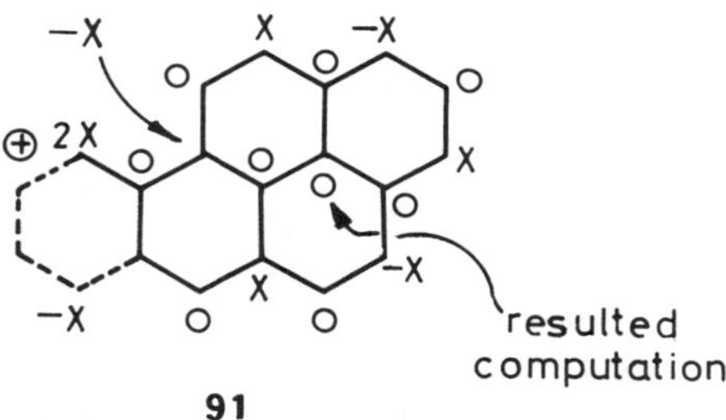

91

5. The value of x is calculated according to the normalization rule which claims that the sum of the squares of all coefficients is equal to one (thus $\sum_i x_i^2 = 1$). Calculation of x gives:

$$7x^2 + 4x^2 = 1 \quad \text{or} \quad x = \frac{1}{\sqrt{11}} \tag{44}$$

therefore a_{or} value at the benzylic position is according to **91** 2x, $a_{or} = 2.(11)^{-1/2} = 0.603$.

The delocalization energy for the carbocation formation is immediately computed using the relationship:

$$\Delta E_{deloc} = 2(1 - a_{or})\beta = 2\left(1 - \frac{2}{\sqrt{11}}\right)\beta = 0.794\beta \tag{45}$$

This value is given in Table 6. As it allows a quantitative correlation with carcinogenic potency for the major part of unsubstituted PAHs, ΔE_{deloc} represents an extremely important and easily accessible prediction element.

It results that the stability of such benzylic carbocations (formed during PAH activation) is essential for the carcinogenic properties of the corresponding PAH, and this rule is also valid for carbocations derived from PAHs which do not possess a true bay-region.

This is the case for cyclopentano(c,d)pyrene (CPP) **84**, which is carcinogenic without possessing a bay-region, actually representing an exception from the bay-region theory. Its activation occurs according to Scheme 18, by epoxidation of the double bond pertaining to the five-membered ring. The arene oxide thus formed undergoes ring opening affording the 3- or 4-pyrenyl carbocation. The 3-pyrenyl carbocation is identical to that formed during BaP activation so that a similar value for ΔE_{deloc} is expected, therefore it represents a carcinogenic species. For the 4-pyrenyl carbocation (see also **93**) a similar calculation as above leads to the following delocalization energy value:

$$x = \frac{1}{\sqrt{87}}; \quad \Delta E_{deloc} = 2\left(1 - \frac{6}{\sqrt{87}}\right)\beta = 0.713\beta \tag{46}$$

This value places the hydrocarbon at the benzo(e)pyrene level of carcinogenicity. It follows

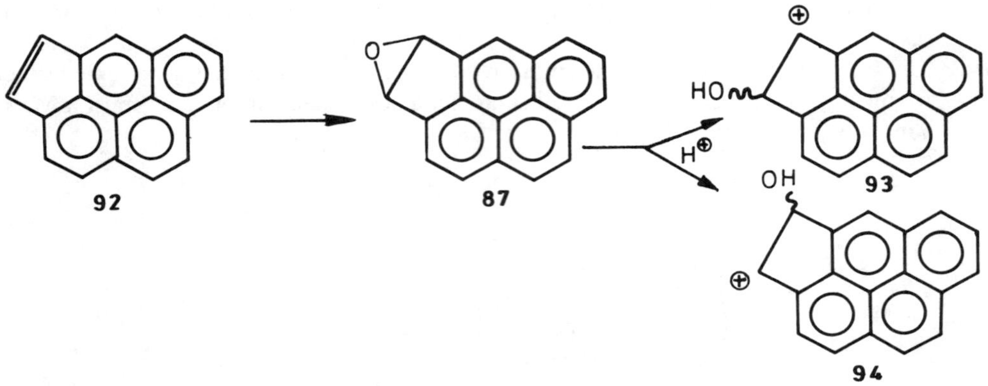

SCHEME 18.   Activation of CPP.

that the ratio between the concentration of the 3- and 4-pyrenyl carbocations formed during activation of this non-bay-region PAH determines its carcinogenicity.

Subsequently, it results that this compound is only an apparent exception from bay-region theory, because the benzylic carbocation is formed easily enough to lend strong carcinogenic character to CPP.

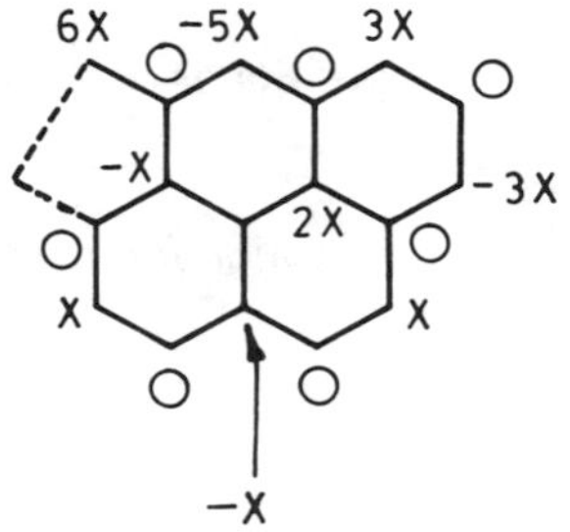

REFERENCES

1. **Arcos, J. C. and Argus, M. F.**, Molecular geometry and carcinogenic activity of aromatic hydrocarbons, *Adv. Cancer Res.*, 11, 305, 1968.
2. **Scribner, J. D. and Süss, R.**, Tumor initiation and promotion, *Int. Rev. Exp. Pathol.*, 18, 137, 1978.
3. **Boyland, E.**, The history and future of chemical carcinogenesis, *Br. Med. Bull.*, 36, 5, 1980.
4. **Ames, B. N., Dunsten, W. E., Yamasaki, E., and Lee, F. D.**, Carcinogens are mutagens: a simple test system combining liver homogenates for activation and bacteria for detection, *Proc. Natl. Acad. Sci. U.S.A.*, 72, 5135, 1973.
5. **McCann, J., Cho, I. E., Yamasaki, E., and Ames, B. N.**, Detection of carcinogens as mutagens in the Salmonella/microsome test: assay of 300 chemicals, *Proc. Natl. Acad. Sci. U.S.A.*, 73, 950, 1975.
6. **Bartsch, H., Malaveille, C., Camus, A. M., Martel-Planche, G., Brun, G., Hautefeuille, A., Sabadie, E., Barbin, A., Kuroki, T., Drevon, C., Piccoli, C., and Montesano, R.**, Validation and comparative studies on 180 chemicals with *S. typhimurium* strains and V79 chinese hamster cells in the presence of various metabolizing systems, *Mutat. Res.*, 76, 1, 1980.
7. **Rinkus, S. J. and Legator, M. S.**, Chemical characterization of 465 known or suspected carcinogens and their correlation with mutagenic activity in the *S. typhimurium* system, *Cancer Res.*, 39, 3289, 1979.

8. **Purchase, I. F. H., Longstaff, E., Ashby, J., Styles, G. A., Anderson, D., Lefebre, P. A., and Westwood, F. R.,** An evaluation of 6 short-term tests for detecting organic chemical carcinogens, *Br. J. Cancer,* 37, 873, 1978.

9. **Zeiger, E.,** Carcinogenicity of mutagens: predictive capability of the Salmonella mutagenesis assay for rodent carcinogenicity, *Cancer Res.,* 47, 1287, 1987.

10. **Williams, G. M.,** DNA reactive and epigenetic carcinogens, in *Mechanisms of Environmental Carcinogenesis,* Barrett, J. C., Ed., CRC Press, Boca Raton, FL, 113, 1987.

11. **Brookes, P. and Lawley, P. D.,** Evidence for the binding of polynuclear hydrocarbons to the nucleic acids of the mouse skin. Relationship between carcinogenic power of hydrocarbons and their binding to deoxyribonucleic acid, *Nature,* 202, 781, 1964.

12. **Pegg, A. E.,** Formation and metabolism of alkylated nucleosides: possible role in carcinogenesis by nitrocompounds and alkylating agents, *Adv. Cancer Res.,* 25, 195, 1978.

13. **Ashurst, S. W., Cohen, G. M., Nesnow, S., Di Giovanni, G., and Slaga, T. J.,** Formation of benzo(a)pyrene-DNA adducts and their relationships to tumor initiation in mouse epidermis, *Cancer Res.,* 43, 1024, 1983.

14. **Jerina, D. M., Sayer, J. M., Agarwal, S. K., Yagi, H., Levin, S., Wood, A. W., Conney, A. H., Preuss-Schwartz, D., Bard, W. M., Pigott, M. A., and Dipple, A.,** in *Biological Reactive Intermediates,* Vol. III, Kocsis, J. J., Jallow, D. J., Witmer, C. M., Nelson, J. O., and Snyder, R., Eds., Plenum Press, New York, 11, 1986.

15. **Barbacid, M.,** *Ras* oncogenes, *Ann. Rev. Biochem.,* 56, 779, 1987.

16. **Bargman, C. I., Hung, M. C., and Weinberg, R. A.,** Multiple independent activations of the *neu* oncogene by a point mutation altering the transmembrane domain of p185, *Cells,* 45, 649, 1986.

17. **Topal, M. D.,** DNA repair oncogenes and carcinogenesis, *Carcinogenesis,* 9, 681, 1988.

18. **Wattenberg, L. W.,** Inhibitors of chemical carcinogenesis, *Adv. Cancer Res.,* 26, 197, 1978.

19. **Lambert, W. C., Andrews, A. D., German, J., et al.,** in *Pathogenesis of Skin Diseases,* Thiers, B. H. and Dobson, R. L., Eds., Churchill Livingstone, New York, 579, 1986.

20. **Gelboin, H. V.,** Benzo(a)pyrene metabolism, activation and carcinogenesis: role and regulation of mixed-function oxidases and related enzymes, *Physiol. Rev.,* 60, 1107, 1980.

21. **Searle, C. E., Ed.,** Chemical Carcinogens, ACS Monogr., 182, Washington, D.C., 1984.

22. **Guengerich, F. B., Ed.,** *Mammalian Cytochromes P-450,* Vol. I, II, CRC Press, Boca Raton, FL, 1987.

23. **Osborne, M. R.,** DNA interactions of reactive intermediates derived from carcinogens, in *Chemical Carcinogens,* Searle, C. E., Ed., American Chemical Society, Monograph, 1984.

24. **Ashurst, S. W. and Cohen, G. M.,** The formation and the persistence of benzo(a)pyrene metabolite — deoxyribonucleoside adducts in rat skin *in vivo, Int. J. Cancer,* 28, 387, 1981.

25. **Di Giovanni, J., Fisher, E. P., and Sawyer, T. W.,** Kinetics of formation and disappearance of 7,12-DMBA-DNA adducts in mouse epidermis, *Cancer Res.,* 46, 4400, 1986.

26. **Yuasa, Y., Srivastava, S. K., Dunn, C. Y., Rhim, J. S., and Aaronson, S. A.,** Acquisition of transforming properties by alternative point mutations within *c-bas/has* protooncogene, *Nature,* 303, 775, 1983.

27. **Ross, W. C. J.,** *Alkylating Agents,* Butterworths, London, 1962.

28. **Lawley, P. D.,** Carcinogenesis by alkylating agents, in *Chemical Carcinogens,* American Chemical Society, Monograph, Vol. I, 483, 1984.

29. **Niculescu-Duvăz, I., Baracu, I., and Balaban, A. T.,** Alkylating agents, in *Chemistry of Antitumor Agents,* Wilman, D., Ed., Blackie and Son, London, 1990.

30. **Lawley, P. D.,** DNA as a target of alkylating carcinogens, *Br. Med. Bull.,* 36, 19, 1980.

31. **Haynes, R. H.,** Influence of repair processes on radiobiological survival curves, in *Cell Survival After Low Doses of Radiations,* Gray, L. H., Ed., 6th Memorial Conf., John Wiley & Sons, London, 197, 1975.

32. **Nebold, R. F. and Brookes, P.,** Exceptional mutagenicity of benzo(a)pyrene diol epoxide in cultured mammalian cells, *Nature (London),* 260, 52, 1976.

33. **Simon, Z.,** Lethal mutation hypothesis for the mechanisms of action of cytosolic alkylating agents, *J. Theor. Biol.,* 8, 193, 1965.

34. **Lawley, P. D.,** Approaches to chemical dosimetry in mutagenesis and carcinogenesis: the relevance of reaction of chemical mutagens and carcinogens with DNA, in *Chemical Carcinogens and DNA,* Vol. I, Grover, P., Ed., CRC Press, Boca Raton, FL, 1, 1980.

35. **Lawley, P. D. and Martin, C. N.,** Molecular mechanisms in alkylation mutagenesis. Induced reversion of bacteriophage T4rIIAP72 by EMS in relation to extent and mode of ethylation of purines in bacteriophage DNA, *Biochem. J.,* 145, 85, 1975.

36. **Druckerey, H.,** Quantitative aspects in chemical carcinogenesis, in *Potential Carcinogenic Hazards from Drugs,* UICC Monography, No. 7, Truhaut, R., Ed., Springer-Verlag, Heidelberg, 60, 1967.

37. **Bardos, T. J., Datta-Gupta, N., Herborn, P., and Triggle, D. J.,** A study of comparative chemical and biological activities of alkylating agents, *J. Med. Chem.,* 8, 167, 1965.

38. **Price, C. C., Gaucher, G. M., Koneru, P., Shibakawa, R., Sowa, J. R., and Yamaguki, M.,** Mechanisms of action of alkylating agents, *Ann. N.Y. Acad. Sci.,* 163, 593, 1969.

39. **Williamson, E. E. and Witten, B.,** Reaction mechanism of some aromatic nitrogen mustards, *Cancer Res.,* 27, 33, 1967.
40. **Sawiki, E., Bender, F. P., Hauser, T. R., Wilson, R. M., and Meeker, J. E.,** Five methods for the spectrophotometric determination of alkylating agents including extremely sensitive autocatalytic methods, *Anal. Chem.,* 35, 1479, 1963.
41. **Spears, C. P.,** Nucleophilic selectivity ratios of model and clinical alkylating agents by 4-(4'-nitrobenzyl)pyridine competition, *Mol. Pharmacol.,* 19, 496, 1981.
42. U.S. Department of Health and Human Services, Fourth Ann. Rep. on Carcinogens (NTP-85002), 1985.
43. **Johnstone, T. P. and Montgomery, J. A.,** Relationship of structure to anticancer activity and toxicity of the nitrosoureas in animal systems, *Cancer Treat. Rep.,* 70, 13, 1986.
44. **Badea, F.,** *Reaction Mechanisms in Organic Chemistry,* Ed. Ştiinţifică, Bucureşti, 1971.
45. **Pearson, R. G.,** *Hard and Soft Acids and Bases,* Dowden Huchinson and Ross, Stroudsbourg, PA, 1973.
46. **Ho, T. L.,** *Hard and Soft Acids and Bases Principle in Organic Chemistry,* Academic Press, New York, 1977.
47. **Pullman, A. and Pullman, B.,** Electrostatic effect of macromolecular structure on the biochemical reactivity of the nucleic acids. Significance for chemical carcinogenesis, *Int. J. Quantum Chem.,* 7, 245, 1980.
48. **Pullman, B.,** Aspects of the macromolecular structure of the nucleic acids, *Ann. N.Y. Acad. Sci.,* 367, 181, 1981.
49. **Singer, B.,** Sites in nucleic acids reacting with alkylating agents of differing carcinogenicity and mutagenicity, *J. Toxicol. Environ. Health,* 2, 1279, 1977.
50. **Price, C. C., Gaucher, G. M., Koneru, P., Shibakawa, R., Sowa, J. R., and Yamaguchi, M.,** Relative reactivities for monofunctional nitrogen mustards alkylation of nucleic and components, *Biochem. Biophys. Acta,* 166, 327, 1968.
51. **Lyle, T. A., Royer, R. E., Daub, G. H., and Vander Jagt, D. L.,** Reactivity-selectivity properties of reactions of carcinogenic electrophiles and nucleosides: influence of pH on site selectivity, *Chem. Biol. Interact.,* 29, 197, 1980.
52. **Lavery, R. A., Pullman, A., and Pullman, B.,** The electrostatic molecular potential of yeast t-RNA[Phe]. The potential due to the phosphate backbone, *Nucleic Acid Res.,* 8, 1069, 1980.
53. **Bodell, W. J., Tokuda, K., and Ludlum, D. B.,** Differences in DNA methylation products formed in sensitive and resistant human glioma cells treated with *N*-(2-Chlorethly)-*N*-nitrosourea, *Cancer Res.,* 48, 4489, 1988.
54. **Leo, A., Panthananickal, A., Hansch, C., Theiss, J., Shimkin, M., and Andress, A. W.,** A comparison of mutagenic and carcinogenic activities of aniline mustards, *J. Med. Chem.,* 24, 859, 1981.
55. **Hopfinger, A. J. and Potenzone, R., Jr.,** Ames test and antitumor activity of 1-(1-phenyl)-3,3-dialkyl-triazenes, *Mol. Pharmacol.,* 21, 187, 1982.
56. **Sugiura, K. and Goto, M.,** Mutagenicities of styrene-oxide derivatives on bacterial test systems: relationship between mutagenic potencies and chemical reactivity, *Chem. Biol. Interact.,* 35, 71, 1981.
57. **Hansch, C., Venger, B. H., Hathaway, G. J., and Amrein, Y. U.,** Ames test of 1(X-phenyl)-3,3-dialkyl-triazenes, *J. Med. Chem.,* 22, 473, 1979.
58. **Hansch, C., Venger, B. H., and Panthananickal, A.,** Mutagenicity of substituted (*o*-phenyldiamine) platinum dichlorides in the Ames test. A quantitative structure activity study, *J. Med. Chem.,* 23, 459, 1980.
59. **Dun, W. J., III and Wold, S.,** The carcinogencity of *N*-nitroso compounds: a SIMCA pattern-recognition-study, *Bioorg. Chem.,* 10, 29, 1981.
60. **Thomson, C. and Reynolds, C.,** A theoretical study of *N*-nitrosoamine metabolites. Possible alkylating species in cancerogenesis by *N,N*-dimethyl nitrosoamine, *J. Quantum Chem.,* 30, 751, 1986.
61. **Frecer, V. and Miertus, S.,** Theoretical study of *N*-nitrosoureas and mechanism of their carcinogenic effect, *Neoplasma,* 36, 257, 1989.
62. **Loew, G. H., Poulsen, M. T., Spangler, D., and Kirkjian, E.,** Mechanistic structure-activity studies of carcinogenic dialkylnitrosoamines, *Int. J. Quantum Chem., Quantum Biology Symp.,* 10, 201, 1983.
63. **Klopman, G., Kalos, A. N., and Rosenkrantz, H.,** A computer automated study of the structure-mutagenicity relationships of non-fused ring nitroarenes and related compounds, *Mol. Toxicol.,* 1, 61, 1987.
64. **Yuta, K. and Jurs, P. C.,** Computer assisted structure-activity studies of chemical carcinogens — aromatic amines, *J. Med. Chem.,* 24, 241, 1981.
65. **Miller, K. J., Rein, F. H., Taylor, E. R., and Kowalczyk, P. J.,** Generation of nucleic acid structures and binding of molecules to DNA, *Ann. N.Y. Acad. Sci.,* 439, 64, 1984.
66. **Rogers, K. S. and Cammarata, A.,** Superdelocalizability and charge density. A correlation with partition coefficients, *J. Med. Chem.,* 12, 692, 1969.
67. **Nagata, C., Fukui, K., Yonezawa, T., and Tagashira, Y.,** Electronic structure and carcinogenic activity of aromatic compounds, *Cancer Res.,* 15, 233, 1955.
68. **Lewis, D. F. V.,** Molecular orbital calculations and quantitative structure-activity relationships for some polyaromatic hydrocarbons, *Xenobiotica,* 17, 1451, 1987.

69. **Smith, I. A., Berger, G. D., Seybold, P., and Serve, M. P.,** Relationships between carcinogenicity and theoretical reactivity indices in polycyclic aromatic hydrocarbons, *Cancer Res.,* 38, 2968, 1978.

70. **Szentpaly, L.,** Carcinogenesis by polycyclic aromatic hydrocarbons: a multilinear regression on new type PMO indices, *J. Am. Chem. Soc.,* 106, 6021, 1984.

71. **Schmidt, O.,** Characterisierung der einfachen und Krebs erzeugenden aromatischen Kohlenwasserstoffe durch die Dichteverteilung bestimmer Valenzelectronen, *Z. Phys. Chem.,* 42, 83, 1939.

72. **Dipple, A., Moschel, R. C., and Bigger, A. H.,** Polynuclear aromatic carcinogens, in *Chemical Carcinogens,* Searle, C. E., Ed., American Chemical Society Monograph, Vol. 1, 41, 1984.

73. **Pullman, A.,** Structure electronique et activité cancerogène des hydrocarbures aromatiques, *Bull. Soc. Chim. Fr.,* 595, 1954.

74. **Pullman, A. and Pullman, B.,** Electronic structure and carcinogenic activity of aromatic molecules. New developments, *Adv. Cancer Res.,* 3, 117, 1955.

75. **Mainster, M. A. and Memory, J. D.,** Superdelocalizability indices and the Pullman theory of chemical carcinogens, *Biochim. Biophys. Acta,* 148, 605, 1967.

76. **Zahradnik, R.,** Quantum chemical studies of chemical-carcinogens, *Neoplasma,* 10, 581, 1963.

77. **Veljkovic, V. and Lalovic, D. A.,** Theoretical prediction of carcinogenicity by quasi-valence number, *Experentia,* 33, 1228, 1977.

78. **Miertus, S. and Majek, P.,** Calculation of reactivity indices for benzo(a)anthracene and benzo(a)pyrene and their approximative models of complex with enzyme epoxidase, *Neoplasma,* 28, 441, 1981.

79. **Simon, Z., Balaban, A. T., Ciubotariu, D., and Balaban, T. S.,** QSAR for carcinogenesis by polycyclic aromatic hydrocarbons and derivatives in terms of delocalization energy, minimal steric differences and topological indices, *Rev. Roum. Chimie,* 30, 385, 1985.

80. **Bingham, R. C., Dewar, M. I. S., and Lo, D. H.,** Ground state of molecule, XXV. MINDO/3 an improved version of MINDO semi-empirical SC-FMO method, *J. Am. Chem. Soc.,* 97, 1285, 1975.

81. **Byung, K. P., Moon, H., and Sung, T. D.,** Finding of a characteristic reactive region common to some series of chemical carcinogens, *Bull. Korean Chim. Soc.,* 6, 103, 1985.

82. **Borgen, A. H., Darvey, N., Castagnoli, N., Crocker, T. T., Rasmussen, R. E., and Wang, I. Y.,** Metabolic conversion of BaP by syrian hamster liver microsomes and binding of metabolites to DNA, *J. Med. Chem.,* 16, 502, 1973.

83. **Jerina, D. M., Lehr, R., Schaefer-Ridder, M., Yagi, H., Karle, J. M., Thakker, D. R., Wood, A. H., Lu, A. Y. H., Ryan, D., West, S., Levin, W., and Conney, A. H.,** Bay-region epoxides of dihydrodiols: a concept explaining the mutagenic and the carcinogenic activity of benzo(a)pyrene and benzo(a)anthracene, in *Origins of Human Cancer,* Hiat, H., Watson, J. D., and Winstin, I., Eds., Cold Spring Harbor, New York, 639, 1977.

84. **Jerina, D. M. and Lehr, R. E.,** The bay-region theory. A quantum mechanical approach to aromatic hydrocarbons induced carcinogenicity, in *Microsomes and Drug Oxidations,* Ulrich, V., Roots, I., Hilderbrandt, A., and Eastbrook, R. W., Eds., Pergamon Press, Elmsford, NY, 709, 1978.

85. **Dipple, A.,** Formation metabolism and mechanism of action of polycyclic aromatic hydrocarbons, *Cancer Res. (Suppl.),* 43, 2422s, 1983.

86. **Loew, G. H., Philips, J., Wong, J., Hjelmeland, L., and Pack, G. R.,** Quantum chemical studies of the metabolism of polycyclic aromatic hydrocarbons. Bay-region activity as a criterion for carcinogenic potency, *Cancer Biochem. Biophys.,* 2, 113, 1978.

87. **Loew, G. H., Wong, J., Philips, J., Hjelmeland, L., and Pack, G. R.,** Quantum chemical studies of the metabolism of benzo(a)pyrene, *Cancer Biochem. Biophys.,* 2, 123, 1978.

88. **Loew, G. H., Boray, S. S., and Ferrell, J. E., Jr.,** Quantum chemical studies of polycyclic aromatic hydrocarbons and their metabolites: correlations to carcinogenicity, *Chem. Biol. Interact.,* 26, 75, 1979.

89. **Fujimoto, H. and Fukui, K.,** Intermolecular interactions and chemical reactivity, in *Chemical Reactivity and Reaction Paths,* Klopman, G., Ed., John Wiley & Sons, New York, 23, 1974.

90. **Seybold, P. G., Vestewig, R., and Schribner, J. D.,** Relationships between carcinogenicity, mutagenicity and theoretical reactivity indices for polycyclic aromatic hydrocarbons, *Int. J. Quantum. Chem. Quantum Biology Symp.,* 8, 401, 1981.

91. **Seybold, P. G.,** Steric and electronic determinants of carcinogenicity in polycyclic aromatic hydrocarbons: use in short term tests, in *Polynuclear Aromatic Hydrocarbons: Chemistry, Characterization and Carcinogenesis,* Cooke, M. and Dennis, A. J., Eds., Battelle Press, Columbus, OH, 1986, 839.

92. **Fu, P. P., Harvey, R. G., and Beland, F.,** Molecular orbital theoretical prediction of the isomeric products formed from reactions of arene oxides and related metabolites of polycyclic aromatic hydrocarbons, *Tetrahedron,* 34, 857, 1978.

93. **Selkirk, J. K.,** Comparison of epoxide and free-radical mechanisms for activation of benzo(a)pyrene by Sprague-Dawley rat liver microsomes, *J. Natl. Cancer Inst.,* 64, 771, 1980.

94. **Marnett, L. J.,** Peroxyl free radicals: potential mediators of tumor initiation and promotion, *Carcinogenesis,* 8, 1365, 1987.

95. **Miyashita, Y., Seri, T., Takahashi, Y., and Daiba, S. T.,** Computer assisted structure-carcinogenicity studies on polycyclic aromatic hydrocarbons by pattern recognition methods, *Anal. Chim. Acta,* 133, 603, 1981.

96. **Andreozzi, P., Hofinger, A. I., and Klopman, G.,** Theoretical study of *N*-nitrosoamines and their presumed proximate carcinogens, *Cancer Biochem. Biophys.,* 4, 209, 1980.

97. **Mohammed, S. N. and Hopfinger, A. J.,** Chemical reactivity of a methyldiazonium ion with nucleophilic centers of DNA bases, *J. Theor. Biol.,* 87, 41, 1980.

98. **Loew, G., Poulsen, M. T., Spangler, D., and Kirkjan, E.,** Mechanistic structure-activity studies of carcinogenic dialkyl nitrosoamines, *Int. J. Quantum Chem.,* 10, 201, 1983.

99. **Wood, A. W., Chang, R. L., Levin, W., Yagi, H., Thakker, D. R., Jerina, D. M., and Conney, A. H.,** Differences in mutagenicity of the optical enantiomers of the diastereoisomeric benzo(a)pyrene-7,8-diol-9,10-epoxides, *Biochem. Biophys. Res. Commun.,* 77, 1389, 1977.

100. **Wood, A. W., Chang, R. L., Levin, W., Lehr, R. E., Schaefer-Ridder, M., Karle, J. M., Jerina, D. M., and Conney, A. H.,** Mutagenicity and cytotoxicity of benz(a)anthracene diol-epoxides and tetrahydroepoxides: exceptional activity of the bay-region 1,2-epoxides, *Proc. Natl. Acad. Sci. U.S.A.,* 74, 2745, 1977.

101. **Ferrel, J. E. and Loew, G.,** Mechanistic studies of arene oxide and diol-epoxide rearrangement and hydrolysis reaction, *J. Am. Chem. Soc.,* 101, 1385, 1979.

102. **Whalen, D. L., Ross, A. M., Yagi, H., Karle, J. M., and Jerina, D. M.,** Stereoelectronic factors in the solvolysis of bay-region diol-epoxides of polynuclear aromatic hydrocarbons, *J. Am. Chem. Soc.,* 100, 5218, 1978.

103. **Whalen, D. L., Rose, A. M., Montemerano, J. A., Thakker, D. R., Yagi, H., and Jerina, D. M.,** General acid catalysis in the hydrolysis of BaP-7,8-diol-9,10-epoxides, *J. Am. Chem. Soc.,* 101, 5086, 1979.

104. **Yagi, H., Thakker, D. R., Hernandez, O., Koreeda, M., and Jerina, D. M.,** Synthesis and reactions of highly mutagenic 7,8-diol-9,10-epoxides of the carcinogen benzo(a)pyrene, *J. Am. Chem. Soc.,* 99, 1604, 1977.

105. **Becker, A. R., Janusz, J. M., Rogers, D. Z., and Bruice, T. C.,** Structural features which determine the carcinogenesis-mutagenesis rate of acid- and water-mediated solvolysis of arene oxides and nucleophilic attack upon diol-epoxides bay-region and non-bay-region tetrahydroepoxides and K-region and non-K-region arene oxides, *J. Am. Chem. Soc.,* 100, 3244, 1979.

106. **Dewar, M. J. S.,** *The Molecular Orbital Theory of Organic Chemistry,* McGraw Hill-Book, New York, 1969.

107. **Jeffrey, A. M., Jeannette, K. W., Blobstein, S. H., Weinstein, I. B., Beland, F. A., Harvey, R. G., Kasai, H., Miura, I., and Nakanishi, K.,** Benzo(a)pyrene nucleic acid derivative found *in vivo*: structure of a benzo(a)pyrene tetrahydrodiolepoxide — guanosine adduct, *J. Am. Chem. Soc.,* 98, 5714, 1976.

108. **Latif, F., Moschel, R. O., Hemminki, K., and Dipple, A.,** Styrene-oxide as a stereochemical probe for the mechanism of aralkylation at different sites on guanosine, *Chem. Res. Toxicol.,* 1, 354, 1988.

109. **Geacintov, N. E., Yoshida, N., Ibanez, V., and Harvey, R.,** Noncovalent interactive binding of 7,8-dihydroxy-9,10-benzo(a)pyrene to DNA, *Biochem. Biophys. Res. Commun.,* 100, 1569, 1981.

110. **Gupta, S. C., Pohl, T. M., Friedman, S. L., Whalen, D. L., Yagi, H., Jerina, D. M.,** Guanosine-5-monophosphate catalyzed hydrolysis of diastereoisomeric benzo(a)pyrene-7,8-diol-9,10-epoxides, *J. Am. Chem. Soc.,* 104, 3101, 1983.

111. **Geacintov, N. E., Yoshida, H., Ibanez, V., and Harvey, R.,** Non-covalent binding of 7β, 8α-dihydroxy-9α, 10α-epoxytetrahydrobenzo(a)-pyrene to DNA and its catalytic effect on hydrolysis of the diolepoxide to tetrol, *Biochemistry,* 21, 1864, 1982.

112. **Michaud, D. P., Gupta, S. C., Whalen, D. L., Sayer, D. L., Jerina, D. M., and Jerina, J. M.,** Effect of pH and salt concentration on the hydrolysis of benzo(a)pyrene-7,8-diol-9,10-epoxides catalyzed by DNA and polyadenieic acid, *Chem. Biol. Interact.,* 44, 41, 1983.

113. **Melikian, A. A., Leszczynska, J. M., Amin, S., Hecht, S. S., Hoffman, D., Pataki, G., and Harvey, R. G.,** Rates of hydrolysis and extent of DNA bindings of 5-methylchrysene dihydrodiols epoxides, *Cancer Res.,* 45, 1990, 1985.

114. **Stoica, G., Safirman, C., Arnăutu, M., Voiculetz, N., and Niculescu-Duvăz, I.,** Mechanisms of carcinogenesis inhibition. I. Direct interaction between carcinogenesis inhibitors and B(a)P diol-epoxides, *Rev. Roum. Biochem.,* 24, 245, 1987.

115. **Melikian, A. A., Amin, S., Huie, K., Hecht, S. S., and Harvey, R. G.,** Reactivity with DNA bases and mutagenicity toward *S. typhimurium* of 5-methylchrysene diol-epoxide enantiomers, *Cancer Res.,* 48, 1781, 1988.

116. **Whalen, D. L., Montemarano, J. A., Thakker, D. R., Yagi, H., and Jerina, D. M.,** Changes of mechanisms and product distributions in the hydrolysis of benzo(a)pyrene-7,8-diol-9,10-epoxide metabolites induced by changes in pH, *J. Am. Chem. Soc.,* 99, 5522, 1977.

117. **Moore, P. D., Koreeda, M., Wislocki, P. G., Levin, W., Conney, A. H., Yagi, H., and Jerina, D. M.,** in *Drug Metabolism Concepts,* Jerina, D. M., Ed., American Chemical Society, ACS, Symp. Ser., Washington, 44, 127, 1977.
118. **Jerina, D. M., Sayer, J. M., Yagi, H., Croisy-Delcey, M., Ittah, Y., Thakker, D. R., Wood, A. W., Levin, W., and Conney, A. H.,** in *Biological Reactive Intermediates,* Vol. II, Part A, Plenum Publishing, 1982.
119. **Yagi, H., Hernandez, O., Jerina, D. M.,** Synthesis of ($\pm$)7β, 8α-dihydroxy-9β,10β-epoxy-7,8,9,10-tetrahydrobenzo(a)pyrene, a potential metabolite of the carcinogene BaP with stereochemistry related to the antileukemic triptolides, *J. Am. Chem. Soc.,* 97, 6881, 1975.
120. **Thakker, D. R., Yagi, H., Whalen, D. L., Levin, W., Wood, A., Conney, A. H., and Jerina, D. M.,** in *Environmental Health Chemistry,* McKineey, J. D., Ed., Ann Arbor, 383, 1980.
121. **Whalen, D. L., Ross, A. M., Montemarano, J. A., Thakker, R. D., Yagi, H., and Jerina, D. M.,** General acid catalysis in the hydrolysis of benzo(a)pyrene-7,8 diol-9,10-epoxides, *J. Am. Chem. Soc.,* 101, 5086, 1979.
122. **Geacintov, N. E., Yoshida, N., Ibanez, V., and Harvey, R.,** Noncovalent interactive binding of 7,8-dihydroxy-9,10-epoxy-benzo(a)pyrene to DNA, *Biochem. Biophys. Res. Commun.,* 100, 1569, 1981.
123. **Kootstra, A., Hass, B., and Slaga, T. J.,** Reaction of benzo(a)pyrene diol-epoxides with DNA and nucleosomes in aqueous solutions, *Biochem. Biophys. Res. Commun.,* 94, 1432, 1980.
124. **McLeod, M. C. and Selkirk, J. K.,** Covalent intercalative binding of BaP-9,10-diol-7,8-epoxy to DNA, AACR Abstr., *Cancer Res. (Suppl.),* 42, 61, 1982.
125. **Meehan, T., Gamper, H., and Becker, J. H.,** Characterization of reversible physical binding of benzo(a)pyrene to DNA, *J. Biol. Chem.,* 257, 10479, 1982.
126. **Hecht, S. S., Melikian, A. A., and Amin, S.,** Methylchrysene as probe for the mechanism of metabolic activation of carcinogenic methylated polynuclear aromatic hydrocarbons, *Acc. Chem. Res.,* 19, 174, 1986.
127. **Ibanez, W. I., Geacintow, N. E., Gagliano, A. G., Brandi, S., and Harvey, R. G.,** Physical binding of tetrols derived from 7,8-diol-9,10-epoxy-BaP to DNA, *J. Am. Chem. Soc.,* 102, 5661, 1982.
128. **Gamper, H. B., Tung, A. S., Straub, K., Barthotomew, J. C., and Calvin, M.,** A DNA strand scission by benzo(a)pyrene diol-epoxides, *Science,* 197, 671, 1977.
129. **Safirman, C., Stoica, G., Lupu, F., Voiculetz, N., and Niculescu-Duvǎz, I.,** The *in vitro* screening of the cancerogenesis inhibitors acting by the inhibition of the microsomal PAH activation systems, *Neoplasma,* 34, 261, 1987.
130. **Dipple, A.,** Reactive metabolites of carcinogens and their interactions with DNA, in *Chemical Carcinogens,* Vol. 5, Politzer, P. and Martin, F. J., Jr., Eds., Elsevier, 1988, 32.
131. **Moschel, R. C., Hudgins, W. R., and Dipple, A.,** Selectivity in nucleoside alkylation and aralkylation in relation to chemical carcinogenesis, *J. Org. Chem.,* 44, 3324, 1979.
132. **Moschel, R. C., Hudgins, W. R., and Dipple, A.,** Aralkylation of guanosine by the carcinogen *N*-nitroso-*N*-benzyl-urea, *J. Org. Chem.,* 45, 533, 1980.
133. **Dipple, A., Moschel, R. C., and Hudgins, W. R.,** Selectivity of alkylation and aralkylation of nucleic acid components, *Drug Metabol. Rev.,* 13, 249, 1982.
134. **Moschel, R. C., Hudgins, W. R., and Dipple, A.,** Substituent-induced effects on the stability of benzylated guanosines: model systems for the factor influencing the stability of carcinogen — modified nucleic acids, *J. Org. Chem.,* 49, 363, 1984.
135. **Moschel, R. C., Hudgins, W. R., and Dipple, A.,** Reactivity effects on site selectivity in nucleoside aralkylation: a model for the factors influencing the sites of carcinogen-nucleic acid interactions, *J. Org. Chem.,* 51, 4180, 1986.
136. **Mureşan, Z., Stoica, A., Stafidov, N., and Voiculetz, N.,** Inducible high-affinity binding site for benzo(a)pyrene in cytosol from rat liver, *Neoplasma,* 34, 523, 1987.
137. **Collins, S. and Marletta, M.,** Carcinogen-binding proteins. High affinity binding sites for BaP in mouse liver distinct from the Ah receptor, *Mol. Pharmacol.,* 25, 353, 1984.
138. **Jerina, D. M. and Daly, J. W.,** Oxidation of carbon, in *Drug Metabolism from Microbe to Man,* Parke, D. V. and Smith, R. L., Eds., Taylor and Francis, London, 1976, 13.
139. **Conney, A. H.,** Induction of microsomal enzymes by foreign chemicals and carcinogenesis by polycyclic aromatic hydrocarbons, *Cancer Res.,* 42, 4875, 1982.
140. **Osborne, M. R.,** Carcinogenicity indices in polycyclic hydrocarbons, *Cancer Res.,* 39, 4760, 1979.
141. **Silverman, B. D.,** Molecular conformation and polycyclic aromatic hydrocarbons carcinogenesis, in *Computer Simulation of Carcinogenic Processes,* Silverman, B. D., Ed., CRC Press, Boca Raton, FL, 1988, 91.
142. **Silverman, B. D. and Lowe, J. P.,** Carcinogenicity of methylated hydrocarbons: effect of methylation on the calculated diol-epoxide reactivity, *Cancer Biochem. Biophys.,* 6, 89, 1982.
143. **Poulsen, M. T. and Loew, G. H.,** Quantum chemical studies on methyl and fluro-analogs of chrysene: metabolic activation and correlation with carcinogenic activity, *Cancer Biochem. Biophys.,* 5, 81, 1981.

144. **Smith, J. A. and Seybold, P. G.,** Methylbenz(a)anthracenes: correlation between theoretical reactivity indices and carcinogenicity, *Int. J. Quantum Chem. Symp.,* 5, 311, 1981.
145. **Allinger, N. L. and Spraque, J. T.,** Calculation of the structure of hydrocarbons containing delocalized electronic systems by the molecular mechanics method, *J. Am. Chem. Soc.,* 95, 3893, 1973.
146. **Loew, J. P. and Silverman, D. B.,** Predicting carcinogenicity of polycyclic aromatic hydrocarbons, *Acc. Chem. Res.,* 17, 332, 1984.
147. **Fu, P. P., Beland, A., and Yang, S. K.,** Cyclopenta-polycyclic aromatic hydrocarbons: potential carcinogens and mutagens, *Carcinogenesis,* 1, 725, 1980.
148. **Roberts, J. D. and Caserio, M. C.,** *Modern Organic Chemistry,* W. A. Benjamin, New York, 1967, 560.
149. **Levin, W., Wood, A. W., Chang, R. L., Kumar, S., Yagi, H., Jerina, D. M., and Conney, A. H.,** Tumor initiating activity of benz(a)acridine and twelve of its derivatives on mouse skin, *Cancer Res.,* 43, 4625, 1983.
150. **Wood, A. W., Chang, R. L., Levin, W., Kumar, S., Shirai, N., Jerina, D. M., Lehr, E. E., and Conney, A. H.,** Bacterial and mammalian cell mutagenicity of four optically active bay-region 3,4-diol-1,2-epoxides and other derivatives of the nitrogen heterocycle dibenz(e,h)acridine, *Cancer Res.,* 46, 2760, 1986.
151. **Chang, R. L., Levin, W., Wood, A. W., Shirai, N., Ryan, A. J., Duke, C. C., Jerina, D. M., Holder, G. M., and Conney, A. H.,** High tumorigenicity of the 3,4-dihydrodiol of 7-methylbenz(c)acridine in mouse skin and in newborn mice, *Cancer Res.,* 46, 4552, 1986.
152. **Parks, W. C., Schurdak, M. E., Randerath, K., Maher, V. M., and McCormick, J. J.,** Human cell mediated cytotoxicity, mutagenicity and DNA adduct formation of 7-H-Dibenzo(c,g)carbazole and its *N*-methyl derivative in diploid human fibroblasts, *Cancer Res.,* 46, 4706, 1986.
153. **Lehr, R. E. and Jerina, D. M.,** Aza polycyclic aromatic hydrocarbon carcinogenicity: prediction of reactivity of tetrahydrobenzo-ring-epoxide derivatives, *Tetrahedron Lett.,* 24, 27, 1983.
154. **Lowe, J. P. and Silverman, B. D.,** Heteroatom effects in chemical carcinogenesis: effects of ring heteroatoms on ease of carbocation formation, *Cancer Biochem. Biophys.,* 7, 53, 1983.
155. **Imamura, A., Seiji, T., and Kanda, K.,** Molecular orbital study on the metabolic pathway through the diol-epoxide forms of carcinogenic benzene in comparison with benzo(a)pyrene, *J. Theor. Biol.,* 135, 205, 1988.
156. **Thakker, D. R., Lewin, W., Yagi, H., Conney, A. H., and Jerina, D. M.,** in *Biological Reactive Intermediates,* Vol. II, Part A, Plenum Publishing, 1982, 525.
157. **Dix, T. A., Fontana, R., Panthani, A., and Marnett, L. J.,** Hematin-catalyzed epoxidation of 7,8-dihydroxy-7,8-dihydrobenzo(a)pyrene by polyunsaturated fatty acids hydroperoxides, *J. Biol. Chem.,* 260, 5358, 1985.
158. **Preuss-Schwartz, D., Nimeshem, A., and Marnett, L. J.,** Peroxyl radical and cytochrome P-450 dependent metabolic activation of (+)-7,8-dihydroxy-7,8-dihydrobenzo(a)pyrene in mouse skin *in vitro* and *in vivo, Cancer Res.,* 49, 1732, 1989.
159. **Slaga, T. J., Gleason, G. L., DiGiovanni, J., Sukumaran, K. B., and Harvey, R. G.,** Potent tumor-initiating activity of the 3,4-dihydrodiol of 7,12-dimethylbenzo(a)anthracene in mouse skin, *Cancer Res.,* 39, 1934, 1979.
160. **Buenning, M. K., Wislocki, P. G., Lewin, W., Yagi, H., Thakker, D. R., Akagi, H., Koreeda, M., Jerina, D. M., and Conney, A. H.,** Tumorigenicity of the optical enantiomers of the diastereoizomeric benzo(a)pyrene 7,8-diol-9,10-epoxides in newborn mice: exceptional activity of (+)7β,8α-dihydroxy-9α, 10α-epoxy-7,8,9,10-tetrahydrobenzo(a)pyrene, *Proc. Natl. Acad. Sci. U.S.A.,* 75, 5358, 1978.
161. **Neidle, S., Subbiah, A., Cooper, C. S., and Riberio, O.,** Molecular structure of (±)-7α,8β-hydroxy-9β,10β-epoxy-7,8,9,10-tetrahydrobenzo(a)pyrene; an X-ray crystallographic study, *Carcinogenesis,* 1, 249, 1980.
162. **Glusker, J. P.,** X-ray-crystallographic studies on carcinogenic polycyclic aromatic hydrocarbons and their derivatives, in *Polycyclic Hydrocarbons and Cancer,* Vol. 3, Ts'o, P.O.P., Ed., Academic Press, New York, 1980.
163. **Neidle, S., Cooper, C. S., and Ribeiro, O.,** The molecular structure of (±)-8α,9β,10β,11α-tetrahydroxy-8,9,10,11-tetrahydrobenzo(a)anthracene; an X-ray crystallographic analysis, *Carcinogenesis,* 2, 445, 1981.
164. **Lehr, R. E., Schaefer-Ridder, M., and Jerina, D. M.,** Synthesis and reactivity of diol-epoxides derived from non K-region trans-dihydrodiols of benzo(a)anthracene, *Tetrahedron Lett.,* 6, 539, 1977.
165. **Zacharias, D. E., Glusker, J. P., Fu, P. P., and Harvey, R. C.,** Molecular structures of the dihydrodiols and diol-epoxides of carcinogenic polycyclic aromatic hydrocarbons. X-ray crystallographic and NMR analysis, *J. Am. Chem. Soc.,* 101, 4043, 1979.
166. **Bühler, D. R., Unlu, F., Thakker, D. R., Slaga, T. J., Newman, M. S., Levin, W., Conney, A. H., and Jerina, D. M.,** Metabolism and tumorigenicity of 7-,8-,9- and 10-fluorobenzo(a)pyrenes, *Cancer Res.,* 42, 4779, 1982.

167. **Kinoshita, I., Konieczny, M., Santella, R., and Jeffrey, A. M.,** Metabolism and covalent binding to DNA of 7-methylbenzo(a)pyrene, *Cancer Res.,* 42, 4032, 1982.

168. **Kapitulnik, J., Wislocki, P. G., Levin, W., Yagi, H., Thakker, D. R., Akagi, G., Koreeda, M., Jerina, D. M., and Conney, A. H.,** Marked differences in the carcinogenic activity of optically pure (+) and (−) *trans*-7,8-dihydroxy-7,8-dihydrobenzo(a)pyrene in newborn mice, *Cancer Res.,* 38, 2661, 1978.

169. **Harvey, G. G. and Dunne, F. B.,** Multiple regions of metabolic activation of carcinogenic hydrocarbons, *Nature,* 273, 566, 1978.

170. **Yeh, C. Y., Fu, P. P., Beland, F. A., and Harvey, R. G.,** Application of CNDO/2 theoretical calculations to the interpretation of the chemical reactivity and biological activity of the *syn* and *anti* diolepoxides of BaP, *Bioorg. Chem.,* 7, 497, 1978.

170a. **Karle, J. M., Mahl, H. D., Jerina, D. M., and Yagi, H.,** Synthesis of dihydrodiols from chrysene and dibenzo(a,h)anthracene, *Tetrahedron Lett.,* 4022, 1977.

171. **Sukuraman, K. B. and Harvey, R. G.,** Synthesis of *trans*-3,4-hydroxy-3,4-dihydro-7,12-dimethyl-benzo(a)anthracene, a highly carcinogenic metabolite of 7,12-DMBA, *J. Am. Chem. Soc.,* 101, 1353, 1979.

172. **Wood, A., Chang, R. L., Levin, W., Ryan, D. E., Thomas, P. E., Croisy-Delcey, M., Itah, Y., Yagi, H., Jerina, D. M., and Conney, A. H.,** Mutagenicity of the dihydrodiols and bay-region diolepoxides of benzo(c)phenanthrene in bacterial and mammalian cells, *Cancer Res.,* 40, 2876, 1980.

173. **Levin, W., Wood, A. W., Chang, R. L., Itah, Y., Delcey, M., Yagi, H., Jerina, D. M., and Conney, A. H.,** Exceptionally high tumor-initiating activity of benzo(c)phenanthrene bay-region diol-epoxide on mouse skin, *Cancer Res.,* 40, 3910, 1980.

174. **Levin, W., Chang, R. L., Wood, A. W., Thakker, D. R., Yagi, H., Jerina, D. M., and Conney, A. H.,** Tumorigenicity of optical isomers of the diastereoisomeric bay-region 3,4-diol-1,2-epoxides of benzo(c)phenanthrene in murine tumor models, *Cancer Res.,* 46, 2257, 1986.

175. **Agarwal, S. K., Sayer, J. M., Yeh, H. J. C., Pannell, L. K., Hilton, B. D., Digott, M. A., Dipple, A., Yagi, H., and Jerina, D. M.,** Chemical characterization of DNA adducts derived from the configu-rationally isomeric benzo(c)phenanthrene-3,4-diol-1,2-epoxides, *J. Am. Chem. Soc.,* 109, 2497, 1987.

176. **Slaga, T. J., Bresnik, W. J., Gleason, G., Levin, W., Yagi, H., Jerina, D. M., and Conney, A. H.,** Marked differences in skin tumor initiating activities of the optical enantiomers of the diastereoisomeric benzo(a)pyrene 7,8-diol-9,10-epoxides, *Cancer Res.,* 39, 67, 1979.

177. **Marquardt, H., Baker, S., Tiernay, B., Grover, P. L., and Sims, P.,** Induction of malignant trans-formation and mutagenesis by dihydrodiols derived from 7,12-dimethylbenz(a)anthracene, *Biochem. Bio-phys. Res. Commun.,* 85, 357, 1978.

178. **Hecht, S. S., Rivenson, A., and Hoffmann, D.,** Tumor initiating activity of dihydrodiols formed meta-bolically from 5-methylchrysene, *Cancer Res.,* 40, 1380, 1980.

179. **Coombs, M. M., Bhatt, T. S., Kissonerghis, A. M., and Vose, C. W.,** Mutagenic and carcinogenic metabolites of the carcinogen 15,16-dihydro-11-methylcyclopenta(a)phenanthrene-17-one, *Cancer Res.,* 40, 882, 1980.

180. **La Voie, E. J., Tulley-Freiler, N., Bedenko, V., and Hoffmann, D.,** Mutagenicity tumor initiating activity and metabolism of methylphenanthrenes, *Cancer Res.,* 41, 3441, 1981.

181. **Iyer, R. R., Lyga, J. W., Secrist, J. A., Daub, G. H., and Slaga, T. J.,** Comparative tumor initiating activity of methylated benzo(a)pyrene derivatives in mouse skin, *Cancer Res.,* 40, 1073, 1980.

182. **Huberman, E. and Slaga, T. J.,** Mutagenicity and tumor initiating activity of fluorinated derivatives of 7,12-dimethyl-benz(a)anthracene, *Cancer Res.,* 39, 411, 1979.

183. **Yang, S. K., Chou, M. W., and Roller, P. P.,** Potential proximate carcinogens of 7,12-dimethyl-benz(a)anthracene: characterization of two metabolically formed *trans*-3,4-dihydrodiols, *J. Am. Chem. Soc.,* 101, 237, 1979.

184. **Chiu, P. L., Fu, P. S., and Yang, S. K.,** Stereoselectivity of rat liver microsomal enzymes in the metabolism of 7-fluorobenz(a)anthracene and mutagenicity of metabolites, *Cancer Res.,* 44, 562, 1984.

185. **Hamarnik, K., Chiu, P. L., Chou, M. W., Fu, P. P., and Yang, S. K.,** in *Polynuclear Aromatic Hydrocarbons: Formation, Metabolism and Measurement,* Cooke, M. and Dennis, A. J., Eds., Batelle, Columbus, OH, 1983, 583.

186. **Lehr, R. E., Kumar, S., Levin, W., Wood, A. W., Chang, R. L., Buening, M. K., Conney, A. H., Thakker, D. R., Yagi, H., and Jerina, D. M.,** B(e)P dihydrodiols and epoxides: chemistry, mutagenicity and tumorigenicity, Dennis, A., Bjorseth, A., Eds., Fourth Int. Symp. Polynuclear Aromatic Hydrocarbons, Columbus, OH, 1980.

187. **Yagi, H., Thakker, D. R., Lehr, R. E., and Jerina, D. M.,** Benzo-ring diol-epoxides of benzo(e)pyrene and triphenylene, *J. Org. Chem.,* 44, 3439, 1979.

188. **MacLeod, M. C., Cohen, G. M., and Selkirk, J. K.,** Metabolism and macromolecular binding of the carcinogen benzo(a)pyrene and its relatively inert isomer benzo(e)pyrene by hamster embryo cells, *Cancer Res.,* 39, 3463, 1979.

189. **McLeod, M. C., Levin, W., Conney, A. H., Lehr, R. E., Mansfield, B. K., Jerina, D. M., and Selkirk, J. K.,** Metabolism of benzo(a)pyrene by rat liver microsomal enzymes, *Carcinogenesis*, 1, 165, 1980.

190. **Wood, A. W., Levin, W., Thakker, D. R., Chang, R. L., Ryan, D. E., Thomas, P. E., Dansette, P. M., Whittaker, N., Turujman, S., Lehr, R. E., Kumar, S., Jerina, D. M., and Conney, A. H.,** Biological activity of benzo(e)pyrene: an assessment based on mutagenic activities and metabolic profiles of the polycyclic hydrocarbon and its derivatives, *J. Biol. Chem.*, 254, 4408, 1979.

191. **Chang, R. L., Levin, W., Wood, A. W., Yagi, H., Tada, M., Vyas, K. P., Jerina, D. M., and Conney, A. H.,** Tumorigenicity of enantiomers of chrysene-1,2-dihydrodiol and the diastereomeric bay-region chrysene-1,2-diol-3,4-oxides on mouse skin and in the newborn mice, *Cancer Res.*, 43, 192, 1983.

192. **McLeod, M. C. and Selkirk, J. K.,** Covalent intercalative binding of BaP-9,10-diol-7,8-epoxide to DNA, AACR Abstr., *Cancer Res. (Suppl.)*, 42, 61, 1982.

193. **Vigny, P., Ginot, Y. M., Kindts, M., Cooper, C. S., Grover, P. L., and Sims, P.,** Fluorescence spectral evidence that benzo(a)pyrene is activated by metabolism in mouse skin to a diol-epoxide and a phenol-epoxide, *Carcinogenesis*, 1, 945, 1980.

194. **Glusker, J. P.,** *Polycyclic Hydrocarbons and Cancer*, Academic Press, New York, 1982, 61.

195. **Armstrong, R. N., Levin, W., Ryan, D. E., Thomas, P. E., Mah, H. D., and Jerina, D. M.,** Stereoselectivity of rat liver cytochrome P-450c on formation of benzo(a)pyrene-4,5-oxide, *Biochem. Biophys. Res. Commun.*, 190, 1077, 1981.

196. **Wood, A. W., Chang, R. L., Huang, M. T., Levin, W., Lehr, W., Kumar, S., Thakker, D. R., Yagi, H., Jerina, D. M., and Conney, A. H.,** Mutagenicity of BaP and triphenylene tetrahydroepoxides and diol-epoxides in bacterial and mammals cells, *Cancer Res.*, 40, 1985, 1980.

197. **La Voie, E. J., Hecht, S. S., Amin, S., Bedenko, V., and Hoffmann, D.,** Identification of mutagenic dihydrodiols as metabolites of benzo(j)-fluoranthene and benzo(k)fluoranthene, *Cancer Res.*, 40, 4528, 1980.

198. **Perin-Roussel, O., Croisy-Delcey, M., Mispelter, J., Saguem, S., Chalvet, O., Ekert, B., Fouquet, J., Jaquignon, P., Lhoste, J. M., Muel, B., and Zajdela, F. E.,** Metabolic activation of dibenzo(a,e)fluoranthene a nonalternant carcinogenic polycyclic hydrocarbon in liver homogenates, *Cancer Res.*, 40, 1742, 1980.

199. **Hutchins, D. A., Skipper, P. L., Naylor, S., and Tannenbaum, S. R.,** Isolation and characterization of the major fluoranthene hemoglobin adducts formed *in vivo* in the rat, *Cancer Res.*, 48, 4756, 1988.

200. **Goldstein, B. D.,** Hematotoxicity in human, *J. Toxicol. Environ. Health*, 2 (Suppl.), 1, 1977.

201. **Rinsky, R. A., Smith, A. B., Hornung, R., Filloun, T., Young, R. J., Okun, A. H., and Landrigan, P. J.,** Benzene and leukemia. An epidemiologic risk assessment, *N. Engl. J. Med.*, 316, 1044, 1987.

202. **Kawanishi, S., Inoue, S., and Kawanishi, M.,** Human DNA damage induced by 1,2,4-benzenetriol, a benzene metabolite, *Cancer Res.*, 49, 164, 1989.

203. **Greenlee, W. F., Gross, E. A., and Irons, R. D.,** Relationship between benzene toxicity and the disposition of ^{14}C-labeled benzene metabolites in the rat, *Chem. Biol. Interact.*, 33, 285, 1981.

204. **Arfellini, G., Grilli, S., Colacci, A., Mazullo, M., and Prodi, G.,** *In vivo* and *in vitro* binding of benzene to nucleic acids and proteins of various rat tissues and mouse organs, *Cancer Lett.*, 28, 159, 1985.

205. **Aleksejczyk, R. A., Berchtold, G. A., and Braun, A. G.,** Benzene diol epoxide, *J. Am. Chem. Soc.*, 107, 2554, 1985.

206. **Wood, A. W., Levin, W., Chang, R., Thuang, M., Ryan, D. E., Thomas, P. E., Lehr, R. E., Kumar, S., Koreeda, M., Akagi, H., Dansette, P., Yagi, H., Jerina, D. M., and Conney, A. H.,** Mutagenicity and tumor initiating activity of cyclopenta(c,d)-pyrene and structurally related analogs, *Cancer Res.*, 40, 642, 1980.

207. **Gold, A., Nesnow, S., Moore, M., Garland, H., Curtis, G., Howard, B., Graham, D., and Eisenstadt, E.,** Mutagenesis and morphological transformation of mammalian cells by a non bay-region polycyclic cyclopenta(c,d)pyrene (CP) and its 3,4-oxide, *Cancer Res.*, 40, 4482, 1980.

208. **Reardon, D. B., Bigger, A. H., Strandberg, G., Yagi, H., Jerina, D. M., and Dipple, A.,** Sequence selectivity in the reaction of optically active hydrocarbon dihydrodiol-epoxide with rat *H-ras* DNA, *Chem. Res. Toxicol.*, 2, 12, 1989.

209. **Szentpaly, L.,** The MCS-model of chemical initiation of cancer, *Int. J. Quantum Chem., Quantum Biol. Symp.*, 12, 287, 1985.

210. **Szentpaly, L., Parkanyi, C.,** The MCS model of chemical initiation of cancer: PPP calculations on methylated and *N*-heteroaromatic polycycles, *J. Mol. Struct.*, 151, 245, 1987.

211. **Seybold, P. G.,** Topological influence on carcinogenicity of aromatic hydrocarbons. II. Substituent effects, *Int. J. Quantum Chem., Quantum Biol. Symp.*, 10, 103, 1983.

212. **Coulson, A. A., O'Leary, B., and Mallion, R. B.,** Hückel theory for organic chemists, Academic Press, London, 1978.

213. **Streitwieser, A., Jr.,** *Molecular Orbital Theory for Organic Chemists,* John Wiley & Sons, New York, 1962.
214. **Heilbronner, E. and Bock, H.,** Das HMO-Modell und seine Anwendung, *Verlag Chemic,* GmbH, Weinheim/Berstr., 3 vol., 1970.

Chapter 4

TOPOLOGICAL CORRELATIONS AND CANCER

Alexandru T. Balaban

TABLE OF CONTENTS

I. CHEMICAL FORMULAS AND TOPOLOGY

Chemical structures are expressed by formulas. One and the same molecular formula (e.g., $C_{20}H_{42}$) can correspond to many different substances called isomers, having different arrangements of atoms in molecules, i.e., different structures; in the case of the above simple saturated hydrocarbon devoid of rings there are 3,396,844 possible isomers.[1]

Structural formulas of organic compounds indicate by lines covalent bonds (electron pairs shared by two atoms) and include stereochemical information: configuration in chiral molecules and data about diastereomerism such as (1) *cis/trans* orientation of groups in molecules possessing rings or double bonds, as well as (2) configurations of polychiral molecules.

If in organic formulas we leave out information about stereochemistry and if all hydrogen atoms are also left out, we obtain the so called constitutional formula. This formula can be modeled by a molecular graph (hydrogen-suppressed graph) wherein the points (vertices) symbolize atoms, and the lines (edges) symbolize covalent bonds. For the above example one may write 366,319 different constitutional formulas. It can be seen that leaving out stereoisomerism leads to considerable simplification.[1a]

The nature of the nonhydrogen atoms is specified for each vertex; two vertices may be bonded by a single, double or triple bond (edge); this type of graph where multiple edges are allowed is called a multigraph.

The problem in quantitative structure-activity relationships (QSAR) or quantitative structure-property relationships (QSPR) is that biological activities or physicochemical properties of substances are measured on continuous numerical scales (and form a set which can be ordered according to the corresponding measured values), whereas chemical structures expressed by their constitutional formulas or molecular graphs, are discrete entities without an apparent ordering criterion. Acyclic structures such as the molecular graphs of saturated hydrocarbons (alkanes) can be perceived as more or less branched, but this is a qualitative rather than a quantitative notion.

It will not be disputed that branching increases (Figure 1) for the three isomeric pentanes C_5H_{12} in the order: *n*-pentane (**1**) < 2-methylbutane **2** < 2,2-dimethylpropane **3**. However, in other cases the ordering is not evident; which of the heptane isomers **4** to **7** is more branched and which is less branched? In cyclic systems the situation is even more complicated. For dealing with such problems, a topological approach based upon graph theory was developed.

Another incentive for devising topological approaches is the problem of chemical information storage and retrieval. More than ten million structures have been prepared and are indexed in the Beilstein, Gmelin, and Chemical Abstracts databases, and each year about a half a million new structures are added. By means of molecular formulas (such as $C_8H_8O_4$ for aspirin, $C_6H_{14}O_6S$ for Myleran) one may easily obtain a lexicographic indexing. However, isomerism complicates the picture. At present, complicated nomenclature rules are applied for discriminating isomers but these rules are arbitrary, complex and differ according to the nomenclature system (IUPAC, Chemical Abstracts, Wiswesser Line Notation,[2] etc.). Recently, several topological systems have been proposed in the hope to devise molecular identification numbers,[3-6] as will be shown in Section IV.

Topological information is equivalent to knowing only adjacency relationships between atoms (or graph vertices), ignoring provisionally the stereochemical, i.e., the geometrical, arrangement of atoms in molecules.

II. TOPOLOGICAL AND GRAPH-THEORETICAL INTERMEZZO

In a graph, the number of edges meeting at a vertex is called the *degree* of that vertex. The number of edges separating two vertices along the shortest path between them is called

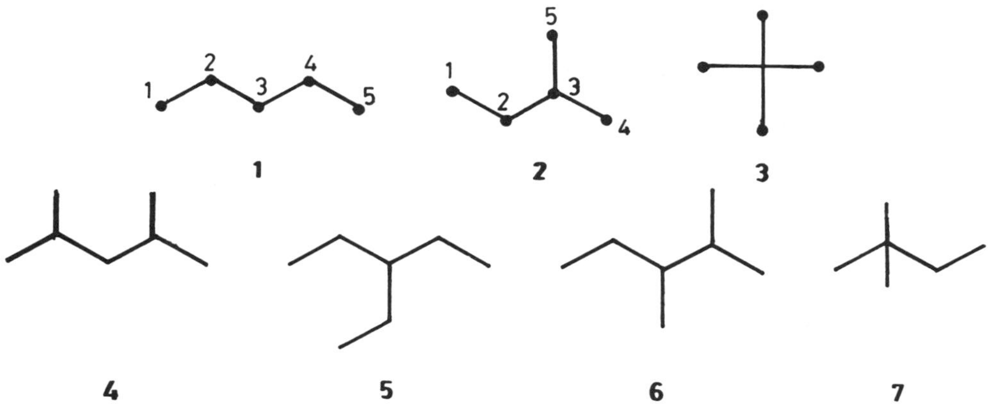

FIGURE 1.   Molecular graphs of the three isomers of pentane (**1** to **3**) and of four from the heptane isomers (**4** to **7**).

FIGURE 2.   For 2-methylbutane (arbitrary numbering of carbon atoms), the adjacency matrix **A** with vertex degrees v_i, and the distance matrix **D** with distance sums s_i.

the topological *distance* between the two vertices. Two vertices connected by an edge are said to be *adjacent* and, according to the preceding definition, are at distance 1. A graph devoid of cycles is called a *tree*.

The *adjacency matrix* **A** of a graph has as entry a_{ij} for row i and column j a digit 1 if vertices i and j are adjacent and a zero if not. The *distance matrix* **D** of a graph has as entry d_{ij} the topological distance between vertices i and j. As examples, **A** and **D** for graph **2** are shown in Figure 2 with vertices numbered arbitrarily. It is easy to see that both are symmetrical matrices because $a_{ij} = a_{ji}$, $d_{ij} = d_{ji}$. Each of these matrices uniquely characterizes the given graph. Knowing one of these matrices, it is possible to reconstruct the given graph.

The sums over rows or vertices are the vertex *degrees* v_i for **A**, and the *distance sums* s_i for **D**. Irrespective of the arbitrary vertex numbering, v_i and s_i are *graph invariants* for each vertex.

A graph or tree wherein no two vertices are equivalent (i.e., no vertex invariants are equal except for cases of accidental degeneracy) are called *identity graphs* (or *trees*, respectively).

The largest distance between two vertices in a graph is called the *graph diameter*.

A graph wherein the vertices or edges are labeled (e.g., by coloring, symbolizing the different nature of heteroatoms) is called a *chromatic graph*.

III. DESCRIPTION OF SELECTED TOPOLOGICAL INDICES

One can associate with any graph one or several numbers obtained from its vertex invariants according to definite mathematical formulas or algorithms; such numbers are

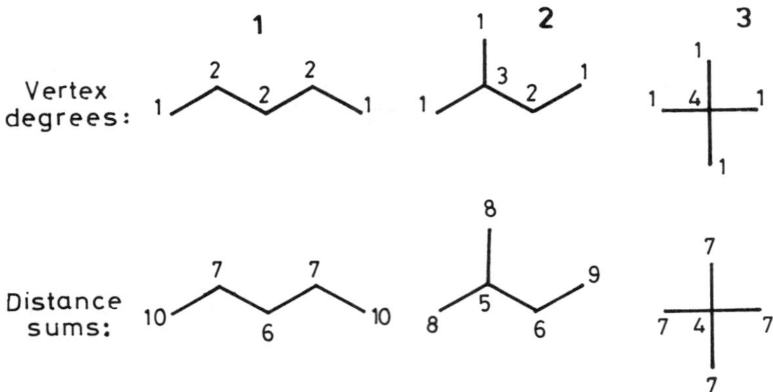

FIGURE 3.   Vertex degrees and distance sums (local graph invariants, LOVIs) for the three pentane isomers **1** to **3**.

called *topological indices* (TIs). In most cases these TIs present *degeneracy*, i.e., two or more different graphs have the same TI; it is possible to construct the TI from the graph, but is no longer possible to retrieve the graph from the value of the TI.

In the series of isomeric pentanes **1** to **3** as in any tree, the sums of vertex degrees are identical, $\Sigma_i\, v_i = 2q$, where q is the number of edges, as seen in Figure 3.

On summing all distance sums and dividing the total by two, one obtains w, the oldest TI, devised in 1944 to 1945 by H. Wiener:[7-9]

$$w = \sum_i \sum_j d_{ij}/2 = \sum_i s_i/2$$

thus for the graphs **1**—**3** their Wiener indices are 20, 18, and 16, respectively.

Another TI, denoted by M, was proposed by the Zagreb group,[10] and results on summing the squares of vertex degrees: $M = \Sigma_i\, v_i^2$; for the three isomeric pentanes, their indices M are 14, 16 and 20, respectively.

One can see that with increasing branching the former index decreases and the latter index increases. Both these TIs, however, are rather primitive and have a high degeneracy.

An index with excellent qualities was proposed by M. Randić.[11,12] and is called molecular connectivity: the inverse square root of the product of vertex degrees for the two endpoints of each edge is summed over all graph edges:

$$\chi = \sum_{\text{edge } i-j} (v_i v_j)^{-1/2}$$

In practice, meaningful correlations have been made with χ along with other parameters such as hydrophobicity, etc.

In the alkane series, the degeneracy of this index starts with octanes: the same value of χ is found for 3- and 4-methylheptanes, and similarly for 3,4-dimethylhexane and for 3-ethyl-2-methylpentane. Three types of refinements for this index were recently proposed:

1.   On considering the edge $i-j$ as the simplest case of a path with length equal to one in the molecular graph, and on extending the summation over all possible paths with length h, one obtains:

$$^h\chi = (v_i v_j \ldots v_{h+1})^{-1/2}$$

In practice, meaningful correlations have been made for $h \leqslant 5$.[13]

TABLE 1
Valence Delta ($^v\delta$)

Atom	Group	$^v\delta$	Atom	Group	$^v\delta$
$C(sp^3)$	$-CH_3$	1	$N(sp^3)$	$-NH_2$	3
	$-CH_2-$	2		$-NH-$	4
	$-CH-$	3		$-N-$	5
	$-C-$	4			
$C(sp^2)$	$=CH_2$	2	$N(sp^2)$	$=NH$	4
	$=CH-$	3		$=N-$	5
	$=C-$	4	$N(sp)$	$\equiv N$	5
$C(sp)$	$\equiv CH$	3	P	$-PH_2$	0.33
	$\equiv C-$	4		$-PH-$	0.44
				$-P-$	0.56
$O(sp^3)$	$-OH$	5		$=P-$	2.22
	$-O-$	6			
$O(sp^2)$	$=O$	6	F	$-F$	7
S	$-SH$	0.56	Cl	$-Cl$	0.78
	$-S-$	0.67	Br	$-Br$	0.26
	$-SS-$	0.89			
	$=S-$	1.33	I	$-I$	0.16
	$=S=$	2.67			

From Kier, L. B., Hall, L. H., Murray, W. F., and Randić, M., *J. Pharm. Sci.*, 64, 1971, 1985. With permission.

2. For molecules with heteroatoms, Kier and Hall[13,14] adapted Randić's index by replacing the vertex degree with valence delta values $^v\delta$:

$$^v\delta = (^vZ - h)/(Z - {^vZ} - 1)$$

where Z is the atomic number (total number of electrons) of the neutral heteroatom, ^vZ is the number of valence electrons, and h is the number of hydrogen atoms suppressed. Thus, every carbon atom in benzene has $^v\delta = 3$, and in cyclohexane $^v\delta = 2$.

Table 1 presents for some functional groups the corresponding $^v\delta$ values. It can be seen that there is a large difference between first-row atoms and heavier atoms, i.e., between nitrogen, oxygen, fluorine and the corresponding counterparts, namely phosphorus, sulfur and chlorine, respectively. A third refinement, the molecular identification numbers ID, will be described later in Section IV.

Bonchev and Trinajstić[15,16] applied information theory for characterizing molecular structures and, in particular, for reducing the degeneracy of TIs. Thus, the high degeneracy of the Wiener index is due to the fact that sums of entries d_{ij} in the distance matrix **D** may coincide although the summands differ. If a certain topological distance d_i appears $2a_i$ times

TABLE 2
Informational Indices for Graphs 1-3

1	**2**	**3**
d_i 1 2 3 4	d_i 1 2 3	d_i 1 2
a_i 4 3 2 1	a_i 4 4 2	a_i 4 6
$I_D^w = 20 \log_2 20 - 6 \log_2 2 - 6$ $\log_2 3 - 4 \log_2 4 = 62.929$	$I_D^w = 18 \log_2 18 - 8 \log_2 2 - 6$ $\log_2 3 = 57.549$	$I_D^w = 16 \log_2 16 - 12 \log_2 2 = 52.0$
$\bar{I}_D^w = 62.929/20 = 3.146$	$\bar{I}_D^w = 57.549/18 = 3.197$	$\bar{I}_D^w = 52/16 = 3.25$
$I_D^E = 10 \log_2 10 - 4 \log_2 4 - 3$ $\log_2 3 - 2 \log_2 2 = 18.464$	$I_D^E = 10 \log_2 10 - 8 \log_2 4 - 2$ $\log_2 2 = 15.219$	$I_D^E = 10 \log_2 10 - 4 \log_2 4 - 6$ $\log_2 6 = 9.71$
$\bar{I}_D^E = 18.464/10 = 1.846$	$\bar{I}_D^E = 15.219/10 = 1.522$	$\bar{I}_D^E = 9.71/10 = 0.971$

in the distance matrix **D** (in this symmetrical matrix, each entry is repeated twice), then the Wiener index can also be expressed as w = $\Sigma_i d_i a_i$. By means of formulas such as:

$$I_D^w = w\log_2 w - \sum_i a_i d_i \log_2 d_i$$

$$\bar{I}_D^w = I_D^w/w = - \sum_i a_i \frac{d_i}{w} \log_2 \frac{d_i}{w}$$

one can calculate in bits the information content I_D^w and the mean information content $\bar{I}_D^w$ on realized distances.

By means of the following formulas:

$$\bar{I}_D^E = \frac{n(n-1)}{2} \log_2 \frac{n(n-1)}{2} - \sum_i a_i \log_2 a_i$$

$$I_D^E = \frac{2}{n(n-1)} \bar{I}_D^E = \sum_i - \frac{2d_i}{n(n-1)} \log_2 \frac{2d_i}{n(n-1)}$$

one calculates the information content, and the mean information content, respectively, on the distribution of distances in the given graph. All these informational indices are expressed in bits. For the three isomeric pentanes we obtain the data shown in Table 2; taking into account that in the distance matrix we have n(n − 1) entries, $\Sigma_i a_i = n(n-1)/2$:

Another idea due to Bonchev and Trinajstić[17] was to combine several TIs into a "superindex" for reducing the degeneracy.

By means of two axioms and six theorems, Bertz[18] defined rigorously the branching of graphs and introduced "graph derivatives" as the simplest indices for evaluating quantitatively the branching of trees. As one vertex is added to a graph, the new graph in which the atom has been affixed to the precursor atom with the higher degree is the more branched; a branching index B_M for a graph M formed by joining two subgraphs R and S (with branching indices B_R and B_S, respectively) by a bond between atoms of R and S having (before bonding) degrees r and s is:

$$B_M = B_R + B_S + r + s$$

For methane and ethane, $B_M = 0$ by definition. In general, the branching index B_M of a graph M is equal to the number of pairs of adjacent lines in M, i.e.,

$$B_M = \sum_i \binom{d_i}{2} = \sum_i \frac{d_i(d_i - 1)}{2}$$

where d_i is the degree of the ith vertex.

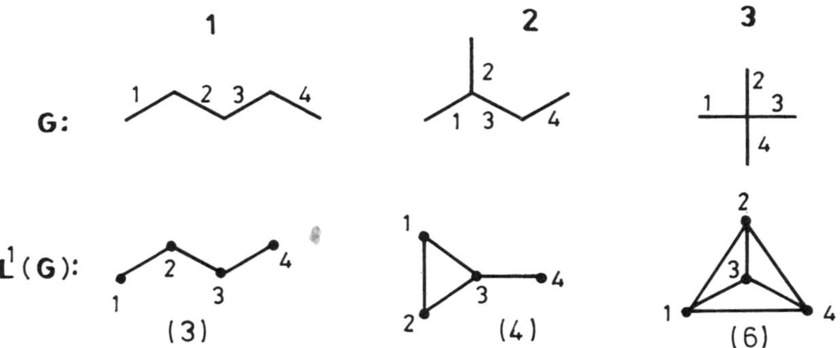

FIGURE 4. The three isomeric pentanes **1** to **3** (G) with arbitrary numbering of lines, their line graphs (first graph derivatives) $L^1(G)$, and in brackets the numbers of lines in $L^1(G)$.

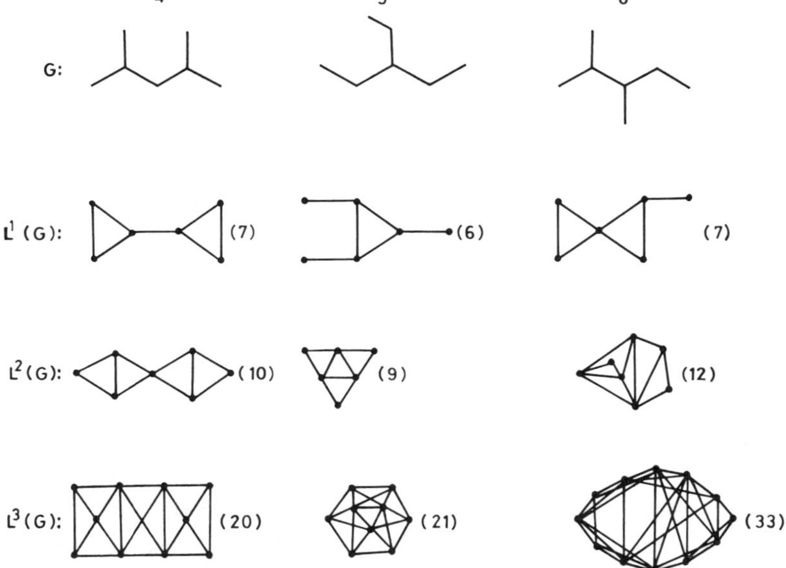

FIGURE 5. The first three graph derivatives for three of the isomeric heptanes **4** to **6**; numbers of lines are indicated in brackets.

Should B_M not be sufficient, one proceeds by iteration: B_M, the number of pairs of adjacent lines in a graph G, is equal to the number of lines in its *line graph*, or *derivative graph*, or *graph-theoretical first derivative*. To construct this derivative graph, one represents the lines of the given graph G by points and connects two such points with a line when the lines they represent are adjacent. By repeating this procedure *n* times, one obtains the *nth iterated line graph*, or *graph-theoretical nth derivative*, $L^n(G)$. The number of lines in $L_n(G)$ is denoted by $L^n(G)$ and is written in brackets in Figures 4 and 5.

The first derivative is sufficient for differentiating the three isomeric pentanes **1** to **3**, as seen in Figure 4; the second derivative differentiates the two isomeric hexanes **4** and **6** which have identical values for $L^1(G)$, as see in Figure 5. It may be observed also that the ordering of the three isomeric hexanes **4** to **6** according to $L^2(G)$ is different from the final ordering according to $L^n(G)$ where n ≥ 3.

Several topological indices were proposed and explored in Bucharest; they will be presented in the following pages.

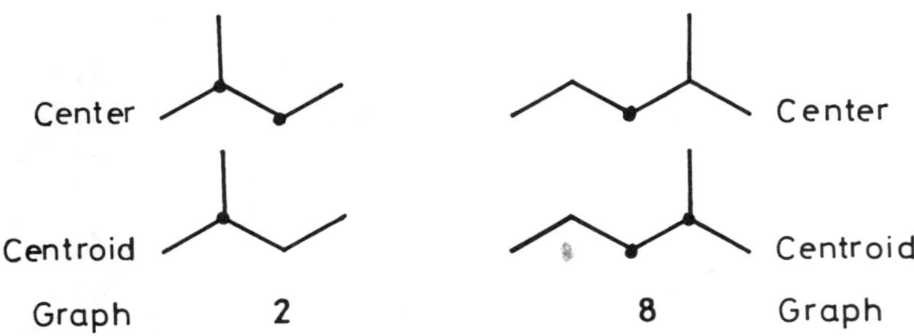

FIGURE 6.   Examples of graph centers and centroids for 2-methylbutane (**2**) and 2-methylpentane (**8**).

For *centric TIs*[19] it can be proved that for acyclic graphs (trees) the distance sum has minimal values for one vertex or a pair of adjacent vertices; one calls the vertex (vertices) with minimal distance sums the *centroid* of the tree.

Also, for trees one defines the *center,* which is either a vertex or a pair of adjacent vertices, by removing stepwise all vertices of degree one (endpoints). Alternatively, one can define for each vertex i its eccentricity e_i as the maximal distance to any other vertex j:

$$e_i = \max d_{ij}$$

Now, if one compares the eccentricity of all vertices in a tree, the center is defined by the minimax condition:

$$e_i = \min$$

The center and the centroid may not coincide, as shown in Figure 6 for graphs **2** and **8**, but they may coincide as in the case of graphs **1** and **3**.

If the numbers of endpoints removed at each step in finding the graph center are denoted by r_i (where r_i is the number of endpoints in the given tree, and the final value r_f is either 1 or 2, depending on whether the center is a vertex or a pair of vertices) and if n is the total number of vertices, $\sum_i r_i = n$, and the centric index is given by

$$B = \sum_i r_i^2$$

In order to define the "topological shape" of the tree, one can normalize this centrix index relative to the least branched tree (chain, $C = 0$), and the most branched tree (star-graph consisting of one center vertex and $n - 1$ endpoints, $C = 1$):

$$C = (B - 2n + [1 - (-1)^n]/2)/2$$

For graphs containing cycles, the generalized center (polycenter) is defined recursively by applying to vertices and edges (on the basis of the vertex distance matrix and the analogous edge distance matrix) three criteria in order as follows:[20,21]

1.   Minimum eccentricity: $e_i = \min$ (as the center for trees)
2.   Minimum distance sum: $s_i = \min$ (as the centroid for trees)
3.   Minimum number K of occurrence of the largest distance: $K_{max,i} = \min$

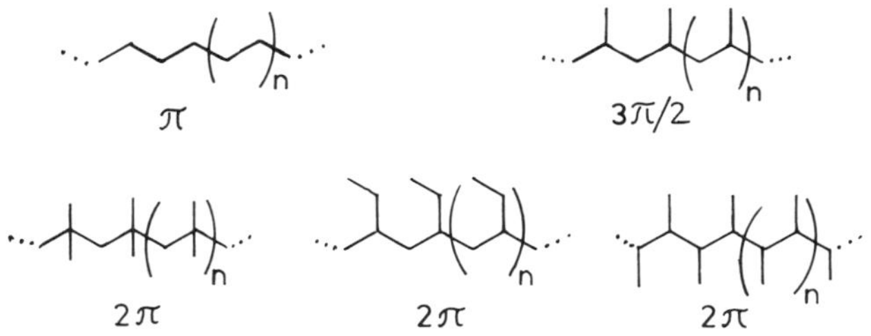

FIGURE 7.   Infinite nonbranched and branched graphs ($n \rightarrow \infty$); under each graph the corresponding J value is shown.

(if the largest distance d_{max} occurs the same number of times for several vertices, the distance d_{max-1} is considered and so on).

One obtains vertex and edge equivalence classes which are ranked centrically starting with rank zero for the most central class. These rankings serve as criteria for the next iteration according to rank sums.

The *mean square (topological) distance*[22] is defined as:

$$D = \left[\sum_{ij} d_{ij}^2 / n(n-1) \right]^{1/2}$$

For trees (acyclic graphs), one can calculate the *endpoint mean square distance*[22] by modifying the above formula so as to take into account only the r_1 endpoints and their mutual distances $d_{1,ij}$:

$$D_1 = \left(\sum_{ij} d_{1,ij}^2 / r_1(r_1-1) \right)^{1/2}$$

The centric indices and the mean distances can be correlated satisfactorily with properties which depend on branching, such as the octane numbers of alkanes.[23] These TIs suffer, however, from the drawback of high degeneracy.

A newer TI with a very low degeneracy was devised with the purpose of defining more precisely the "topological shape" of molecules, and called *average distance sum connectivity*:[22,24-29]

$$J = \frac{q}{q - n + 2} \sum_{\text{edge } ij} (s_i s_j)^{-1/2}$$

The denominator is the number q of edges and the numerator is higher by one than the cyclomatic number of the graph (this number indicates the minimal number of edges that have to be removed for converting the given graph into a tree). The summation formula resembles Randić's formula being over all edges i to j in the graph, but instead of taking the degrees as vertex invariants (they can be combined in carbon compounds only in 10 modes because the vertex degrees can only be the integers 1 to 4), one takes the distance sums which have no limitation whatsoever.

The index was designed so as not to automatically increase with the number n of vertices like practically all TIs (the exception is C): when the number n of carbon atoms in a linear (normal) alkane increases infinitely as in poly(ethene), index J tends toward $\pi = 3.14$; for an infinitely long poly(propene), $J = 3\pi/2$; for infinitely long poly(isobutene), poly-(1-butene) or poly-(2-butene), $J = 2\pi$ (Figure 7). However, when each vertex of the alkane except the endpoints has degree 3 or 4 then J increases indefinitely when n increases.[28]

Therefore it is usually necessary, in correlations using J, to additionally introduce the

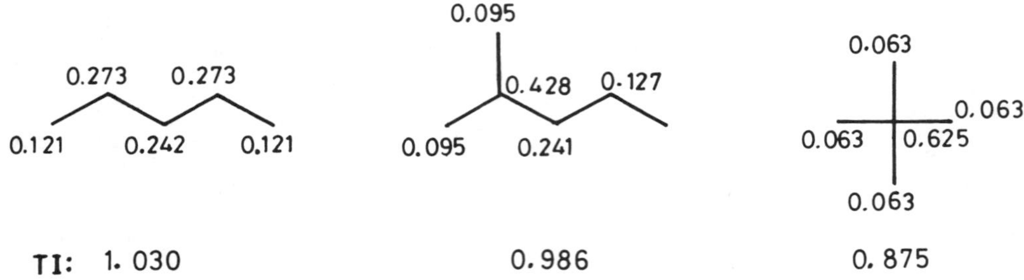

FIGURE 8.   AZV-LOVIs and the topological index (TI) obtained by their simple summation for the three pentane isomers **1** to **3**.

number n in biparametric equations of vertices. For molecules with heteroatoms, the nature of the heteroatom is taken into account either by means of its electronegativity or of its steric parameters; an example will be discussed at the end of Chapter 6.

For molecules containing multiple bonds, each double bond can be treated as two single bonds, and each triple bond as three single bonds in the evaluation of J. Alternatively, one may use a conventional bond order b (b = 1.5 for aromatic bonds; b = 1,2,3 for single, double, and triple bonds, respectively) in the topological distance d = 1/b for the respective bond(s).[26]

Interestingly, the intermolecular ordering of all isomeric alkanes up to, and including, heptanes is the same according to the Bertz graph derivatives as the order based on the index J.[18]

A different approach for reducing the degeneracy of TIs was to design new vertex invariants (in the place of vertex degrees or distance sums which can take only integer values).

One type[29] of local vertex invariants (LOVI) was obtained as solutions of a system of n linear equations obtained either from the adjacency matrix **A** or from the distance matrix **D**: on the main diagonal a vector P_i is introduced and as the free term for each equation, another vector Q_i (i = 1 to n) appears; the matrix is interpreted as the system of n linear equations, whose unknowns are the LOVIs x_i (i = 1 to n). Then this system of n equations with n unknowns x_i is solved. The two vectors P and Q may be constants (0,1, the number n of vertices, n^2, etc.) or graph-theoretical data (e.g., the corresponding vertex degrees v_i or distance sum s_i) or chemical data (e.g., the atomic number Z_i of the atom symbolized by the corresponding vertex). The combination: matrix-vector P-vector Q is indicated by the respective symbols, e.g., AZV, DSN, A1N, ANN^2, etc.

Then the LOVIs are converted into a TI by means of a global operation such as simple summation, summation of squares, Randić-type formulas, etc.

Figure 8 presents as examples the AZV-LOVIs and the TI resulted by their simple summation for the three isomers of pentane **1** to **3**.

Other types of vertex invariants are based on information on distances. So far, informational theoretic approaches have been used for the reduction of degeneracy of TIs at the global level, but less at the local invariant level: one exception consisted in LOVIs proposed by Raychaudhury and Basak[30-32] (first order topological information content, or vertex distance complexity, and its normalized version[32a]). In order to replace a crude operation (summing up all distances j into the distance sum s_i) by a more refined one, we first convert the distance vector (sequence of distances j = 1 to the graph diameter) into a LOVI by means of information theory, and then use the resulting LOVIs with various formulas for obtaining new TIs.[33] The new LOVIs are the mean local information on the magnitude of distances:

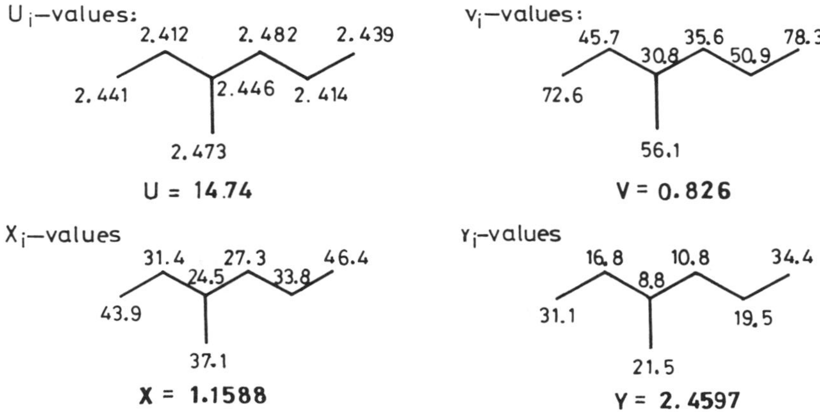

FIGURE 9.   For the smallest identity tree (3-methylhexane), four LOVIs (u_i, v_i, x_i, y_i) and the corresponding TIs: U, V, X, Y.

$$u_i = - \sum_j \frac{j}{s_i} \log_2 \frac{j}{s_i};$$

the local information on the magnitude of distances:

$$v_i = s_i \log_2 s_i - u_i;$$

the mean extended local information on distance magnitude:

$$y_i = - \sum_j j \log_2 j;$$

and the extended local information on distance magnitude:

$$x_i = s_i \log_2 s_i - y_i$$

Figure 9 presents these four local vertex invariants for the identity tree with seven vertices.

For obtaining new TIs it was proposed to apply a formula analogous to that used for J:

$$U = \frac{q}{q - n + 2} \sum_{\text{edge } ij} (u_i u_j)^{-1/2}$$

$$V = \frac{q}{q - n + 2} \sum_{\text{edge } ij} (v_i v_j)^{-1/2}$$

$$X = \frac{q}{q - n + 2} \sum_{\text{edge } ij} (x_i x_j)^{-1/2}$$

$$Y = \frac{q}{q - n + 2} \sum_{\text{edge } ij} (y_i y_j)^{-1/2}$$

Index U decreases with increasing branching and increases fast with increasing n; the remaining TIs have an opposite variation, as indicated for two isomeric pentanes **1** and **2** in Figure 10.

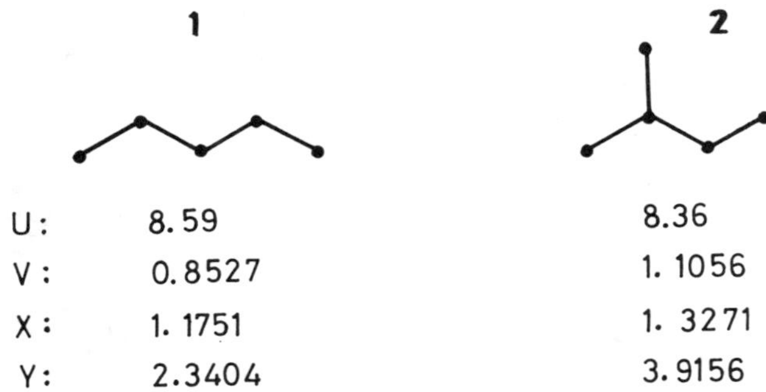

U:	8.59	8.36
V:	0.8527	1.1056
X:	1.1751	1.3271
Y:	2.3404	3.9156

FIGURE 10.   Topological indices U, V, X, Y for two isomers of pentane.

When the number n of vertices increases towards infinity, V, X and Y decrease slowly toward zero, therefore these three indices should be used, like J, in biparametric correlations along with n.

A third type of LOVIs is based on the idea[34] that the vertex degrees reflect only the immediate neighbors of a vertex, while distance sums place the major contribution on the most distant vertices. In the new type of LOVI, remote vertices should have a nonzero, but a lower contribution to the "regressive connectivity" of a given vertex. This can be achieved by means of new matrices: entries b_{ij} in the branching matrix **B** are defined as sums of vertex degrees for all vertices situated at distance $j - 1$ from vertex i (i.e., the sums of vertex degrees for all vertices on the jth layer around vertex i). Evidently, the entries b_{ij} on the first column represent the vertex degrees. Matrix **B** has $i_{max} = n$ rows and $j_{max} = 1 + d_{max}$ columns, where d_{max} is the graph diameter, i.e., the maximum distance in the graph. For the three isomeric pentanes the **B**-matrices are shown in Figure 11.

Local vertex invariants BR_i (regressive vertex degrees) may be obtained from the B-matrix by two operations denoted by (1) and (2).

$$BR_i^{(1)} = \sum_j j^{-3} b_{ij}; \qquad BR_i^{(2)} = \sum_j 10^{1-j} b_{ij}$$

In Figure 11, the upper LOVI values correspond to the former and the lower values to the latter operator.

From each type of LOVI, three TIs may be obtained:

$$BY^{(1)} = 2nq \left(\sum_i BR_i \right)^{-1}; \qquad BY^{(2)} = 2nq \sum_i BR_i; \qquad BY^{(3)} = 2nq \left[\sum_i (BR_i)^{2-1/2} \right]$$

Thus, with $BR_i^{(2)}$ as LOVI, the three TIs for the three isomeric pentanes are shown in Table 3. It can be seen that with increasing branching, $BY^{(2)}$ decreases while $BY^{(3)}$ increases. Bond multiplicity and the presence of heteroatoms may be taken into account by suitable additional factors introduced into the formulas for BY.

We conclude here the enumeration of selected TIs. Other, more detailed data may be found in various reviews on TIs;[35-49] among these, a few deal especially with correlations involving biological, biochemical or pharmacological data.

Randić's ID numbers[3] are defined by weighting each edge e of a graph according to the degrees v_i, v_j of its endpoints (i,j) by a factor:

$$g(e) = (v_i v_j)^{-1/2}$$

We thus obtain the *connectivity ID number*, if instead of summing these weights for all

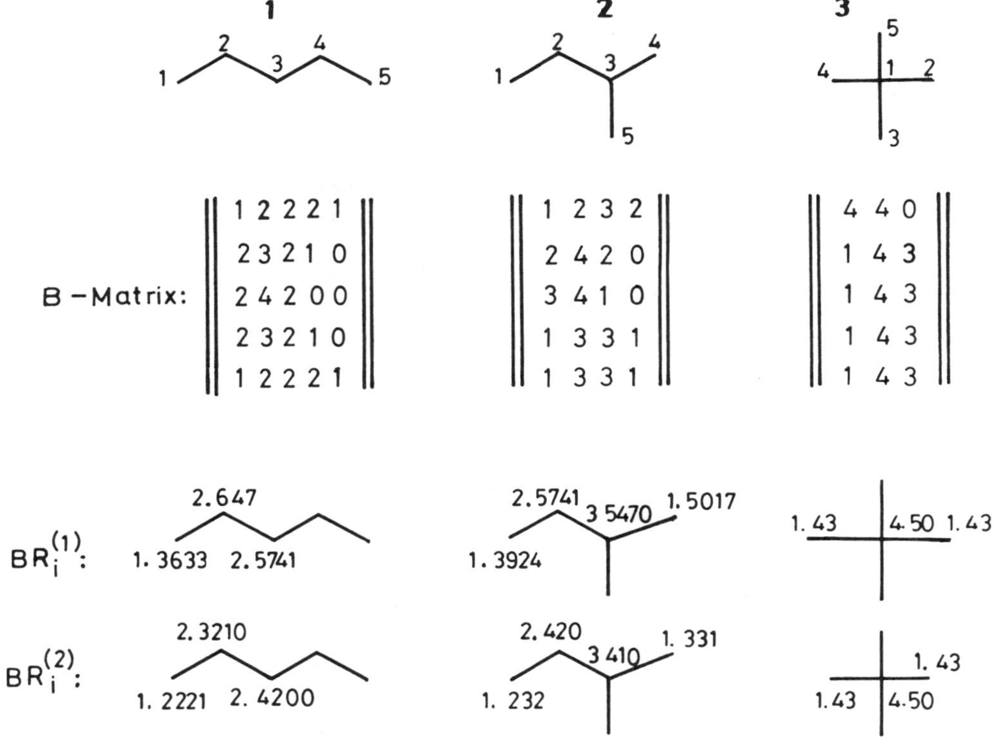

FIGURE 11.   **B**-Matrices for the three pentane isomers (**1** to **3**) and LOVIs (regressive vertex degrees) $BR_i^{(1)}$ and $BR_i^{(2)}$; vertices without LOVI values have equivalent vertices elsewhere.

TABLE 3
Indices $BY^{(1)}$ — $BY^{(3)}$ for Graphs 1—3

Graph	$BY^{(1)}$	$BY^{(2)}$	$BY^{(3)}$
1	3.9100	9.5062	4.4292
2	3.8070	9.7240	4.7482
3	3.6548	10.1200	5.2478

edges, one sums them for all paths in the graph, i.e., continuous chains of edges without any repeating edges. Having observed that the reduction of degeneracy is not complete, Randić proposed *prime ID numbers*[6] replacing the vertex degrees by the first ten prime numbers between 1 and 23 so that the 10 possible bond types have the weights indicated in the third column of Table 4.

These ID numbers have low degeneracy. In the alkane series, the degeneracy starts with 15 carbon atoms for the connectivity ID number and with 20 carbon atoms for the prime ID numbers. An even less degenerate ID number was devised independently by Szymanski et al.[50] and by Balaban[51] on replacing the vertex degrees in the preceding formula by distance sums. Unlike the preceding two ID numbers, these weighted ID numbers show no clustering around the values corresponding to the ten possible classes according to Table 4, and have no degeneracy for alkanes or trees with up to 20 vertices; however, tricyclic graphs with six vertices do lead to degeneracies.

TABLE 4
Edge Weights for ID Numbers
According to Bond Types, i.e., to
the Vertex Degrees of the Two
Endpoints

	Edge weight for ID numbers	
Bond type	**Connectivity**	**Prime**
1;1	$1^{-1/2}$	$1^{-1/2}$
1;2	$2^{-1/2}$	$2^{-1/2}$
1;3	$3^{-1/2}$	$3^{-1/2}$
1;4	$4^{-1/2}$	$5^{-1/2}$
2;2	$4^{-1/2}$	$7^{-1/2}$
2;3	$6^{-1/2}$	$11^{-1/2}$
2;4	$8^{-1/2}$	$13^{-1/2}$
3;3	$9^{-1/2}$	$17^{-1/2}$
3;4	$12^{-1/2}$	$19^{-1/2}$
4;4	$16^{-1/2}$	$23^{-1/2}$

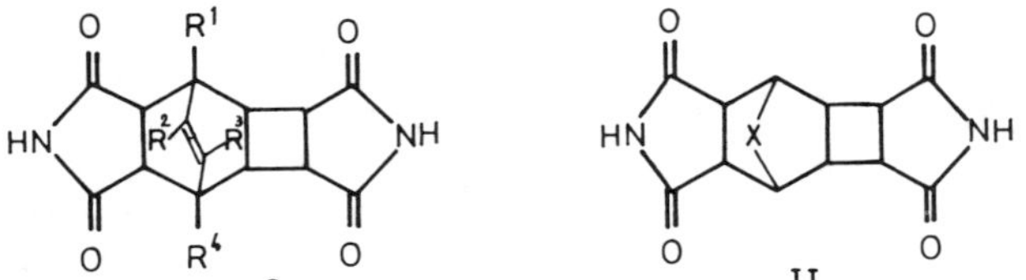

FIGURE 12. Basic molecular skeletons for mitindomides I and II.

IV. QSAR STUDIES OF MITINDOMIDES (ANTITUMOR COMPOUNDS)

Carter, Trinajstić and Nikolić[52] investigated nine antitumor agents synthesized recently by Bryce-Smith and co-workers (mitindomides I and II, Figure 12*) attempting to find QSAR between their experimental activities expressed as ID_{50} values (in $\mu mol/L$) against two types of tumors (V79 and P388), as seen in Table 5. The lower the experimental data, the more active the compound: inactive compounds are indicated by i. For heteroatoms, weighting was also performed by valencies similar to data of Kier and Hall (Table 1), leading to two sets of calculated values according to degrees, or to valence-weighted degrees.

It may be observed that satisfactory correlations exist for activity against V79 tumors: the lower the ID number, the higher the activity. For skeleton I, the order of calculated ID numbers using valences coincides with the experimental order; the calculated threshold separating active from inactive compounds is 37.133. The four active compounds are also distinguished by lower ID numbers calculated using vertex degrees, but their ordering does not match that found experimentally. The activity against P388 tumors is also mirrored by calculated ID values for skeleton II but the number of compounds is too small for meaningful correlations.

---

* So far, graphs were denoted by boldface Arabic numbers; henceforth, chemical formulas will be denoted by Roman numbers.

TABLE 5

Anti-Tumor Activities of Compounds I and II vs. Degree-ID or Valence-ID Numbers

Comp.		R^1	R^2	R^3	R^4	Exp. data[a]		I		II	
						V 79	P388	Degree	Valence	Degree	Valence
I	1	H	H	H	H	16	i	42.311	36.830	38.123	33.337
	2	H	Me	H	H	27	i	42.359	37.080	38.103	33.422
	3	Me	H	H	Me	26	i	42.179	36.955	38.076	33.507
	4	Me	Me	H	H	28	i	42.306	37.133	38.082	33.494
	5	H	Me	Me	H	i	28	42.417	37.318	38.084	33.499
	6	H	i-Pr	H	H	i	i	42.555	37.220	38.199	33.483
II	7	$X = 0$				—	19	—	—	38.073	33.957
	8	$X = CH_2CH_2$				—	34	—	—	38.124	34.027
	9	$X =$ none				—	4.1	—	—	37.468	33.324

[a] Experimental data are ID_{50} values (μM); when $ID_{50} > 100$, the compound is inactive (i).

V. AUTOCORRELATIONS AND CARCINOGENIC ACTIVITIES

Another method for handling molecular structures is the autocorrelation of the distribution of a property; this can be studied on the topological (constitutional) or on the geometrical (tri-dimensional) structure. The latter approach defines molecules in physical rather than topological terms, so that the properties can be seen as a function of three-dimensional coordinates of various atoms.[53-55]

In comparing molecules, one proceeds similarly to the comparison between two objects in the macromolecular world, e.g., a horse and a cow: we try to superimpose the head, the legs etc., i.e., common parts of the object that have the same function. In comparing two steroid molecules, one superimposes rings A, B, C, and D of one molecule on rings A, B, C, and D of another molecule. In the framework of topological methods, this method is the basis of the Free-Wilson and MTD methods. Even without knowing the detailed structure of the receptor, or of the structure responsible for the activity, one can thus obtain significant correlations.

An autocorrelation vector is constructed for various molecules (the learning set) on the basis of a set of properties (vertex connectivity, van der Waals volume and electronegativity of each atom as well as its increment to the total hydro/lipophilicity, type of atom, i.e., carbon/noncarbon or hydrogen-bonding ability) defined in Boolean manner, i.e., by 0/1 digits.

The points representing the molecules are distributed in a multidimensional vector space. The biological property associated with each molecule then determines a grouping of certain points according to this property, e.g., carcinogenic ability. For recognizing structure-activity correlations, pattern recognition techniques and principal component analysis (PCA) or linear discriminant analysis (LDA) were applied.

Thus, 209 molecules tested for their carcinogenicity were studied by PCA and they were projected on the plane determined by the (first) two principal factors; the first factor accounts for 51% of the variance and the second for 19%; polyaromatics form a well-defined family in this representation. In a similar study by LDA, with 12 variables included in the discriminant function, the percentage of good recognition is 83.7% and the breakdown according to the numbers of (misclassified molecules/numbers of molecules in the family) is:

		Good recognition
Aromatic amines	(9/33)	72.7%
Alkyl halides	(1/15)	93.3%
Nitroaromatics	(3/17)	82.4%

		Good recognition
Miscellaneous	(2/12)	83.3%
Nitrogen compounds	(2/9)	77.7%
N-Nitroso compounds	(3/21)	85.7%
Polyaromatics	(3/29)	89.7%
Ethers-epoxides-carbamates	(7/18)	61.1%
Diazo compounds	(2/11)	81.8%
Natural compounds	(1/36)	97.2%
Fungal toxins	(0/4)	100.0%
Heterocyclics	(1/4)	75.0%
Total	(34/209)	83.7%

VI. THE DARC/PELCO METHOD

The DARC/PELCO method, introduced by J. E. Dubois and co-workers,[1c,56] is based upon the simultaneous representation of (1) all structures S for which one wishes to correlate structural variations with variations in property (activity or information I), and of (2) population P which contains these structures.

Each structure S is formally assimilated to a chromatic graph whose vertices represent nonhydrogen atoms and whose edges represent the covalent bonds between these atoms. In this graph one has to distinguish the focus (FO) consisting of an atom, a bond or a group of atoms characterizing a series of compounds and the environment (E) consisting of the remaining atoms and bonds that are concentrically organized around the focus and ordered according to priority rules. The structures are placed in an ordered space called hyperstructure (HS) which has an associated graph whose every vertex represents a studied structure and whose edges represent the topochromatic distances between these structures.

HS provides two tools:[57] (1) the population trace TR(P), a graph that regroups all the ordered sites appearing at least once in the environments of all the structures in P, and characterizes space HS where the structures of P and those predictable from P are located and (2) the topochromatic vector $\vec{T}(E)$, a Boolean vector associated with the environment of each structure, indicating the presence or absence of each ordered site. This vector provides a quantitative expression of the structure of the compound in a population characterized by its trace; it accounts directly for the overall topology and chromaticity (nature of bonds and atoms, geometrical and stereochemical data) of the structures described, and retains the local information. This tool allows the rapid retrieval of the structure by a simple procedure.

The topochromatic vectors $\vec{T}(E)$ and the information I are used to establish a relationship between the information associated with the environment I(E) and the vector I(m) characterizing the information and resulting from the study of m compounds:

$$I(E) = \langle \vec{T}(E) | \vec{I}(m) \rangle$$

The information I(x) obtained from a structure x is calculated from the information $I(x_o)$ corresponding to the reference structure whose environment is reduced to hydrogen atoms:

$$I(x) = I(x_0) + I(E)$$

Thus it is possible to start from properties of known structures, and to predict those of unknown structures.

Comparisons between the DARC/PELCO method and the use of the molecular connectivity χ were carried out by two independent groups[58,59] leading to divergent conclusions for QSAR in antimicrobial activities of halogenated phenols.

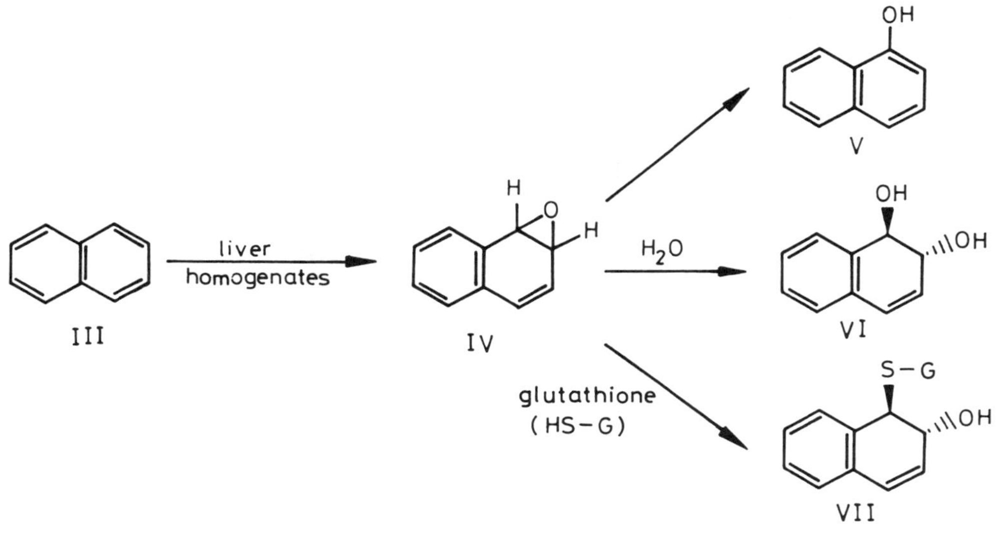

FIGURE 13. For the simplest PAH, naphthalene (III), for example, the enzymatic epoxidation to IV is followed by ring opening of the oxiranic (epoxidic) ring leading to phenolic or alcoholic groups.

VII. TOPOLOGY AND CARCINOGENICITY OF POLYCYCLIC AROMATIC HYDROCARBONS

It is now well established that the polycyclic aromatic hydrocarbons (PAHs) are a major cause of human cancers. Benzo(a)pyrene (BaP, IX) is formed in various pyrolytic/combustion processes of organic compounds (thermoelectric power stations, cigarette smoke, exhaust gases in all vehicles) in large amounts. It was estimated that in the U.S. alone 1300 tons of BaP per year are released into the atmosphere. Along with dibenzo(a,h)anthracene (x), these two PAHs were identified as the major carcinogens in coal tar in the early 1930s, but the mechanism of metabolic activation was elucidated later beginning with the late 1960s. These studies were connected with a molecular rearrangement known as the "NIH shift" because it was discovered by a team of chemists (B. Witkop, J. W. Daly, D. M. Jerina, S. Udenfriend, H. Yagi) at the National Institutes of Health in Bethesda, MD.

The detoxification and excretion of xenobiotic aromatics is activated by nonspecific monooxygenases (involving cytochromes P-450 which are localized in the cellular endoplasmic reticulum of kidney, lung, intestine, skin and especially liver).

Thus naphthalene, III, the simplest PAH, is first converted into an arene oxide (epoxide or oxirane, IV): this may undergo spontaneous isomerization via carbocations to α-naphthol, V (whereby oxiranic hydrogens may undergo NIH-shift scrambling), hydrolysis to a *trans*-1,2-dihydrodiol, VI, catalyzed by the enzyme epoxide hydrase, or conversion into the glutathione conjugate, VII which is water-soluble; the last process is catalyzed by glutathione-S-epoxide transferase.

One of the earliest attempts to correlate structure with potential carcinogenic activity of PAHs is the K-region theory,[61] ascribing the activity to regions with high olefinic character such as the 9,10-double bond in phenanthrene. On the other hand, the presence of an L-region indicates deactivation; the earliest correlations were quantum chemical calculations with π-electron densities in these regions exemplified for benzo(a)anthracene, VIII.

Pullman and Pullman's[61] calculations claimed satisfactory correlations; more recently Herndon[62] found some correlations between the so called experimental Iball carcinogenicity index and the K-region localization energy. However, the K-region epoxides are less active than the parent hydrocarbons. In the mid-1970s Jerina and co-workers[63,64] advanced the bay-

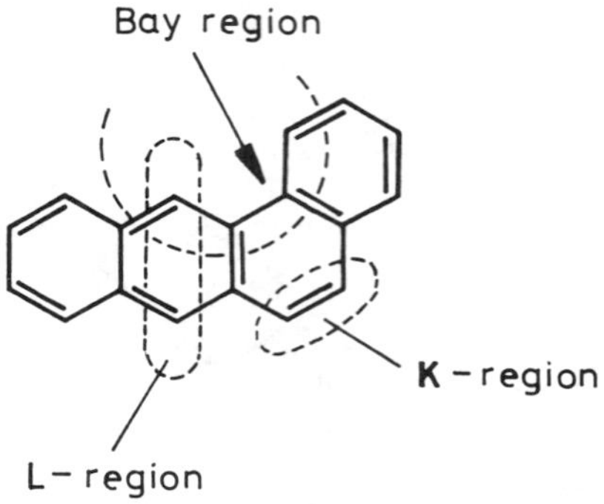

FIGURE 14.   For benz(a)anthracene VIII, for example, the bay-region as well as the K- and L-regions are shown.

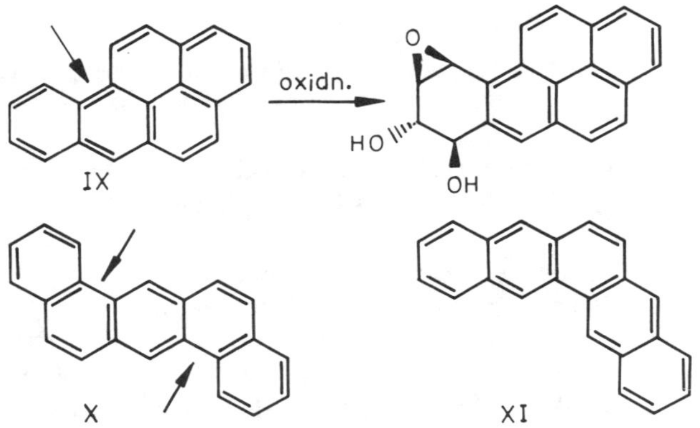

FIGURE 15.   Metabolic activation of benzo(a)pyrene, BaP (IX) to the bay-region diol-epoxide; bay-regions in BaP (IX) and in dibenz(a,h)anthracene (X) are indicated by arrows; the pentaphene XI has no bay-region.

region theory: a PAH has a bay-region if a concave region is adjacent to one benzenoid ring, as in VIII, IX, X, but not in XI. It may be observed that very often a K-region is on the other side of a bay-region.

The presence of a bay-region seems to be a necessary but insufficient condition for a PAH to possess carcinogenic activity. Practically all-known carcinogenic PAHs have bay regions, but many other PAHs with one or more bay-regions are not carcinogenic. Certainly, additional factors are also required. The presence of other substituents (methyl, fluoro) strongly influences the carcinogenicity, as shown for benz(a)anthracene VIII where substituents block, decrease or enhance carcinogenicity.

The ultimate carcinogen is the diol-epoxide at the benzo ring adjacent to the bay-region; the exocyclic 2-amino groups of guanine residues in DNA or RNA are nucleophilic enough to become covalently attached to these ultimate carcinogens by ring opening of the oxirane ring. The structure of the covalently bound nucleotide from the bay-region diol-epoxide of benzo(a)pyrene and poly(guanosine) is shown in XII. The ring opening of the oxirane on attack of the nucleophile HNu (the guanosine residue), involves a quasi-cationic transition state, where the positive charge (which needs not be fully formed) is stabilized by benzylic conjugation and by proximity of the aromatic ring characterizing the bay-region.

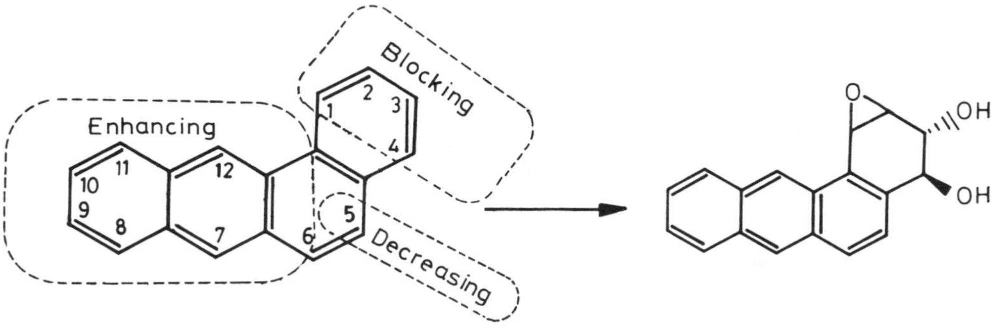

FIGURE 16. Positions of substituents in benz(a)anthracene which block, decrease or enhance the metabolic activation to the carcinogenic diol-epoxide.

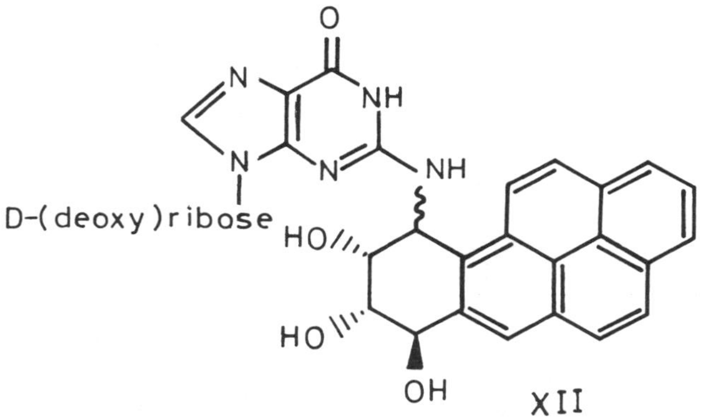

FIGURE 17. Product (XII) formed from guanosine and the BaP-diol-epoxide.

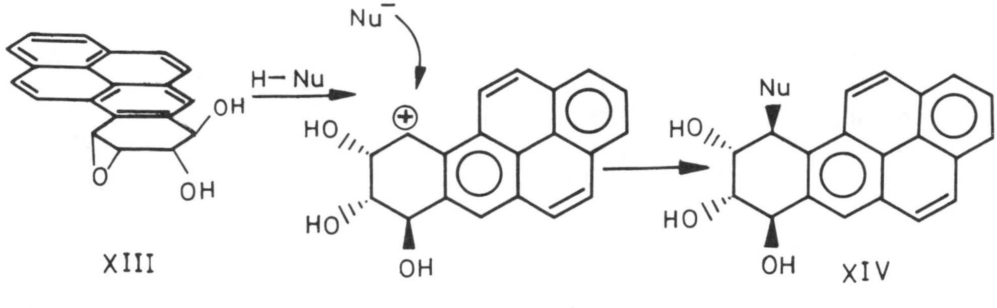

FIGURE 18. Nucleophilic attack by a generalized nucleophile H—Nu on the bay-region diol-epoxide XIII of BaP.

The mechanism of the ring opening during the bonding of the ultimate carcinogen to DNA is shown in general form in Scheme XIII and XIV; XII is a particular case of XIV.

Deviations from planarity, induced by substituents such as the methyl in the highly carcinogenic 5-methylchrysene, XV, may also play a part (by contrast, the unsubstituted chrysene and its other four monomethyl-derivatives are weakly carcinogenic); only in the 5-methyl-derivative is steric hindrance present. Thus, the methyl group enhances the kinetic stabilization of the positive charge adjacent to the bay-region.

Apart from quantum-chemical calculations which indeed show a high degree of stabi-

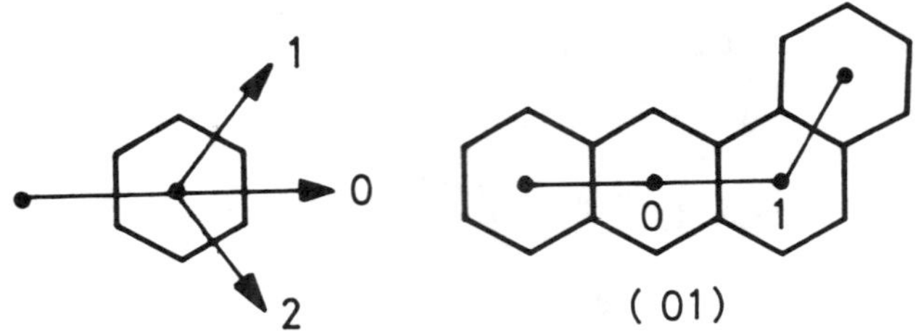

FIGURE 19.   Enhancement of the reactivity of 5-methylchrysene due to steric hindrance around the bay-region.

FIGURE 20.   Annelation of a terminal benzenoid ring in a PAH may occur in three directions, denoted by 0, 1, or 2; these digits allow an unambiguous coding of cata-condensed PAHs, as shown for benz(a)anthracene and its dualist graph.

lization for the bay-region cations, topological correlations between chemical structure and the carcinogenicity of PAHs were also published.

For topological specification of the structure of PAHs several systems were proposed from which we shall mention only four:

1. The very first system was proposed by Balaban and Harary;[65-67] and can be used for cata-condensed systems (catafusenes), i.e., those PAHs which have no carbon atom common to three benzo rings; when such carbon atoms do exist, the system is peri-condensed (perifusene). Annelating a benzene ring to yield a catafusene may occur in three ways, specified by digits 0, 1, 2 for 180°, 120° or 240° angles, respectively. The structure of the catafusene is uniquely determined by its *dualist graph,* whose vertices are the centers of the hexagons and whose edges correspond to condensed hexagons (i.e., hexagons sharing two carbon atoms). Thus, dualist graphs of catafusenes are trees while those of perifusenes have three-membered rings; unlike usual graphs where the length and direction of edges do not matter, they do matter in dualist graphs. A unique code is attached to a dualist graph by the convention that the direction of annelation from one end of the nonbranched catafusene to the other be specified by the digits 0, 1, 2 which on being read sequentially afford the smallest number; thus the dualist graph of benz(a)anthracene VIII is coded by 01 (and not by 02, 10 or 20, which are the three other possibilities, because these correspond to larger numbers). For branched catafusenes, the branch digits are included in brackets according to other conventions.[67]

For a series of cata- and perifusenes, using the above coding, Balasubramanian, Kaufman, Koski and Balaban[68] published the first paper aiming at the enumeration of all possible PAHs possessing bay-regions. A computer program for generating all possible cata-condensed PAHs and selected perifusenes was elaborated and implemented for PAHs with up to nine benzenoid rings. In the paper,[68] all PAHs with bay-regions and up to six benzenoid rings are presented. Bay-regions are detected by

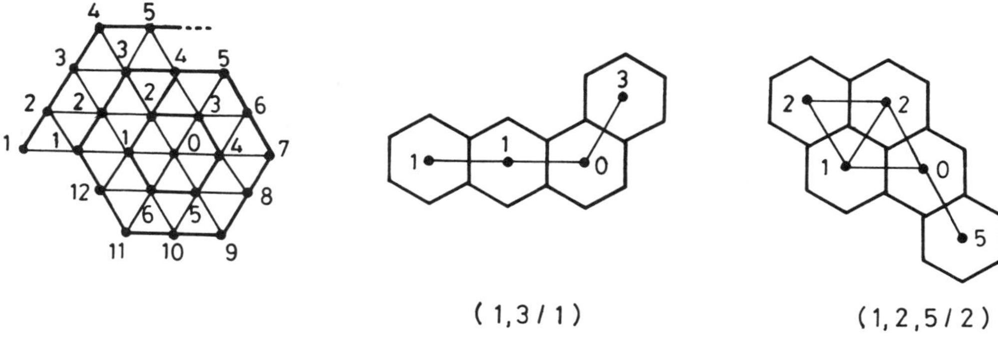

(1,3 / 1)   (1,2,5 / 2)

FIGURE 21.   Topological centric coding of PAHs by means of their dualist graphs: vertices of these dualist graphs (except for the center denoted by zero and absent from the final notation) are arranged in shells around the center, and separated by slashes for each shell; examples are benz(a)anthracene and benzo(a)pyrene with their coding.

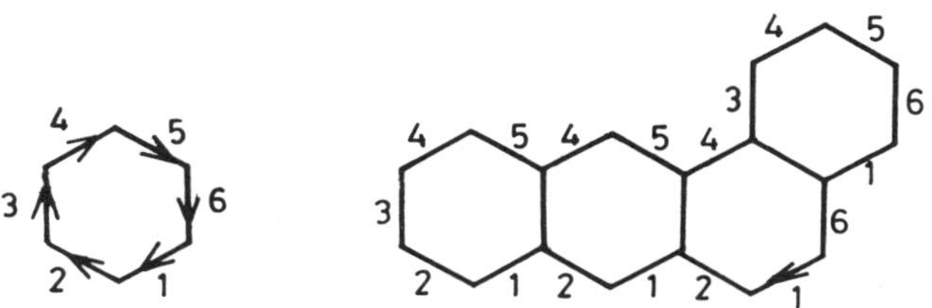

FIGURE 22.   Conventions for coding edge directions in PAHs (left-hand formula); application for the boundary code of benz(a)anthracene, starting with the edge bearing an arrow because in this case the minimal number is obtained.

scanning the code from left to right; a bay is present if the code of the i-th vertex is 1 or 2, and the degree of the ith vertex, or the vertices two edges away from the i-th vertex, is 1.

2.   Recently, this code was modified by Knop et al.[69,69a] for also including pericondensed systems. The digits are now 1, 2, 4, and they represent the ordering in the three directions: 60° to the left (2), straightforward (1) and 60° to the right (4). These digits are summed in pericondensed systems so that if there are hexagons in all three directions, then the entry is maximum, i.e., 7. If there are no hexagons in any of three directions, the entry is zero. The code for PAHs can never start with a zero. This coding procedure has been implemented by a computer program.

3.   Any PAH (catafusene or perifusene) may be coded according to Bonchev and Balaban[70] using the topological center of the dualist graph of the PAH. One finds this center according to a definite algorithm, and lists the other vertices by their numbers in successive shells around the center. The PAH is depicted so as to have two vertical C-C bonds for each ring; then its dualist graph will cover a position of the triangulated plane. The superposition is done according to certain rules leading to the minimal numbers in various shells around the center (denoted by zero, and not explicitly indicated in the code); the occupied vertices of the triangulated plane are specified in each shell in increasing order, and separated by slashes.

4.   For a PAH written as indicated above with two vertical C-C bonds for each ring, all edges are oriented according to one of three possible orientations;[71] if a sense is assigned to any line, then there are six possibilities of labeling the contour of any PAH; this observation was used by Balaban[71] and later by Trinajstić and co-workers[72-76] for specifying the structure of a PAH by its boundary code (again with the convention of

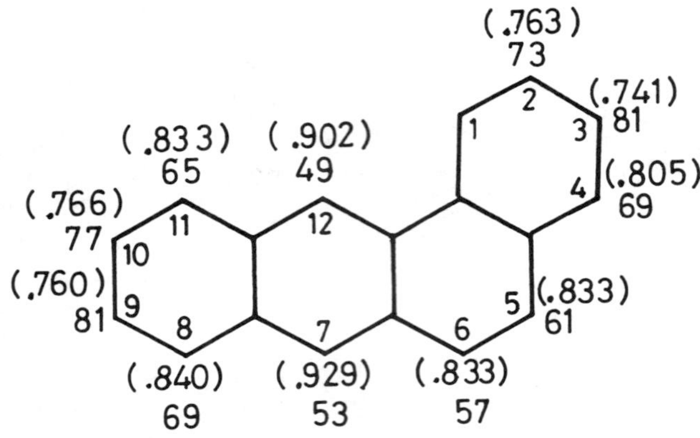

FIGURE 23.   For benz(a)anthracene with the IUPAC numbering of CH groups (inner numbers), the distance sums s_i (outer integer numbers) correlate well with ΔE_{deloc} (in brackets).

starting the code at a vertex leading to the minimal number). A computer program was developed and applied for generating all PAHs; in particular, it was possible to identify all PAHs with bay-regions.[74-76] Thus benz(a)anthracene has the boundary code 121212345454345616. The results of the two computer programs coincide insofar as the former[68] also counted helicenes (geometrically nonplanar PAHs) while the latter program[74-76] excluded them. Phenyltriazenes and *para*-triazeno-benzoic acids have tumor-inhibiting properties; topological correlations[31,51a] rationalized their activities: thus the information content accounts for 80% of the variance for triazeno-benzoic acids.[32]

VIII. TOPOLOGY AND MUTAGENICITY

Chapter 1 contained a detailed discussion of quantum-mechanical methods for calculating ΔE_{deloc} in carbocations derived from diol-epoxides of PAHs. It was shown by Lowe and Silverman[77] that good correlations exist between ΔE_{deloc} and tumor-initiating activities of monomethylderivatives or monoaza-derivatives derived from such PAHs as benzo(a)pyrene or benzo(a)anthracene.

A fairly simple correlation was found by Seybold[78] between the distance sums (which can be regarded as LOVIs) and the relative stabilities of carbocations which in turn determine the carcinogenic activities of ultimate carcinogens (PAH diol-epoxides).

Thus, benz(a)anthracene presents the ΔE_{deloc} (β units) indicated in brackets and the distance sums indicated outside the rings; numberings of the various positions are indicated inside the rings. It is apparent that the highest ΔE_{deloc} values correspond to the lowest distance sums, in positions 7 and 12. A negative correlation coefficient r = 0.869 was found. Substitution by methyl or hydroxy groups at positions with the highest distance sums lead to the highest carcinogenic activities. Also, ring fusion effects on carcinogenicity show good correlations with topological data of the edge on which a benzenoid ring is added.[78]

The ''graph distance complexity'' is a TI proposed by Raychaudhury, Basak et al.[30-32] It is based on the distances in a graph, and is obtained from the value of the ''vertex distance complexity'' which is a measure of the information content of a vertex on the basis of the distances of all vertices from that vertex.

Klopman and Raychaudhury used the above LOVI for identifying regions (or substructures) in the molecules (or molecular graphs) which may be used to determine mutagenic properties in nonfused-ring aromatic compounds. A training set of 200 compounds (114 actives and 86 inactives) were screened for mutagenicity using *Salmonella typhimurium* strain TA100 without S9 activation and the result was expressed as revertants/nmol.[79]

Chemical structures included nitro-, amino-, ether-, halo-, carboxy-, hydroxy- and formyl-derivatives of benzene and biphenyl as well as systems containing more than one of the above substituents; 183 of the 200 compounds were classified correctly by using the KLN algorithm, and only two of the misclassified compounds are highly mutagenic.

The test set consisted of 33 more compounds (20 active and 13 inactive), and it was found that 28 of these compounds, including all those that were highly mutagenic were classified correctly.[79]

An excellent review was published by Klopman and co-workers[80] on QSAR for mutagens and carcinogens, emphasizing correlations using physical property variables (hydrophobicity according to Hansch, steric parameters) or using pattern recognition techniques (SIMCA method which employs Hansch parameters, the ADAPT program which was developed by Jurs, Enslein's approach, and Klopman's CASE program which are both based on substructures. These aspects are treated in more detail in Chapter 3. Here it should be mentioned that the CASE program shows that additional features (presence of bay-region *and* a few other structural conditions) are necessary and sufficient for carcinogenic activity of polycyclic aromatic hydrocarbons. A recent paper[81] describes new vertex indices (distance exponent indices) or previously described indices (vertex distance complexity or its normalized counterpart) used for correlating the antileukemic activity of 9-anilinoacridines (100 compounds in the training set and 50 compounds in the test set) identifying quite effectively the biologically relevant vertices.

REFERENCES

1. **Balaban, A. T., Ed.,** *Chemical Applications of Graph Theory,* Academic Press, London, 1976.
1a. **Read, A. C.,** Enumeration of acyclic chemical compounds, *Chemical Applications of Graph Theory,* Balaban, A. T., Ed., Academic Press, London, 1976, 24.
1b. **Balaban, A. T.,** Enumeration of cyclic graphs, *Chemical Applications of Graph Theory,* Academic Press, London, 1976, 163.
1c. **Dubois, J. E.,** Ordered chromatic graphs and limited environment concepts, *Chemical Applications of Graph Theory,* Balaban, A. T., Ed., Academic Press, London, 1976, 333.
2. **Wiswesser, W. J.,** *A Line-Formula Chemical Notation,* Crowell, New York, 1954.
3. **Randić, M.,** On molecular identification numbers, *J. Chem. Inf. Comput. Sci.,* 24, 164, 1984.
4. **Randić, M.,** Graph-theoretical approach to structure-activity studies: search for optimal antitumor compounds, in *Molecular Basis of Cancer. Part A. Macromolecular Structure, Carcinogens, and Oncogens,* Rein, R., Ed., Alan R. Liss, New York, 1985, 309.
5. **Randić, M., Brissey, G. M., Spencer, R. B., and Wilkins, C. L.,** Use of self-avoiding paths for characterization of molecular graphs with multiple bonds, *Comput. Chem.,* 4, 27, 1980.
6. **Randić, M.,** Prime molecular identification numbers, *J. Chem. Inf. Comput. Sci.,* 26, 134, 1986.
7. **Wiener, H.,** Structural determination of paraffin boiling points, *J. Am. Chem. Soc.,* 69, 17, 1947.
8. **Wiener, H.,** Correlation of heats of isomerization, and differences in heats of vaporization of isomers, among paraffin hydrocarbons, *J. Am. Chem. Soc.,* 69, 2636, 1947.
9. **Wiener, H.,** Influence of interatomic forces on paraffin properties, *J. Chem. Phys.,* 15, 766, 1947.
10. **Gutman, I., Ruščić, M., Trinajstić, N., and Wilcox, C. F., Jr.,** Graph theory and molecular orbitals. XII. Acyclic polyenes, *J. Chem. Phys.,* 62, 3339, 1975.
11. **Randić, M.,** On characterization of molecular branching, *J. Am. Chem. Soc.,* 97, 6609, 1975.
12. **Randić, M.,** Graph-theoretical analysis of structure-property and structure-activity correlations, *Int. J. Quantum Chem., Quantum Chem. Symp.,* 5, 245, 1978.
13. **Kier, L. B., Hall, L. H., Murray, W. F., and Randić, M.,** Molecular connectivity. I. Relation to nonspecific local anesthesia, *J. Pharm. Sci.,* 64, 1971, 1985.
14. **Kier, L. B., Murray, W. J., Randić, M., and Hall, L. H.,** Molecular connectivity. V. Connectivity series concept applied to density, *J. Pharm. Sci.,* 65, 1226, 1976.

15. **Bonchev, D. and Trinajstić, N.,** Information theory, distance matrix, and molecular branching, *J. Chem. Phys.,* 67, 4517, 1977.
16. **Bonchev, D. and Trinajstić, N.,** On topological characterization of molecular branching, *Int. J. Quantum Chem., Quantum Chem. Symp.,* 12, 293, 1978.
17. **Bonchev, D., Mekenyan, O., and Trinajstić, N.,** Isomer discrimination by topological information approach, *J. Comput. Chem.,* 2, 127, 1981.
18. **Bertz, S. H.,** Branching in graphs and molecules, *Discrete Appl. Math.,* 19, 65, 1988.
19. **Balaban, A. T.,** Chemical graphs. Part 34. Five new topological indices for the branching of tree-like graphs, *Theor. Chem. Acta (Berlin),* 53, 355, 1979.
20. **Bonchev, D., Balaban, A. T., and Randić, M.,** The graph center concept for polycyclic graphs, *Int. J. Quantum Chem.,* 19, 61, 1981.
21. **Bonchev, D., Mekenyan, O., and Balaban, A. T.,** Iterative procedure for the generalized graph center in polycyclic graphs, *J. Chem. Inf. Comput. Sci.,* 29, 91, 1989.
22. **Balaban, A. T.,** Topological indices based on topological distances in molecular graphs, *Pure Appl. Chem.,* 55, 199, 1983.
23. **Balaban, A. T. and Moţoc, I.,** Chemical graphs. Part 36. Correlations between octane numbers and topological indices of alkanes, *Math. Chem. (MATCH),* 5, 197, 1979.
24. **Balaban, A. T.,** Highly discriminating distance-based topological index, *Chem. Phys. Lett.,* 89, 399, 1982.
25. **Balaban, A. T.,** Chemical graphs, Part 48. Topological index J for heteroatom-containing molecules taking into account periodicities of element properties, *Math. Chem. (MATCH),* 21, 115, 1986.
26. **Balaban, A. T. and Filip, P.,** Computer program for topological index J, *Math. Chem. (MATCH),* 16, 183, 1984.
27. **Balaban, A. T. and Quintas, L. V.,** The smallest graphs, trees, and 4-trees with degenerate topological index J, *Math. Chem. (MATCH),* 14, 213, 1983.
28. **Balaban, A. T., Ionescu-Pallas, V., and Balaban, T. S.,** Asymptotic values of topological indices J and J′ (average distance sum connectivities) for infinite acyclic and cyclic graphs, *Math. Chem. (MATCH),* 17, 121, 1985.
29. **Filip, P. A., Balaban, T. S., and Balaban, A. T.,** A new approach for devising local graph invariants: derived topological indices with low degeneracy and good correlation ability, *J. Math. Chem.,* 1, 61, 1987.
30. **Raychaudhury, C., Ray, S. K., Ghosh, J. J., Roy, A. B., and Basak, S. C.,** Discrimination of isomeric structures using information theoretic topological indices, *J. Comput. Chem.,* 5, 581, 1984.
31. **Ray, S. K., Basak, S. C., Raychaudhury, C., Roy, A. B., and Ghosh, J. J.,** A quantitative structure-activity relationship study of tumor-inhibitory triazenes using bonding information content and lipophilicity, *IRCS Med. Sci.,* 10, 933, 1982.
32. **Ray, S. K., Basak, S. C., Raychaudhury, C., Roy, A. B., and Ghosh, J. J.,** The utility of information content, structural information content, hydrophobicity and Van der Waals volume in the design of barbiturates and tumor-inhibitory triazenes, *Arzneim. Forsch.,* 33, 352, 1983.
32a. **Klopman, G. and Raychaudhury, C.,** Vertex indices of molecular graphs in structure-activity relationships: a study of the convulsant-anticonvulsant activity of barbiturates and the carcinogenicity of unsubstituted polycyclic aromatic hydrocarbons, *J. Chem. Inf. Comput. Sci.,* 30, 12, 1990.
33. **Balaban, A. T. and Balaban, T. S.,** New vertex invariants and topological indices of chemical graphs based on information on distances, *J. Math. Chem.,* in press.
34. **Diudea, M. V., Minailiuc, O., and Balaban, A. T.,** Molecular topology. IV. Regressive vertex degrees (new graph invariants) and derived topological indices, *J. Comput. Chem.,* in press.
35. **Sabljić, A. and Trinajstić, N.,** QSAR — the role of topological indices, *Acta Pharm. Jugosl.,* 31, 189, 1981.
36. **Stankevich, M. I., Stankevich, I. V., and Zefirov, N. S.,** Topological indices in organic chemistry, *Usp. Khim.,* 57, 337, 1988.
37. **Hansen, P. J. and Jurs, P. C.,** Chemical applications of graph theory. Part I. Fundamentals and topological indices, *J. Chem. Educ.,* 65, 574, 1988.
38. **Rouvray, D. H.,** The challenge of characterizing branching in molecular species, *Discrete Appl. Math.,* 19, 317, 1988.
39. **Rouvray, D. H.,** The modelling of chemical phenomena using topological indices, *J. Comput. Chem.,* 8, 470, 1987.
40. **Rouvray, D. H.,** The prediction of biological activity using molecular connectivity indexes, *Acta Pharm. Jugosl.,* 36, 239, 1986.
41. **Rouvray, D. H.,** Predicting chemistry from topology, *Sci. Am.,* 254, No. 9, 40, 1986.
42. **Balaban, A. T., Chiriac, A., Moţoc, I., and Simon, Z.,** *Steric Fit in Quantitative Structure-Activity Relations,* Lecture Notes in Chemistry No. 15, Springer-Verlag, Berlin, 1980, 22.
43. **Balaban, A. T., Moţoc, I., Bonchev, D., and Mekenyan, O.,** Topological indices for structure-activity correlations, *Top. Curr. Chem.,* 114, 21, 1983.
44. **Rouvray, D. H. and Balaban, A. T.,** Chemical applications of graph theory, in *Applications of Graph Theory,* Wilson, R. J. and Beineke, L. W., Ed., Academic Press, London, 1979, 177.

45. **Trinajstić, N.,** *Chemical Graph Theory,* Vol. 2, CRC Press, Boca Raton, FL, 1983, 105.

46. **Balaban, A. T.,** Applications of graph theory in chemistry, *J. Chem. Inf. Comput. Sci.,* 25, 334, 1985.

47. **Kier, L. B. and Hall, L. H.,** *Molecular Connectivity in Chemistry and Drug Research,* Academic Press, New York, 1976.

48. **Kier, L. B. and Hall, L. H.,** *Molecular Connectivity in Structure-Activity Analysis,* Research Studies Press, Letchworth, England, 1986.

49. **Bonchev, D.,** *Theoretic Information Indices for Characterization of Molecular Structures,* Research Studies Press, Chichester, England, 1983.

50. **Szymanski, K., Müller, W. R., Knop, J. V., and Trinajstić, N.,** On the identification number for chemical structures, *Int. J. Quantum Chem., Quantum Chem. Symp.,* 20, 173, 1986.

51. **Balaban, A. T.,** Numerical modelling of chemical substances: local graph invariants, and topological indices, in *Graph Theory and Topology in Chemistry,* King, R. B. and Rouvray, D. H., Eds., Elsevier, Amsterdam, 1987, 159.

51a. **Carter, S., Nikolić, S., and Trinajstić, N.,** A QSAR study of the anti-tumoric activity of phenyltriazenes, in *MATH/CHEM/COMP, 1988,* Elsevier, Amsterdam, 1989.

52. **Carter, S., Trinajstić, N., and Nikolić, S.,** A note on the use of ID numbers in QSAR studies, *Acta Pharm. Jugosl.,* 37, 37, 1987.

53. **Broto, P., Moreau, G., and Vandyke, C.,** Autocorrelation of logic or of spatial structures: a means for quantitative comparison, in *QSAR Design of Bioactive Compounds,* Prous, K. M., Ed., Barcelona, 1984, 393.

54. **Henry, D., Jurs, P. C., and Denny, W. A.,** Structure-antitumor activity relationships of 9-anilinoacridines using pattern recognition, *J. Med. Chem.,* 25, 899, 1982.

55. **Jurs, P. C., Chou, J. T., and Yuan, M.,** Computer-assisted structure-activity studies of chemical carcinogens. A heterogeneous data set, *J. Med. Chem.,* 22, 476, 1979.

56. **Dubois, J. E. and Sobel, Y.,** DARC System for documentation and artificial intelligence in chemistry, *J. Chem. Inf. Comput. Sci.,* 25, 326, 1985.

57. **Mercier, C. and Dubois, J. E.,** Comparison of molecular connectivity and DARC/PELCO methods: performance in antimicrobial, halogenated phenol QSARs, *Eur. J. Med. Chem. Ther.,* 14, 415, 1979.

58. **Duperray, B., Chastrette, M., Cohen-Makabeth, M., and Paceco, H.,** Comparative analysis of Hansch, Free-Wilson and DARC/PELCO correlations in a bactericide series — halophenols, *Eur. J. Med. Chem. Ther.,* 11, 323, 1976.

59. **Hall, L. H. and Kier, L. B.,** A comparative analysis of Hansch, Free-Wilson and DARC/PELCO methods in the structure-activity relationship of halogenated phenols, *Eur. J. Med. Chem. Ther.,* 13, 89, 1978.

60. **Tang, Wing-Sum and Griffin, G. W.,** *Metabolic Activation of Polynuclear Aromatic Hydrocarbons,* Pergamon Press, Oxford, 1979.

61. **Pullman, A. and Pullman, B.,** Electronic structure and carcinogenic activity of aromatic molecules, *Adv. Cancer Res.,* 3, 117, 1955.

62. **Herndon, W. C.,** Theory of carcinogenic activity of aromatic hydrocarbons, *Trans. N.Y. Acad. Sci.,* 36, 200, 1974.

63. **Jerina, D. M. and Daly, J. W.,** Arene oxides. New aspects of drug metabolism, *Science,* 185, 573, 1974.

64. **Harvey, R. G.,** Activated metabolites of carcinogenic hydrocarbons, *Acc. Chem. Res.,* 14, 218, 1981.

65. **Balaban, A. T. and Harary, F.,** Chemical graphs. V. Enumeration and proposed nomenclature of benzenoid cata-condensed polycyclic aromatic hydrocarbons, *Tetrahedron,* 24, 2505, 1968.

66. **Balaban, A. T.,** Chemical graphs. VII. Proposed nomenclature of branched cata-condensed benzenoid hydrocarbons, *Tetrahedron,* 25, 2949, 1969.

67. **Balaban, A. T.,** Challenging problems involving benzenoid polycyclics and related systems, *Pure Appl. Chem.,* 54, 1075, 1982.

68. **Balasubramanian, K., Kaufman, J. J., Koski, W. S., and Balaban, A. T.,** Graph-theoretical characterization and computer generation of certain carcinogenic benzenoid hydrocarbons and identification of bay-regions, *J. Comput. Chem.,* 1, 149, 1980.

69. **Müller, W. R., Szymanski, K., Knop, J. V., Nikolić, S., and Trinajstić, N.,** On counting polyhex hydrocarbons, *Croat. Chem. Acta,* 62, 481, 1989.

69a. **Müller, W. R., Szymanski, K., Knop, J. V., Nikolić, S., and Trinajstić, N.,** On the enumeration and generation of polyhex hydrocarbons, *J. Comput. Chem.,* 11, 223, 1990.

70. **Bonchev, D. and Balaban, A. T.,** Topological centric coding and nomenclature of polycyclic hydrocarbons. I. Condensed benzenoid systems (polyhexes, fusenes), *J. Chem. Inf. Comput. Sci.,* 21, 2, 1981.

71. **Balaban, A. T.,** Chemical graphs. Part 12. Configurations of annulenes, *Tetrahedron,* 26, 6115, 1971.

72. **Dzonova-Jerman-Blazić, B., and Trinajstić, N.,** Computer-aided enumeration and generation of Kekulé structures in conjugated hydrocarbons, *Comput. Chem.,* 6, 121, 1982.

73. **Dzonova-Jerman-Blazić, B., and Trinajstić, N.,** Application of reduced graph model to the enumeration of Kekulé structures and conjugated circuits of benzenoid hydrocarbons, *Croat. Chem. Acta,* 55, 347, 1982.

74. **Knop, J. V., Szymanski, K., Jeričević, Z., and Trinajstić, N.,** Computer enumeration and generation of benzenoid hydrocarbons and identification of bay-regions, *J. Comput. Chem.,* 4, 23, 1983.

75. **Knop, J. V., Szymanski, K., Jeričević, Z., and Trinajstić, N.,** Computer generation and identification of carcinogenic bay-regions in benzenoid hydrocarbons, *Int. J. Quantum Chem.*, 23, 713, 1983.
76. **Knop, J. V., Müller, W. R., Szymanski, K., and Trinajstić, N.,** *Computer Generation of Certain Classes of Molecules,* Kemija u Industriji, Zagreb, 1985.
77. **Lowe, J. P. and Silverman, B. D.,** Predicting carcinogenicity of polycyclic aromatic hydrocarbons, *Acc. Chem. Res.*, 17, 332, 1984.
78. **Seybold, P. G.,** Topological influences on the carcinogenicity of aromatic hydrocarbons. I. The bay-region geometry, *Int. J. Quantum Chem., Quant. Biol. Symp.*, 10, 95, 1983; II. Substituent effects, *ibid.*, 10, 103, 1983.
79. **Klopman, G. and Raychaudhury, C.,** A novel approach to the use of graph theory in structure-activity relationship studies. Application to the qualitative evaluation of mutagenicity in a series of nonfused ring aromatic compounds, *J. Comput. Chem.*, 9, 232, 1988.
80. **Frierson, M. R., Klopman, G., and Rosenkranz, H. S.,** Structure-activity relationships (SARs) among mutagens and carcinogens: a review, *Environ. Mutagenesis*, 8, 283, 1986.
81. **Raychaudhury, C. and Klopman, G.,** New vertex indices and their applications in evaluating antileukemic activity of 9-anilinoacridines and the activity of 2′,3′-dideoxy-nucleosides against HIV, *Bull. Soc. Chim. Belg.*, 99, 255, 1990.

Chapter 5

QSAR (SAR) MODELS AND THEIR USE FOR CARCINOGENIC POTENCY PREDICTION

Ion Niculescu-Duvăz, Dan A. Ciubotariu, Zeno Simon, and Nicolae Voiculetz

TABLE OF CONTENTS

I. INTRODUCTION

Since the first articles of Hansch,[1] several textbooks on this subject (to mention only two recent ones[2,3]) as well as many reviews appeared, testifying its success for practical drug design.[4,5] A recent review on structure-activity relationships for mutagens and carcinogens may also be cited.[6]

The scope of this section is to analyze the various QSAR techniques examining what can be expected from them in the carcinogen area, taking into account the peculiarities of effector-receptor interactions in this domain. A brief presentation of techniques used for the QSAR analysis and especially for those methods emphasized in this chapter will follow. Some of these procedures were previously reported by the present authors and co-workers.

Several classifications were proposed for structure-activity relationship techniques. Frierson et al.[6] divided them into thermodynamic approaches and connectivity approaches.* The former ones emphasize the physical properties of the molecules and are the basis of "classical" QSAR. The latter point out the atomic or fragment construction of molecules and, while handling nocongenerie databases, often refer only to a classification of compounds into active or inactive ones. Trinajstiĉ et al.[7] classify QSAR approaches into three groups: (1) structure-cryptic, often involving a large number of parameters used in multiparametric linear correlation analysis; (2) structure-implicit, typically quantum chemistry calculations of various degrees of sophistication and (3) structure-explicit, in which structures are characterized by selected structural invariants which are subsequently used for representations of chemical structure (see Figure 1). A criticism of this elegant classification is that no clear distinction between models and methodology was made. For instance, if an extrathermodynamic approach such as that developed by Hansch (using lipophilicity, molar refractivity, Taft parameters) is clearly a cryptic model, the same formalism using MTD or shape descriptors is an explicit one.

Other classifications are also possible. For instance, from the point of view of the sophistication of the computer techniques used, the "classical" Hansch-type QSARs or those using minimal steric (topologic) differences, MTD[8,9] are relatively simple. Methods based upon computation of effector-receptor interaction energies, as the distance geometry approach[10] or the comparative molecular field analysis (CoMFA) method[11] are much more sophisticated. Pattern-recognition methods[12] use logic algebra-based techniques. More recently the methods using dichotomous parameters as independent variables are termed SAR, because no physical meaning could be assigned to the relationship between the value of the obtained endpoint and the dose producing this effect.

The physiological action of drugs is based upon a receptor-effector[13] interaction. If drug transport and decay are not rate-limiting and especially if the receptor-effector equilibrium is measured directly, the structure-activity relationship is actually describing the affinity for the active conformation of the receptor as a function of structural features of effector molecules (expressed explicitly or implicitly by selected physical or structural parameters). In this sense, QSAR and SAR are interesting not only for drug design, but also for the mechanisms of drug-receptor interaction and for the relevant structural features of the receptor site. On the other hand, if predictions for a broad type of activity (such as carcinogenesis as a general phenomenon), based upon several types of mechanisms are needed, success may be expected only from "pattern recognition", or "connectivity" approaches and a contribution to the mechanism of action can hardly be expected.

Even the connectivity methods have apparent serious shortcomings because the mechanisms of action in a structurally heterogenous series of compounds is certainly different, and it is not sure that a combination of "good" descriptors will lead to an active compound. Another criticism consists in the fact that some ambiguity is linked to the concept of chemical

---

* This classification is also used in the present report.

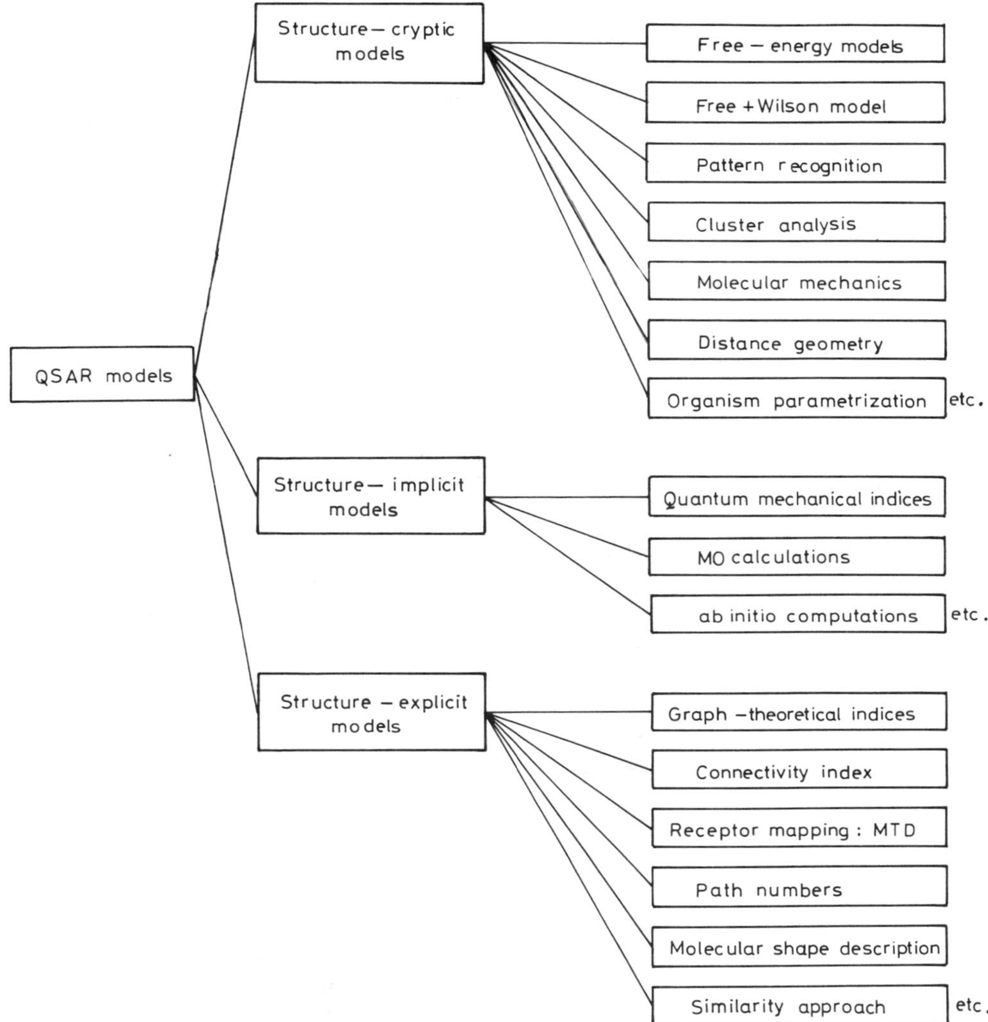

FIGURE 1.   Classification of QSAR techniques according to Trinajstič[7].

structure which in different areas of chemistry is used in different contexts and with different meanings.[14] More important is the fact that topological methods such as the connectivity approach ignore stereochemistry.

II. METHODOLOGY OF QSAR APPROACHES

The methodology employed in the QSAR approaches is of paramount importance for the quality of the expected results. The methodologies employed are summarized in Table 1.

A clear distinction has to be made, however, between the methodology and the computation techniques employed in such approaches. Thus, if in the framework of methodology can be included extrathermodynamic, multiparametric, or connectivity models, each being able to be visualized in 2D- or 3D-spaces, the computation techniques are much more numerous. The techniques most frequently used are multiple regression analysis (MRA) (which in turn can be multiliniar, parabolic, polynomial, transcendental, etc.), cluster anal-

TABLE 1
Methodology of QSAR Approaches[a]

Parameters used	Extrathermodynamic methods and multiparametric analysis	Connectivity methods	2-D or 3-D
Transport:			
π, log P	X	X	X
Electronic:			
Quantum mechanical indices	X	X	X
Steric:			
Topological indices, receptor mapping, path numbers, fragment descriptor, molecular shape descriptors, etc.	X	X	X

[a] From the point of view of mathematical techniques involved, these are multivariate statistical analysis, numerical optimization methods and artificial intelligence pattern recognition procedures.

ysis, factor and discriminant analysis, pattern recognition, etc. In addition to these, a number of statistic methods (more or less method-specific) were developed for evaluating the significance of the correlations thus obtained. However, the most important elements of all these correlational approaches are the parameters (especially the biological ones) employed as database.

This chapter will be organized taking into account the methodologies and the parameters used for predicting carcinogenic properties of various types of chemicals. A brief theoretical description of these approaches is reported.

A. EXTRATHERMODYNAMIC APPROACHES

Modern approaches for the design of bioactive molecules such as drugs, insecticides, herbicides, and fungicides are based on the quantification of bioactivity as a function of molecular structure. The seeds of this concept lie in the work of Meyer[15] and Overton[16] who successfully demonstrated a dependence of bioactivity on the partition coefficient, which is a function of molecular structure. Vital to the development of the field was the concept of the receptor site, adumbrated by the work of Longley stated and developed by Ehrlich (cited after[17]). Biological activity, according to this model, depends on the recognition of a bioactive substrate (*bas*) by a receptor site, followed by binding of the *bas* to the receptor site. The correlation between bioactivity and the configuration of the substrate led to the recognition of the fact that steric effects have a significant contribution to the strength of a *bas* binding.[18]

In a parallel development, the effects of the structure of *meta* or *para*-substituted benzene derivatives on their chemical reactivity and physical properties were expressed and modeled quantitatively by the Hammett equation.[19] The topic is well reviewed by Shorter,[20] who applied the Hammett equation to biological activities, while Zahradnik suggested an alternative analogous equation.[17]

The extrathermodynamic approach to structure-activity correlations was based on the Hammett relationship.

A quantitative relationship was found which expresses the effect exerted by the *para*- and *meta*-substituents of the benzenic nucleus on the reaction center. If, for instance, we represent the logarithm of the hydrolysis rate (k_x) of the ethylic esters of a number of substituted benzoic acids vs. the logarithm of the dissociation constants (K_x = pKa) of their corresponding acids a straight line results. This line could be expressed as:

$$\log k_x = \rho \log K_x + b \tag{1}$$

where ρ and b are regression coefficients.

If we divide both constants with their corresponding values for the unsubstituted congeners, respectively, Equation 1 becomes:

$$\log \frac{k_X}{k_H} = \log \frac{K_X}{K_H} + b \tag{2}$$

Mention should be made that both K and k can be related to free energy.

$$\Delta G = -RT\ln K \tag{3a}$$

$$\Delta G^{\neq} = -RT\ln k \tag{3b}$$

($\Delta G^{\neq}$ being the activation free-energy).

Starting from Equation 2, the electronic effect exerted by a substituent X on the benzoic acid acidity could be defined as:

$$\sigma_x = \log \frac{K_X}{K_H} \tag{4}$$

Therefore, Equation 2 could be rewritten as

$$\log \frac{k_X}{k_H} = \rho\sigma + b \tag{5}$$

This relation is known as the Hammett equation.

Such σ constants were expressed only for *meta*-σ_m- and *para*-σ_p positions because they represent the electronic effect exerted by the substituent X on the reaction center. In *ortho* position the steric effect, existing especially when a bulky substituent is located in this position, disturbs the electronic effect exerted on the reaction center.

A major step forward is due to the work of Hansch and Fujita,[21] who showed that a correlational equation accounting for both electronic and hydrophobic effects would successfully model bioactivities. In later works, steric parameters were included.

The classical Hansch equation expresses the biological activity as a function of the transport (hydrophobicity) parameter (π), the electronic effect (expressed by σ) and the steric parameter (E_s). The equation thus obtained is:

$$-\log c = a_1 + a_2\pi + a_3\sigma + a_4 \cdot E_s \tag{6}$$

where the biological activity is expressed by means of the dose (concentration, c) giving a standard biological effect; a_1, a_2 . . . a_4 are coefficients computed by the multilinear regression technique. This expression involved the following implicit assumptions regarding the mechanism of action of a chemical compound.

1. The transport from the site of entry in the organism to the target takes place across one or more barriers. This step is expressed by means of the parameter $\log P$ (or π); the rate of transport through biological barriers (i.e., membranes) is proportional to this parameter.

2.   Its biological action is expressed following its recognition by a receptor (enzyme). This substrate-receptor interaction is the step triggering the expression of the pharmacological properties.

Any of these steps may be bioactivity-determining. In many cases, the use of transport terms as a parabolic function as in Equation 7 gives better results:

$$-\log c = a_1 + a_2\pi + a_2'\pi^2 + a_3\sigma + a_4E_s \qquad (7)$$

All these equations (Equations 6, 7) employ parameters which have in common an ultimate relation to thermodynamic quantities, even though they cannot be derived directly from the postulates of formal thermodynamics. For this reason they have been called extrathermodynamic quantities and the corresponding equations are linear free-energy relationships.

The basic requirements for a significant QSAR analysis by this procedure are

1.   The investigated compounds should be structural analogs, acting by the same mechanism of action (congeneric database).
2.   Reliable physicochemical or structural parameters should be available for each of them.
3.   The number of congeners must be large enough so that statistical methods are applicable.
4.   The biological assay (used as dependent variable) must be reproducible; this is one of the most critical points of QSAR approaches.

Despite the wide use of the Hansch procedure (a wide range of different parameters being employed) some important limitations may be cited:

1.   Selected parameters are not unique, because different parameters can produce the same results, within the accepted tolerance.[22]
2.   Not all parameters are orthogonal.[23,24] For instance, a certain degree of correlation exists between the hydrophobicity substituent constant π and E_s (steric parameter) and even with some electronic or quantum mechanical parameters, since for polycyclic aromatic hydrocarbons all depends on atomic superdelocalizabilities.[25]
3.   Some parameters have no physical interpretation.
4.   The procedure requires a congeneric database.

Hansch's model is probably the most frequently used in QSAR analysis. However, in some applications the loss of its extrathermodynamic character could be noticed, because despite the maintaining of the computational Hansch formalism, parameters which cannot be considered of a strictly thermodynamic nature were introduced (e.g., some steric parameters, indicator variables, topological indices, etc.).

Thus, although the use of such parameters is entirely justified, the equation is no more a linear free-energy relationship, becoming instead a multiparametric correlation model. The equation of such a model is formally of the same nature, namely:

$$Y_i = a + \sum_{j=1}^{n} b_j P_{i,j} \qquad (8)$$

where Y_i are values of a variable measured for a series of i compounds (e.g., biological activity), and $P_{i,j}$ are independent parameters (factors); a is a constant, and b_j represents the susceptibility of Y_i against a generalized P_j parameter.

This model (as well as Hansch's equation) allows the prediction of the still unknown values of the Y variable when the P parameters can be determined.

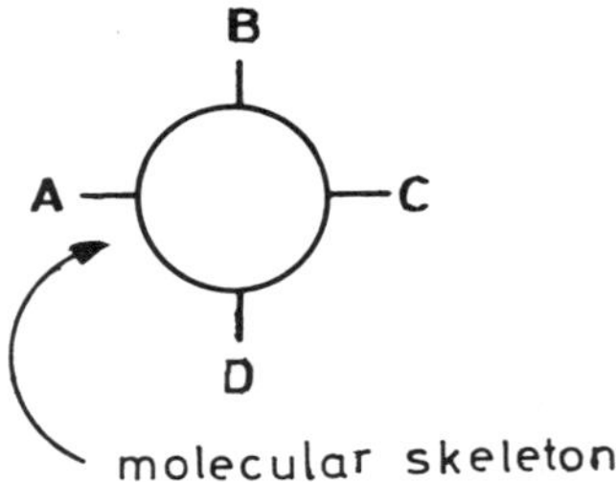

FIGURE 2. Free-Wilson model.

Although formally identical, the two models are conceptually different. The most important parameters used in this type of analysis are described in Section III.

B. CONNECTIVITY METHODS

The axiomatic basis of these methods considers that the chemical and spatial structure of a molecule is responsible for its biological activity. The Free and Wilson model[26] is a typical representative of this concept.

Let us consider a molecule having four different positions A, B, C and D to which various substituents may be attached. It is postulated that the biological activity of this molecule is the sum of the contributions of the four substituents located in positions A, B, C and D, plus the contribution of the molecular skeleton. Generally, the biological activity (BA) of a molecule i with n positions able to be substituted can be written as:

$$BA_i = \text{contribution } 1 + \ldots \text{ contribution } n + \text{contribution of the skeleton} \qquad (9)$$

In a series of i different compounds, the nature of the j substituents located in positions A, B . . . n of each molecule can obviously be different. It is also postulated that the contribution of each substituent to the overall activity of each molecule is independent of the presence or absence of other substituents in the other positions. Finally, a relationship of the following type may be written:

$$BA_i = \sum_j \sum_n a_{a,n} \delta_n + C \qquad (10)$$

where a is the activity contribution of substituent j located at the position n and $\delta_{j,n}$ is an indicator variable having the value 1 if the substituent j is present at the site n and 0 if it is not. The constant C is an average value of the biological activity and is assigned to the molecular skeleton (that has neither substituents, nor hydrogen in the positions of interest). This concept is expressed by the relationship:

$$\sum_n a_{j,n} = 0 \qquad (11)$$

termed restriction equation.

Thus, for a series of m compounds with j substituents in n positions, a system of m equations with $j - n$ unknown variables can be written. It is thus necessary that $m \geq j - n$. The restriction equations are used for obtaining the n additional equations required for solving the system. It is obviously better if the number of compounds exceeds this minimal $j - n$ value strictly needed for solving the system of equations.

The advantage of this procedure consists in the possibility to develop a QSAR analysis

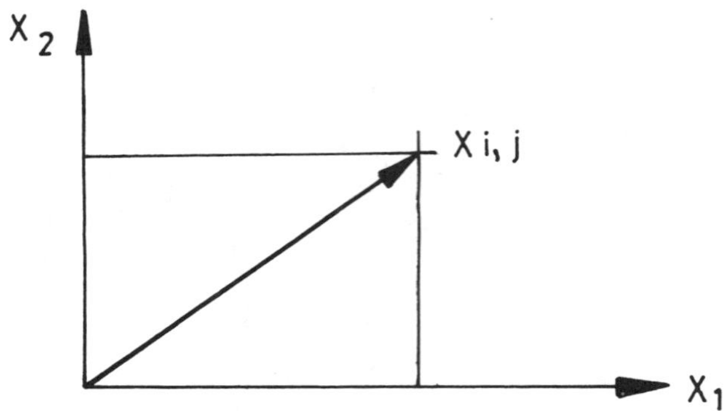

FIGURE 3.   Space of two-dimensional forms.

using a congeneric database without knowing anything about the investigated compounds, except their structure.

The limits of this type of model concern the requirement of a congeneric database (as for extrathermodynamic approach). Also, based on the additivity of the contribution of the substituents to the overall biological activity of a given molecule, the association of other parameters is not justified.

Surprisingly, an equivalence was demonstrated to exist between the Free-Wilson and the Hansch model.[27]

An essentially different approach to QSAR is based on the pattern recognition model. Pattern recognition is an area of artificial intelligence, by means of which a classification is done within a multitude of objects (actually involving a recognition). Let us consider a sample of N objects x_j (j = 1, 2, 3, . . . N), each of them being described by a set of measurable characteristics $x_{i,j}$ (i = 1, 2 . . . n); $x_{i,j}$ represents a pattern and the set $\{x_{i,j}|(i,j)$ $\epsilon 1,2, . . . N\}x\{1,2, . . . n\}$ is termed the pattern space. It follows that every object can be represented by a point in the n-dimensional pattern space. This space is represented for n = 2 in Figure 3.

It is assumed that in this pattern space, the objects similar to one another by respect to a certain property may be grouped distinctly, thus forming domains able to be characterized mathematically.

In practical applications, we are usually concerned with a pattern space with more than two dimensions. The mathematical models employed for solving pattern recognition problems are of either decisional (statistical) or syntactic (linguistic) type. In the classification of biologically active substances the first category of methods is employed.

This methodology developed by Stuper et al.[28] has been intensely used in the last years, especially because of the great advantage that it may be applied to a noncongeneric database. The measurable characteristics of the investigated compounds are expressed by means of the so-called descriptors (actually replacing the parameters from the extrathermodynamic models). However, parameters also specific for Hansch approaches were employed in QSAR analysis developed by pattern recognition methods. An example is the SIMCA-method (Soft Independent Modeling of Class Analogy) developed by Wold and co-workers.[29] In fact, the SIMCA procedure classifies similar compounds based first on activity class, and then computes a correlational equation for each class using the classical parameters employed in extrathermodynamic procedures.

Another computer-assisted approach to QSAR analysis by pattern recognition technique is the ADAPT method (Automated Data Analysis using Pattern Recognition Techniques).

Several excellent reviews on this topic are available.[30,31] In this case, variables are not physicochemical parameters but usually structure descriptors: fragment descriptors, substructure descriptors, environment descriptors, geometric descriptors. They will be discussed further (see Chapter 4, Section D.7).

A method developed on a similar basis by Klopman[32] is the CASE method (Computer Automated Structure Evaluation). The main problem for all QSAR analyses using the pattern recognition technique consists in the appropriate selection of descriptors; it is this selection which actually decides the quality of the computer-afforded solution. Therefore, to improve this choice, the CASE procedure employs several additional preliminary assumptions regarding the structure-activity relationships in the field of the investigated compounds.[33] Both structural descriptors and physicochemical parameters are used; the results obtained can be statistically analyzed.[34]

A similar procedure was developed by Einslein[35-37] which differs from the CASE method by the "descriptor fragment dictionary" it disposes of, as well as by the statistical procedures for evaluating the significance of the contribution of a certain fragment to the overall biological activity.

Within this category of methods for QSAR computations several others may be cited although they are less frequently employed.[38-40]

C. CRITICAL VIEW OF SOME RECENT TYPES OF QSAR-WORKS

Recent work of the group of Hansch studies enzyme-substrate interaction: for a review see Reference 41. Large series of substrates, up to several dozen with a marked congeneric character, were used to set up QSARs with "classical" parameters, such as π (hydrophobicity), σ (Hammett constants) and various indicator variables. They employed interactive stereocomputer graphics as a control of the QSAR results when the X-ray crystallographic structure of the bioreceptor was known. Thus, variables such as hydrophobicity or van der Waals volumes of substituents located at a certain position of the molecular skeleton, which may appear rather suspicious from the point of view of chance correlation (implicitly, this means that the most "successful" position out of several possible has been selected as structural variable) are justified if the substituents in the corresponding position are in contact with a hydrophobic pocket of the enzyme. The interplay between "classical", multiparametric (in the sense of selection of the best group of variables out of several possibilities) QSAR and molecular graphics modeling of enzyme-substrate interactions seem to produce real contributions to the knowledge of the molecular mechanisms in these interactions.

Somewhat opposite regarding the techniques, is the work of the group of Arteca and Mezey.[42] Molecular van der Waals and electrostatic potential surfaces are calculated using quantum chemical methods (for atomic charges) and visualized by molecular modeling techniques. The comparative study of shapes of such molecular potentials, compared with biological activities, should reveal essential features for biological activity. Topology and group theory are used in such studies.[43] Up to now, the method does not seem to have been brought from theoretical principles to a practically usable algorithm and actual applications seem limited to qualitative comparisons of shapes of active molecules.

A promising development seems to be the comparative molecular field analysis.[11] As in the distance geometry method[10] (and in a much more approximate way in the MTD method,[8,9]) the molecules of the QSAR series are allowed to interact with a receptor represented by a "lattice map" of grid points. Superposition of molecules with juxtaposition of pharmacophores is hereby implied. Probe atoms are placed successively at each grid point and the van der Waals (6,12) and electrostatic monopole interaction energies are calculated with each suitably aligned drug molecule. Appropriate multivariate analysis together with "cross-validation" produce a correlational equation as robust as possible with respect to omitting a randomly chosen group of molecules from the studied series. Results of a receptor site model is described by the various types of atoms attributed (by multivariate analysis plus cross-validation) to the grid points. Good results are reported[11] for interaction of steroids to certain hormone binding proteins (about two dozen molecules) and also for other series.[44,45]

A general problem appears for advanced 3D-QSAR methods requiring the calculation of drug receptor and interaction energy, if there are no X-ray studies to describe the receptor site. Namely, this description requires a number of parameters usually much higher than the number of molecules in the QSAR-series. In the CoMFA method these parameters are grid-atom-molecule interaction energies which are "weighted" in a correlational equation by PLS-techniques. This "weighting" (calculation of regressional coefficients) requires an optimization strategy implying some sort of additivity of the multiparametric optimization with respect to the optimization of each singular parameter. Entropy effects, hydration effects, local conformational changes of the receptor site are not included. This assumed additivity may also, sometimes, give a "local" minimum. One may ask if introduction of the initial "receptor maps", as suggested by intuitive considerations or more simple QSAR methods, would not improve the receptor site-model optimization.

An interesting combination of receptor mapping and 3D-techniques is used by the group of Motoc.[46] In a study dealing with features of the binding site of HMG-CoA reductase interaction with substituents of the C_8 position of 9,9-bis(4-fluorophenyl)-3,5-dihydroxy-(8-substituted)-6,8-nonadienoic acid analogs, it was possible to determine the conformation of the inhibitor bound to the enzyme and to derive a reliable 3D-QSAR which relates the inhibitory potency to the shape and size of C_8-substituents. A series of 13 inhibitors was used for the 3D-QSAR. Receptor mapping[47] was used to determine the bioactive conformation in the C_8-region, by comparing three potent inhibitors of the series with the other four potent inhibitors of a somewhat different structure. A probable shape for the C_8-substituent-binding receptor pocket resulted in the union of van der Waals envelopes of the seven potent inhibitors. The 3D-QSAR was devised using two structural parameters, OV and NOV — the volume of the C_8-substituent overlapping with the pocket and the volume protruding into the walls of the pocket, respectively. A cross-validated correlation coefficient r = 0.957 results (13 molecules, 2 structural parameters). The equation well predicts the inhibitory potency for the other five inhibitors. The physical relevance of the binding site model obtained was ascertained by calculating for eight inhibitors (for which NOV = 0) the polarization interaction energy with a methane box of the binding site shape; r = 0.987 was obtained for the inhibitor potency-interaction energy correlations.

It seems that a combination of complementary methods is the best strategy for structure-activity relationships. Computationally sophisticated 3D-techniques for calculating drug molecule-receptor interactions should be the final, most sophisticated, stage. If X-ray crystallographic data for the studied receptor are not available, simple QSAR-techniques (of the Hansch type or MTD) could be useful to provide a start for the receptor model search by more sophiticated techniques. The simpler techniques may also often yield, per se, significant information for the drug-receptor interaction mechanism and for drug design.

III. PARAMETERS AND DESCRIPTORS USED IN THE QSAR ANALYSIS

A review of the parameters employed in QSAR analysis is a compulsory step in the understanding of the conclusions obtained using these types of models. We have to remember that the quality of the results obtained by QSAR analysis is heavily dependent on the parameters and descriptors employed.

A. TRANSPORT PARAMETERS

These were the first parameters used in a QSAR approach by Colander[48] who showed that the transport of a compound through the cell membrane is proportional to log P, where P is the partition coefficient of the respective substance between an organic solvent and water. The most frequently used organic solvent is l-octanol (displaying several advantages, see Reference 27); but data obtained with other organic solvents (cyclohexane, benzene, etc.) have been reported as well. These partition coefficients being actually equilibrium constants, it would not be surprising if free energy relationships between various systems of solvents would exist. The problem was extensively studied[49] and such relationships were demonstrated, for instance:

$$\log P_{benzene} = 1.02(\pm 0.11)\log P_{octanol} + 1.40(\pm 0.14)$$

$$n = 33 \qquad r = 0.962 \qquad s = 0.23 \tag{12}$$

The thermodynamic character further allows the deduction of Hammett-type equations for the partition coefficients, P. By means of these relations a hydrophobicity substituent constant, π, can be defined:

$$\log \frac{P_x}{P_H} = a \cdot \pi \tag{13}$$

where P_H and P_x are partition coefficients of the unsubstituted and substituted congeners, respectively, and a is a proportionality factor.

The most important property of these hydrophobicity substituent constants is their additivity, which allows the computation of log P for any compound, by adding to a congener of known log P the π constants of the necessary substituents taking into account some simple rules for substitution, branching, etc. This additivity is obviously influenced by several factors: electronic and especially steric effects, medium properties, etc. (for instance the lipophilicity decreases sharply for ionized compounds (i.e., $\pi_{COOH} = -0.32$, $\pi_{CO_2^-} = -4.36$). Nevertheless, the constants allow a reasonable, accurate and very simple evaluation of the lipophilicity of any chemical compound. A large number of substituent constants were tabulated.[49,50] Programs for the calculation of these parameters were also developed.[51]

The uptake of a xenobiotic compound in a cell is governed by its lipophilicity. Thus a hydrophilic compound crosses (by passive diffusion) the cell membrane with difficulty, whereas a highly lipophilic one accumulates within; therefore it was logical to assume that there exists a range of optimal lipophilicity (log $P_{optimal}$) favoring the penetration across a cell membrane.

This assumption is supported by the parabolic form obtained often for the equations correlating biological activity with log P:

$$BA_i = a + a_1 \log P + a_1'(\log P)^2 + b + \dots \tag{14}$$

This form allows the computation of log $P_{optimal}$ (log P_o, π_o, etc.) by deriving Equation 14 as a function of log P:

$$\log P_{optimal} = -\frac{a_1}{2a_1'} \tag{15}$$

There are also other ways of expressing this parameter.[52]

B. ELECTRONIC PARAMETERS

This category includes both the parameters of thermodynamic origin described by Hammett's equation and also the quantum-mechanical parameters computed on the basis of completely different concepts.

1. Hammett Substituent Constants

These constants are defined according to Equations 4 and 5. They are actually a measure of the effect exerted by the substituent upon the free enthalpy of activation of the considered compound in a given reaction. This effect exerted by the substituent on the reaction center could be either a "field effect" or an electronic effect transmitted by means of the π and/or σ electrons systems of the molecule or both. The estimation of the "field effect" is difficult. Regarding the purely electronic effect, σ_m estimates the inductive effect of the *meta*-substituent, whereas σ_p estimates both the inductive and mesomeric one. Furthermore, the values of σ_p are more directly dependent of the substituent type and reaction center. Series of σ^- constants (nucleophilic constants) for the case of an electron donating *para*-substituent interacting by trough-resonance with an electronically defficient reaction center as well as electrophilic constants σ^+ (for the case of an electron-withdrawing substituent interacting with an electron-rich reaction center) were defined. Mention should be made that, as expected, electrophilic and nucleophilic σ_m^- and σ_m^+ constants have very close values to the normal σ_m ones. The use of these different types of constants was criticized[53-56] because they express several types of electronic interactions. In order to eliminate the mesomeric component, the utilization of a σ_o constant was suggested, determined on compounds **1**, in which the substituent is separated from the benzenic nucleus by a methylene group.[87]

$$X \text{—} \bigcirc \text{—} CH_2\, CO_2H$$

1

Other tentative methods to improve electronic constants could also be cited,[55] for instance σ^* constant (inductive electronic contribution of aliphatic system,[58,59]), σ_c^* of Yukawa and Tsuno.[60] A number of such constants for a large series of substituents were reported in the literature.

Mention must be made of the strong influence which the primary or secondary steric effects exert upon the values of these constants (steric hindrance of resonance).

A different approach in systems devoid of π-electrons relies on measuring, as a function of the substituent X, the dissociation constants of 4-substituted bicyclo(2.2.2)octane-2-carboxylic acids **2**. Only inductive and/or field effects may operate in such systems, so that this is a reliable method for evaluating these effects.

$$X \text{—} \langle\!\!\!\rangle \text{—} CO_2H$$

2

2. Quantum Mechanical Indices

There are several reasons justifying the use of quantum mechanical indices in QSAR analysis, for instance:

1. As a rule, quantum mechanical methods allow calculations of the reactivity for organic molecules (i.e., both of the rate and of the equilibrium constants) taking into account the topological and spatial structure of the molecule, as well as the π-electron density and the interactions between the π and σ electrons.
2. Quantum mechanics also allows the approximate description of the substrate-receptor interaction, a step of fundamental importance for the expression of the biological properties of a given compound. As the importance of the three-dimensional interaction

TABLE 2
Some of Quantum Mechanical Indices Used in QSAR Analysis

No.	Index (1)	It measures (2)	Could be correlated with: (3)
1.	Energy of the highest occupied molecular orbital, ϵ_{HOMO}	Electronic with drawing capacity	Ionization potential redox potential (plarography), charge transfer complex affinity
2.	Energy of the lowest empty molecular orbital, ϵ_{LEMO}	Electronic removal capacity	Affinity for electrons redox potential
3.	Electron energy, E_π	Total energy of π-electron system	Tautomeric equilibrium
4.	Delocalization energy, ΔE_{deloc}	Ease of a carbocation formation (stability of π-electron system)	Empirical resonance energy
5.	Electronic density, q_r	Electronic charge at the atom r	NMR spectra basicity
6.	Net charge ($\chi_r = n - q_r$)	Difference between the π electrons of the conjugated system and q_r	NMR spectra basicity
7.	Atomic electrophilic superdelocalizability, s_r^R	Corrected electronic density at the atom r	Electrophilic substitution
8.	Atomic nucleophilic superdelocalizability, S_r^N	Corrected electronic density at the atom r	Nucleophilic substitution
9.	Bond order ($P_{r,s}$)	Energy of the π-bond between r and s atoms	Interatomic distance, IR frequencies
10.	Free valence (F_r)	Bond strength	Radicalic reactions

and binding between a substrate and a receptor increases, the weight of the quantum-chemical parameters increases in QSAR analysis. This interaction is described by several theoretical models (Inouye's model, Klopman's, etc.).

The limits imposed by the use of these indices are due to the relatively sophisticated calculations they require, as well as to their quite approximative character.

There are, nowadays, a wide range of procedures for the computation of quantum-mechanical parameters, starting from relatively simple ones, such as Hückel's molecular orbitals method (HMO), to more and more sophisticated methods as Extended Hückel (EHMO), CNDO/2, MINDO/3, MNDO, etc. all being computer-assisted. Several quantum chemical indices more often employed are summarized in Table 2.

Ab initio computations also have to be mentioned as a methodology for obtaining more precise quantum mechanical indices. However, this procedure was used only for simple molecules, because of the high level of sophistication of the mathematical apparatus involved. With the continuous increase of computer power (super-computers), we expect that these *ab initio* methods will become available for carcinogenie molecules in the future.

The more accurate quantum mechanical parameters are calculated using specific techniques for molecular structure optimization by means of modeling packages, using molecular mechanics (software SYBYL, Tripos Associates, Inc., St. Louis, MO, U.S. or WMM Wellcome Molecular Modeling). Quantum mechanical calculations may be initiated from modeling packages, routines currently in use including CNDO, MOPAC and Gaussian 80 (Quantum Chemistry Program Exchange, University of Indiana, U.S.).

Another important problem is the orthogonality of the indices employed in a QSAR analysis. There are theoretical methods described for detection of quantum mechanic descriptors colinearity.[61]

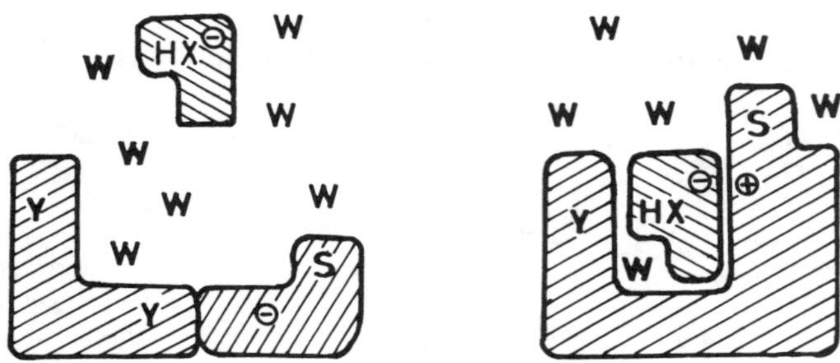

FIGURE 4.   Interaction of a drug molecule with a receptor; w — water molecules; Y, HX, ⊖, ⊕: hydrogen-bonding, polar groups. By interaction with the drug molecule the receptor is forced from the lowest energy to the active conformation. Drug-receptor steric fit is not perfect; a water — w — molecule is enclustered in the drug-receptor complex and the position of the S-receptor group is modified by a local conformational transition produced by steric hindrance.

C. MOLECULAR FEATURES OF RECEPTOR-EFFECTOR INTERACTION AND QSAR

The effector molecule (E) interacts with the biological receptor (R), in the lowest-energy conformation of the latter, and changes hereby this conformation to the physiologically active one (R*). Alternatively, the drug or inhibitor molecule may interact with this inactive lowest-energy conformation preventing the production of the active receptor conformation by interaction with the natural effector (agonic and antagonic actions).[62]

Processes that take place during a drug-receptor interaction are depicted in Figure 4. Various hydration-dehydration processes and conformational changes take place, in addition to the drug (E) receptor (R), interaction, per se:

$$R(aq) + E(aq) \overset{\Delta G}{\rightleftharpoons} R^*E(aq)$$

$$\pm\ H_2O \Updownarrow \Delta G_1 \qquad \Delta G_2 \Updownarrow \pm\ H_2O$$

$$R + E \overset{\Delta G_{int}}{\rightleftharpoons} R^*E$$

$$\Delta G = \Delta G_{int} - \Delta G_1 + \Delta G_2 \tag{16}$$

ΔG_{int} refers to the drug-receptor interaction per se, ΔG_1 and ΔG_2 to hydration processes. Molecular mechanic methods are quite successful in predicting molecular conformations (even conformations of peptidic fragments[63,64]) and they may also be applied for the receptor-effector interaction. One may write:

$$\Delta G_{int} = \Delta U_{R^*E} + \Delta U_{conf} - T\Delta S \tag{17}$$

For calculation of the ΔU_{R^*E} interaction energy, the molecular mechanics methods propose a summation of coulombian, polarization, van der Waals attraction and repulsions and atom-atom interactions. The geometry and nature of the dozens of receptor site atoms are to be known. ΔU_{conf} is the conformational energy change from the inactive (R) to active (R*) conformation. To this, local conformational changes should be added which are forced by steric hindrance (of drug-molecule groups protruding into receptor walls). Steric hindrance will be resolved by conformational changes or bond angle distortions, and not by atomic compressions because van der Waals repulsion potentials are very stiff.

The point is that a large amount of information is required in order to describe the receptor site features which would allow a calculation of the receptor-drug molecule affinity ΔG.

In order to establish a structure-activity relationship, one starts from the information contained in the biological activities and structures of a few dozen studied drug molecules. It is difficult to quantitatively define this information, but the required information is certainly much higher than the one contained in the experimental biological activities studies.[65] One arrives at the chance correlation problem pointed out by Topliss,[66,67] and must recognize that one really needs a bit of luck to obtain a good, realistic, QSAR with a reasonably small number of structural parameters!

As also remarked by Topliss, on the other hand, one should certainly not advocate a rejection of the QSAR and SAR-techniques, but one must be careful with the interpretation of results. There is also the cross-validation technique within the partial least squares method[68] in which the correlational equation is derived omitting a randomly chosen set of compounds, whose potency is predicted from the derived equation. Chance correlations are certainly reduced in this procedure, although it is difficult to say to what extent. With this analysis of receptor-effector interactions in mind, one may wonder about the success, in several QSAR studies, of simple structural parameters such as the Hansch's hydrophobicity.

D. STERIC PARAMETERS

Steric parameters are the third important category of variables employed in free energy linear relationships. Their contribution to the QSAR analysis is of prime importance because they try as accurately as possible to describe the molecular structure (topological, conformational, spatial), which is probably the main element in the substrate-receptor interaction. However, we have to point out that the quantitative expression of the molecular structure is by far one of the most striking problems of modern chemistry. We will review here several of the attempts made to obtain suitable steric parameters.

There are several groups of steric parameters defined on the basis of: (1) chemical reactivities (Taft's E_s parameters and their modifications[69]); (2) van der Waals radii and molecular geometries[70] and (3) a combination of these two sources.[71]

An alternative to these parameters is the use of the topological methods such as DARC/PELCO,[72] topological indices, such as molecular connectivity,[72] (see Chapter 2) minimal steric difference (MTD) method,[73] etc. Steric parameters may also be obtained from force field calculations.

1. Molar Refractivity

MR is one of first parameters introduced by Hansch (1973), as a first-order estimate of steric effects. MR is expressed by the Lorentz-Lorenz equation:

$$MR = \left(\frac{n^2 - 1}{n^2 + 1}\right) \cdot \frac{M}{d} \qquad (18)$$

where n is the refraction index at the sodium D line, M is the molecular weight and d is the density.

2. Taft Parameter and Statistical Analysis of Such Types of Indices

The first generally successful expression of how the steric effect influences organic reactions was deduced by Taft[74,75] according to a suggestion of Ingold. Taft defined the steric constant E_s as:

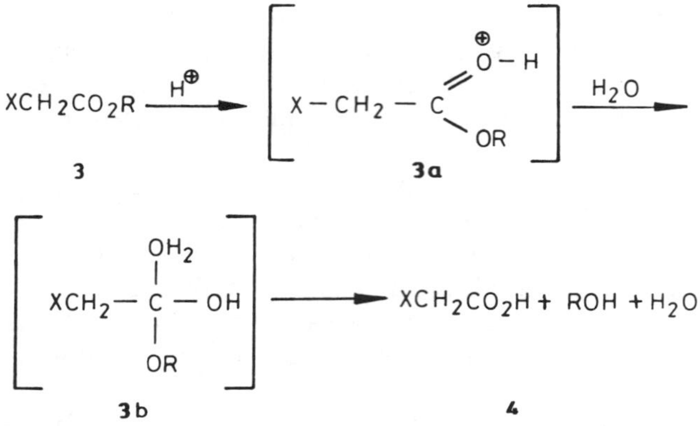

SCHEME 1.   Hydrolysis of aliphatic esters.

$$E_s = \log \left(\frac{k_x}{k_H}\right)_A \qquad (19)$$

where k is the rate constant for the acidic hydrolysis (denoted by A) of esters **3**. The size of X will affect the transition state for the hydration of **3a** formed during hydrolysis and therefore its steric effect will be modeled by E_s. This definition is based on three assumptions: (1) the relative free energies are treated as a sum of independent polar, resonance and steric effects; (2) resonance and steric effects are identical in acid and basic catalysis, (3) since all the original E_s correspond to substituents of the type CH_2X, CHX_2 or CX_3, the resonance factor is considered equal to zero (E_s will be zero when X = H, corresponding to acetic acid esters).[76]

Unfortunately, variations of structure **3** cannot be used to obtain E_s values for many common substituents which are unstable during acid hydrolysis (i.e., X = CN, OR, halogen, NO_2, etc.) The lack of such values for important substituents can be overcome by calculating new values from Equation 20:[77-79]

$$E_s^e = -1.839\, r_{av} + 3.484$$

$$(n = 6;\ r = 0.996;\ s = 0.132) \qquad (20)$$

In this equation, E_s^e is an extended scale of E_s parameters (which holds only for symmetrical substituents such as H, Br, CF_3 or $C(CH_3)_3$) and r_{av} is the average of the minimum and maximum van der Waals radii of the substituent estimated according to Charton.[80]

It must be noted that in Equation 20, only the radius of the first atom has been used to calculate E_s^e for substituents such as OH, OCH_3, SH, SCH_3, and NH_2. Two values of E_s have been calculated for one group such as NO_2 and C_6H_5; in the first the width of the substituents is employed and in the second their thickness.[78] Since one has little or no idea of what to expect in steric effects in biological correlation analysis, one must generally try both parameters to discover which one yields the best fit.[79]

The E_s parameters were introduced in QSAR by Hansch and Hen and have been extensively used (see, for instance, Reference 81). The wide range of applicability of the Taft E_s and extended E'_s parameters is probably the best evidence of their validity; however, several examples of limitations have also been reported.

Two basically different reasons could explain these failures:[76]

1. Either the E_s parameters are not absolutely correctly defined, that is, they may contain not only steric but also inductive, resonance and other types of effects owing to an incorrect separation of these effects in the reference reaction.
2. Or the E_s parameters are correctly defined, reflecting only steric effects, but they are not applicable to all cases since the same substituent can show a completely different "shape" depending upon the reaction or equilibrium considered.

The first assumption has been the major explanation for the discrepancies observed in the QSAR analysis using E_s parameters. Hancock,[82] considering that there may be a contribution of hyperconjugative effects of α-hydrogen atoms in E_s, defined a corrected steric substituent constants E_s^c by the equation:

$$E_s^c = E_s - h(n - 3) \tag{21}$$

where h is a reaction constant for hyperconjugation (taken as -0.306) from quantum chemical calculations by Kreevoy,[83] and n is the number of α-hydrogen atoms.

There are several cases when the use of E_s^c instead of E_s led to a significant increase of correlational index, r. This improvement is limited only to alkyl substituents but on the other hand, Shorter,[69] Charton[84] and Dubois et al.[85] did not find any statistical improvement in the correlations using the E_s^c parameter.

Palm[86] proposed another modified steric parameter considering the contribution of both C-H and C-C bonds involved in hyperconjugation:

$$E_s^o = E_s + 0.33(n_H - 3) + 0.13n_c \tag{22}$$

where n_H is the number of C-H and n_c is the number of C-C bonds.

These indices are also limited only to aklyl groups, and there is no convincing evidence that a statistical improvement of the correlations is obtained.

More recently, Dubois et al.[85,87,88] pointed out that the average procedure used by Taft may introduce errors: consequently, they defined a "revised" Taft steric parameter E'_s suggesting the acid catalyzed esterification of carboxylic acids (at 40°C) as the reference reaction. The E'_s values obtained are similar to E_s except for the bulky substituents. The substituent scale covered by this approach is also limited by the conditions of acid hydrolysis.

The values of these parameters (E_s, E'_s, E_s^e, E_s^c and E_s^o) for common substituents are summarized in Table 3.

Several studies have stressed that E_s parameters are a good representation of geometrical volumes (expressed by van der Waals radii) or they could be related with energies estimated from force field calculations. Thus, Charton proposed the following equation:

$$E_s = \alpha\sigma_I + \beta\sigma_R + \Psi r_v + C \tag{23}$$

where σ_I and σ_R are localized and delocalized effect of substituent constant, r_v is the van der Waals radius and C is a constant. Because σ_I and σ_R are usually small, the equation becomes:

$$E_s = \Psi r_v + C \tag{24}$$

which gives very good correlations. This validates the assumption that the E_s parameter (for CH_2X, CHX_2 and CX_3, respectively) is a linear function of van der Waals radii and that it is independent of electrical effects.[80]

While developing several aspects of steric effects in chemistry (i.e., determination of the nature of the *ortho*-effect, analysis of existing steric scales and determination of a scale

TABLE 3
Values of the Steric Parameter ν for a
Series of Substituents X[18]

X	ν	X	ν
Me	0.52	H	0.00
Et	0.56	F	0.27
Pr	0.68	Cl	0.55
i-Pr	0.76	Br	0.65
Bu	0.68	I	0.78
i-Bu	0.98	FCH_2	0.62
sec-Bu	1.02	$ClCH_2$	0.60
t-Bu	1.24	$BrCH_2$	0.64
Am	0.68	ICH_2	0.67
$sec\text{-}BuCH_2$	1.00	F_2CH	0.68
$i\text{-}PrCH_2CH_2$	0.68	Cl_2CH	0.81
Et_2CH	1.51	Br_2CH	0.89
PhEtCH	1.18	I_2CH	0.97
F_3C	0.90	Cl_3C	1.38
$c\text{-}C_6H_{11}$	0.87	Br_3C	1.56
$c\text{-}C_6H_{11}CH_2$	0.97	I_3C	1.79
C_6H_5[a]	0.57	$ClCH_2CH_2$	0.97
$C_6H_5CH_2$	0.70	$BrCH_2CH_2$	0.93
$C_6H_5CH_2CH_2$	0.70	ICH_2CH_2	0.93
$C_6H_5(Me)CH$	0.99	$MeBr_2C$	1.46
MeO	0.36	MeBrCH	0.75
EtO	0.48	MeClCH	0.70
PrO	0.56	MeNH	0.39
HO	0.32	EtNH	0.59
NC	0.40	PrNH	0.64
H_2N	0.35	BuNH	0.70
O_2N[a]	0.35	AmNH	0.50
i-PrO	0.75	GS	0.60
BuO	0.58	MeS	0.64
i-BuO	0.62	CHO	0.50
s-BuO	0.86	H_2NCO	0.50
t-BuO	1.22	AmO	0.58

[a] Minimal ν.

of steric effects based on van der Waals radii), Charton attempted[84] to avoid the use of a particular chemical reaction for defining a steric substituent constant. He proposed the following expression:

$$\nu_x = r_{V,X} - r_{V,H} = r_{V,X} - 1.20 \qquad (25)$$

In this expression, $r_{V,X}$ is the minimum van der Waals radius[80] for the symmetrical top substituents X, and $r_{V,H}$ is the van der Waals radius for hydrogen ($r_{V,H}$ being 1.20 Å). The ν values thus obtained were used to extend the ν values scale by means of the equation:

$$\log K = \Psi \nu + C \qquad (26)$$

where log K expresses the rates of esterification of substituted carboxylic acids with methanol or ethanol in standard conditions. Some ν indices are summarized in Table 4.

The relationship between Taft's E_s and Charton's ν parameters is a linear one, as shown by the following equation:[79]

TABLE 4
Values[77,87] of the Steric Parameters: E_s(Taft), E'_s (revised),
E_s^w, E_s^c and E_s^o for a Series of Substituents (Standard
Substituent: H)

| Substituents | $-E_s$ | $-E'_s$ | $-E_s^w$ | $-E_s^c$ | $-E_s^o$ |
1.	2.	3.	4.	5.	6.
H	−1.24	−1.12			
Me	0.00	0.00	1.24	1.24	1.24
Et	0.07	0.08	1.31	1.62	1.51
n-Pr	0.36	0.31	1.60	1.91	1.80
i-Pr	0.47	0.48	1.71	2.32	2.09
n-Bu	0.39	0.31	1.63	1.94	1.83
i-Bu	0.93	0.93	2.17	2.48	2.37
t-Bu	1.54	1.43	2.78	3.70	3.38
sec-Bu	1.13	1.00	2.37	2.98	2.77
n-Am	0.40	0.31	1.64	1.95	1.84
3-Am	—	0.97	3.22	3.83	—
$c\text{-}C_5H_{11}$	—	—	2.03	2.64	—
$c\text{-}C_5H_{11}CH_2$	—	—	2.22	2.53	—
C_5H_5	—	2.31	2.01	—	—
$C_5H_5CH_2$	0.38	0.39	1.61	—	—
F	—	−0.57	0.46	—	—
Cl	—	0.02	0.97	—	—
Br	—	0.22	1.16	—	—
I	—	0.50	1.40	—	—
FCH_2	0.24	0.20	1.48	—	1.81
$ClCH_2$	0.24	0.18	1.48	—	1.81
$BrCH_2$	0.27	0.24	1.51	—	1.84
ICH_2	0.37	0.30	1.61	—	—
F_2CH	0.67	0.32	1.91	—	2.57
Cl_2CH	1.54	0.58	2.78	—	3.44
Br_2CH	1.86	0.76	3.10	—	3.76
F_3C	—	—	2.40	—	3.39
Cl_3C	2.06	1.75	3.30	—	4.29
Br_3C	—	—	3.67	—	4.66
$BrCH_2CH_2$	—	—	2.24	2.55	2.43
ICH_2CH_2	—	—	2.26	2.57	2.44
NC	—	—	0.51	—	—
HO	—	—	0.55	—	—
CH_3O	—	—	0.55	—	—
H_2N	1.28	—	1.01	—	—
O_2N	1.28			—	
$HOCH_2$	—	−0.03	1.21	—	1.63
CH_3OCH_2	—	—	1.43	—	1.76

[a]   According to Unger-Hansch 87 model.

$$E_s = -2.062(\pm 0.86)\nu - 0.194(\pm 0.10)$$

$$n = 104 \qquad r = 0.978 \qquad s = 0.250 \tag{27}$$

Many substituents (CN, I, NO_2, OMe, Br, Cl, NH_2, OK, CF_3, etc.) fit this relationship rather poorly (s >0.300) as compared to the standard deviation. Hansch and Ho noted that "any features that these outliers have in common are not obvious, which simply brings out our lack of understanding of steric effects."[79]

All attempts of extending the scale of steric parameters E_s and E'_s are based on the generalization of the correlational analysis models developed between these parameters and

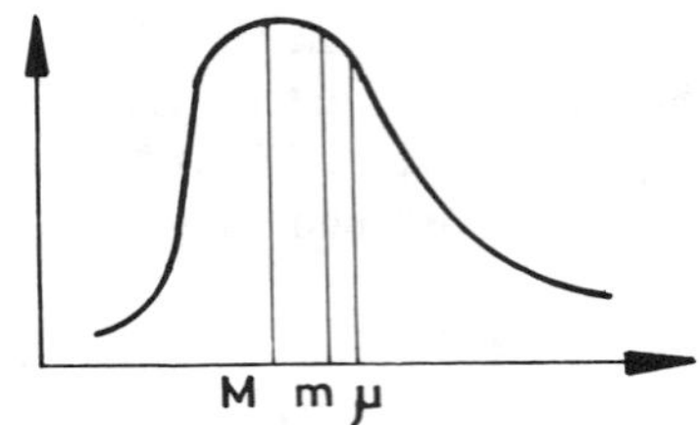

FIGURE 5.   Definition of average (μ), median (m) and modal value for a given distribution.

the van der Waals radii of the substituents (actually, the ν parameters introduced by Charton). Therefore a comparative analysis of their values distribution must be performed, in order to determine whether these populations have the same statistical structure. The relevant statistic parameters are:[89] the median (m), the average (μ), and the modal value (M) of the distributions, the asymmetry coefficient (Pearson), the range of the values, their variance and standard deviation.*

The asymmetry coefficient characterizes both the direction (positive in the example given in Figure 5) and the degree of asymmetry. If the distribution is symmetrical, the average, the median and the modal value are colinear and the asymmetry coefficient is zero. A first indication of the degree of dispersion is given by the range of the values. However, this estimation is not accurate enough, a better evaluation of the dispersion being afforded by the variance of the standard deviation. A high value of this parameter corresponds to a large dispersion of the investigated range of variables. This mode of analysis is extensively discussed in Reference 89.

A statistical analysis of the steric parameters (E_s and ν) is given in Table 5.

The data shown in this table allow a series of interesting inferences. The dispersion range around the average value is twice or even three-fold lower for μ values, than for the E_s values. Resulting, therefore, that the discriminating ability of the parameters as compared to the E_s values, for substituents with similar effects, is significantly lower. Moreover, the symmetry of the distribution of ν values is different from that of the E_s parameters. For all these reasons, the ν parameters are not suited for extending the scale of E_s values. The use of ν values and other parameters based upon r_ν values might lead to a leveling of the expressed effect, or even to unjustified inversions.

The E_s parameters are relatively similar for the dispersion around the average value. The symmetry of distribution is the same (see Table 5), a surprising but accountable inversion occurring for the E_s^c parameter (Table 5, upper half). However, there are significant differences between the substituent structures corresponding to the values of the median, average and modal value.

3. Van der Waals Molecular Descriptors

The recent interest in the van der Waals volume and surface affords an adequate reason for introducing van der Waals molecular descriptors in the treatment of steric effects in chemical structure-biological activity relationship (QSAR).

The intermolecular forces are responsible for most of the physical and chemical properties of matter.[90] Although the exact nature of these forces is very complex, there are no major conceptual difficulties for their treatment. Nevertheless, only semi-quantitative results limited to small molecular systems were obtained. An important element in the study, of intermolecular forces concerns the shape and size of the interacting molecular systems.

---

*   The average coincides with the gravity center of the distribution, the median bisects the area of the distribution and the modal value corresponds to the highest point of the distribution.

TABLE 5
Statistical Analysis of the Taft (E_s, E'_s, E^w_s, E^c_s and E^o_s) and Charton (ν) Parameters[a,b]

Parameters	E_s	E'_s	E^w_s	E^c_s	E^o_s	ν
			Values from Tables 3 and 4			
m	−0.47	−0.39	−1.60	−2.40	−1.97	0.68
μ	−0.74	−0.63	−1.69	−2.26	−2.35	0.76
M	0.08	0.09	−1.43	−2.68	−1.19	0.53
DV	3.67	3.74	3.67	3.83	4.66	1.79
DI	0.86	0.71	1.65	0.68	1.13	0.35
s	0.81	0.77	0.85	0.91	1.04	0.33
C_P	−1.02	−0.94	−0.30	0.46	−1.11	0.70
C_v	−108.40	−122.20	−50.59	−40.42	−44.36	43.26
			Values for a Standard Set of 11 Substituents			
m	−0.39	−0.31	−1.63	−1.94	−1.83	0.68
μ	−0.40	−0.37	−1.64	−2.00	−1.88	0.71
M	−0.37	−0.19	−1.61	−1.81	−1.74	0.62
DV	2.78	2.55	2.78	3.70	3.38	1.24
DI	0.49	0.51	0.49	0.64	0.58	0.25
s	0.71	0.66	0.71	0.95	0.86	0.32
C_P	−0.04	−0.27	−0.04	−0.20	−0.16	0.27
C_v	−178.20	−178.10	−43.46	−47.16	−45.95	45.01

Note: m = median, μ = average value, M = modal value, DV = domain of values (in units); DI = interquartile domain, s = standard deviation(%), C_P = asymmetry coefficient (Pearson), C_v = variation coefficient.

a. Van der Waals Volume

The shape and dimensions of molecules and ions depend on the length of the chemical bonds, the value of the valence angles and the size of the constituent atoms. Usually, atoms are considered to be spheres of radius r^w (the r^w dimension being called the van der Waals radius).

The discussions regarding the van der Waals volume (and surface) must take into account the work of Bondi,[91,92] who developed a suitable procedure allowing the calculation of van der Waals volume, V^w, on the basis of group contributions.

In order to estimate the van der Waals volume a more detailed discussion is required; this is in agreement with the current quantum-mechanical approach.[93]

Let us consider a molecule M made of a number of m atoms, each of them being characterized by a van der Waals radius r_i, where $i = 1,2, \ldots m$. If $V_i(= V^w_i)$ is an atomic van der Waals volume, than it becomes obvious that:

$$r_i = (3V_i/4\pi)^{1/3} \tag{28}$$

Thus, r_i values for any type of atom become available by crystallographic determinations. Assumptions concerning atomic sphericity and centricity are not restrictive; in this regard some alternatives were proposed.[94] The molecular van der Waals volume V^w_M will be composed by the sum of the individual atomic volumes, taking into account that the volumes overlapping (as a result of the intersection of several atomic spheres) must be considered only once. Consequently, V^w_M may be estimated by the following equation:

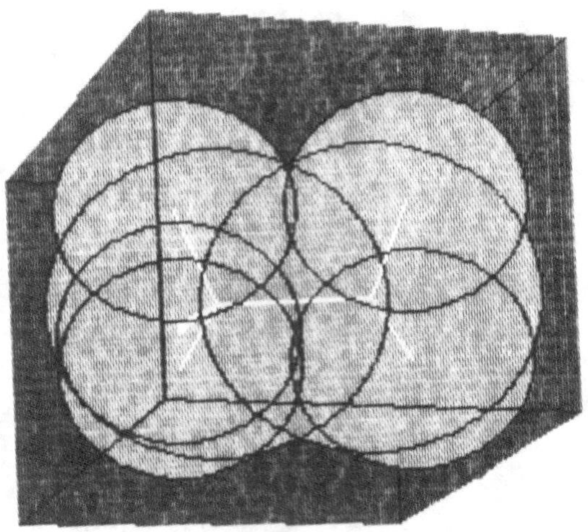

FIGURE 6.   Projection of the eclipsed ethyl radical in the xOy plane.

TABLE 6
Coordinates of the Ethyl Moiety: Eclipsed and Intercalated

Substituent	Atom	Position	X	Y	Z
CH_3-CH_2, ecl.	C	1	0.000	0.000	0.000
	C	2	1.533	0.000	0.000
	H	3	1.913	1.045	0.000
	H	4	−0.380	−0.522	0.905
	H	5	−0.380	−0.522	−0.905
	H	6	1.913	−0.522	0.905
	H	7	1.913	−0.522	−0.905
CH_3-CH_2, intereal	C	1	0.000	0.000	0.000
	C	2	1.533	0.000	0.000
	H	3	1.913	1.045	0.000
	H	4	−0.380	−1.045	0.000
	H	5	−0.380	0.522	−0.905
	H	6	1.913	−0.522	−0.905
	H	7	1.913	−0.522	0.905

$$V_M^w = \sum_{i=1}^{m} V_i - \sum_j (n_j - 1)V_j \tag{29}$$

where n_j is the number of spheres overalpping in the j domain, and V_j is the volume resulted by the intersection. Figure 6 shows a simplified image of the above mentioned situation, i.e., the projection of the eclipsed ethyl radical in the xOy plane (see the coordinates in Table 6). On the basis of Equation 29 the van der Waals volume may be analytically calculated,[95,96] but the algorithms so far available are complicated and time consuming. Therefore, for the calculation of the van der Waals volume (as well as surface) several original techniques were developed by one of us based on the Monte Carlo method.

We consider the "hard spheres" model of a molecule M, with n atoms, in which each atom is represented by a sphere with the center (x_i, y_i, z_i) situated in the equilibrium position of the respective atomic nucleus and with the radius equal to the van der Waals radius, r_i^w. A van der Waals nuclear envelope, Γ, can be uniquely defined as the external surface

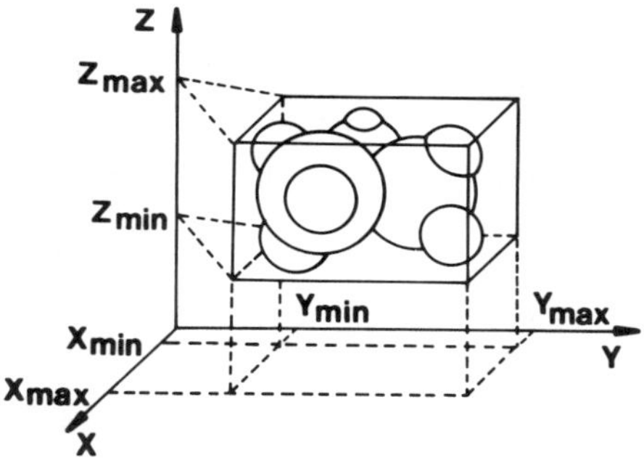

FIGURE 7.   Hard sphere-model.

resulted through the intersection of all the van der Waals spheres associated to the i atoms of the molecule M (as in Figure 7).

The points (x, y, z) situated in the interior of this envelope have to satisfy at least one from the following m inequations:

$$(x_i - x)^2 + (y_i - y)^2 + (z_i - z)^2 \leq (r_i^w)^2, \quad i = 1, 2, \ldots\ldots m \tag{30}$$

Thus, the total volume corresponds to the interior of the van der Waals envelope and represents the van der Waals volume (V_m^w) of the molecule M; V_m^w can be estimated by the Monte Carlo method.[97]

Being given the function $F = f(x,y,z)$ continuous over a closed and limited domain M, we propose to calculate the integral:

$$V^w = \iiint_M f(x,y,z)dx\, dy\, dz = \iiint_M dV \tag{31}$$

where $f(x, y, z)$ is given by the relation (13) and $dxdydz = dV = dM$.*

The integral will be transformed in such a manner that the new integration domain will be contained in a unitary tridimensional cube. By calculating the Jacobian of such a transformation,[98] the integral (31) becomes:

$$V = \iiint_\sigma f'(\xi x, \xi y, \xi z)d\,\xi x d\,\xi y d\,\xi z \tag{32}$$

where $f'(\xi x, \xi y, \xi z) = (A_1 - a_1)(B_1 - b_1)(C_1 - c_1) \cdot f\,[a_1 + (A_1 - a_1)\xi x,$

$$b_1 + (B_1 - b_1)\xi y, c_1 + (C_1 - c_1)\xi z] \tag{33}$$

Introducing the notations:

$$\xi_j = (\xi x, \xi y, \xi z) \text{ and } d\,\theta = d\xi x\xi y\xi z \tag{34}$$

the integral (32) can be written:

$$V = \iiint_\sigma f'(\xi_j)d\vartheta \tag{35}$$

* We implicitly assume that the space within the envelope is isotropic and independent of the nature of atoms.

Since the function f′ is non-negative, the integral (35) may be regarded as representing the volume of a solid in a tridimensional space, in our case the volume V_M^w of the molecule M. Thus, generating on the interval (o, 1) independent sequences ($\xi x,j$, $\xi y,j$, $\xi z,j$) j = 1,2, . . . N of uniformly distributed (pseudoaleatory) numbers, these may be considered as coordinates of the aleatory points $P_j \in \vartheta$ for j = 1,2, . . . N in the tridimensional space. If, from the total of N points, n points belong to the molecule M (otherwise, to the volume V_M^w and N-n points do not belong to this volume, we have:

$$P_j \in \vartheta \text{ for } j = 1,2, \ldots n \tag{36}$$

$$P_j \notin \vartheta \text{ for } j = n + 1, n + 2, \ldots N \tag{37}$$

then for a large enough number of points N, the integral (35) may be approximated as:

$$V^w = \frac{n}{N} \tag{38}$$

For the verification of the conditions (36, 37), the analytical representation of the Γ limits in the ϑ domain is used. If the Γ surface is given by the equation:

$$\varphi(\xi x,j,;\xi y,j,;\xi z,j) = 0 \tag{39}$$

where for $\varphi(P_j) < 0$ the point $P_{j \in \vartheta}$ and for $(P_j) > 0$ the point $P_{j \in \vartheta}$), there is a possibility to verify much more simply and efficiently the conditions (36, 37) by using the relationships (13).

The accuracy of the estimation ϵ (the estimation of the integral (35) with (38) for a given maximum probability 1-ϑ is inversely proportional to the square root of the number N of the aleatory points used:[98]

$$\epsilon = \frac{1}{2\sqrt{\vartheta,N}} \tag{40}$$

The integration by the Monte Carlo method shows a weaker convergence. According to Equation 40, in order to reduce by one order of magnitude (10 times) the error of the estimation ϵ, N has to be increased 100-fold. For instance, for $\epsilon = 0.05$ and $\vartheta = 0.01$, it results that N = 20,000, and for $\epsilon = 0.005$ and $\vartheta = 0.01$, we obtain N = 200,000.

On the basis of the above discussed theoretical considerations, the algorithm MON-CAVE-1 was developed for calculation of the molecular van der Waals volume (V_M^w) (by the Monte Carlo method) for a series of substituents. The results thus obtained are given in Table 7. The calculations were performed using 10,000 aleatory points generated by means of the function RND*, whose statistical quality is excellent. The estimated volumes represent the real volumes with a 99% probability at a confidence level of 95%.

The atomic coordinates of the substituents summarized in Table 7 were calculated by the program QCPE-CORD, using the standard geometric parameters[99] and the Bondi van der Waals radii. For the substituents with conformational mobility, only the minimal and maximal volumes were calculated, corresponding to the most sterically crowded (or compact) structure and to the most extended one, respectively. As expected, the van der Waals volumes of various conformers do not differ significantly; the variations do not exceed the calculated confidence intervals.

---

* RND = random.

TABLE 7
The van der Waals Volumes of the Substituents (X) Calculated by Means of the Program MON-CAVE-1 (in $Å^3$)

X	V^wm/M	var(%V)	SD(%V)	I_{95}(%V)	I_{99}(%V)
Me	26.57	0.06(0.22)	0.24(0.91)	0.17(0.65)	0.25(0.94)
Et	43.51	0.19(0.44)	0.44(1.00)	0.31(0.72)	0.45(1.03)
	43.65	0.32(0.73)	0.56(1.29)	0.40(0.93)	0.58(1.33)
Pr	59.33	0.66(1.11)	0.81(1.37)	0.52(0.87)	0.73(1.23)
	60.71	1.17(1.92)	1.08(1.78)	0.77(1.27)	1.11(1.83)
i-Pr	60.41	0.89(1.48)	0.94(1.56)	0.60(0.99)	0.85(1.40)
	60.53	0.61(1.01)	0.78(1.29)	0.56(0.92)	0.80(1.33)
n-Bu	74.93	0.63(0.84)	0.80(1.06)	0.57(0.76)	0.82(1.09)
	77.25	0.60(0.77)	0.77(1.00)	0.55(0.72)	0.79(1.03)
i-Bu	76.54	1.37(1.79)	1.17(1.53)	0.74(0.97)	1.05(1.37)
	77.30	1.56(2.01)	1.25(1.61)	0.89(1.15)	1.28(1.66)
s-Bu	76.73	1.83(2.39)	1.35(1.77)	0.86(1.12)	1.21(1.58)
	76.99	1.99(2.58)	1.41(1.83)	1.01(1.31)	1.45(1.88)
t-Bu	77.14	2.13(2.76)	1.46(1.83)	0.93(1.20)	1.31(1.70)
	77.47	2.15(2.78)	1.47(1.90)	1.13(1.46)	1.64(2.12)
n-Am	90.10	1.32(1.45)	1.15(1.26)	0.82(0.90)	1.18(1.30)
	94.66	1.10(1.17)	1.05(1.11)	0.75(0.79)	1.08(1.14)
sBuCH$_2$	93.21	1.35(1.45)	1.16(1.25)	0.83(0.89)	1.19(1.28)
	94.20	1.75(1.86)	1.32(1.40)	095(1.00)	1.36(1.44)
i-Am	88.99	2.11(2.37)	1.45(1.63)	1.04(1.17)	1.49(1.68)
	93.54	2.00(2.14)	1.42(1.51)	0.90(0.96)	1.27(1.36)
Et$_2$CH	91.51	2.58(2.81)	1.60(1.75)	1.02(1.11)	1.44(1.57)
	92.25	2.16(2.35)	1.47(1.60)	1.65(1.79)	2.42(2.62)
c-C$_6$H$_{11}$	99.72	1.05(1.05)	1.02(1.03)	0.73(0.73)	1.05(1.06)
C-C$_6$H$_{11}$CH$_2$	116.78	2.54(2.17)	1.59(1.36)	1.14(0.98)	1.64(1.40)
	116.97	2.05(1.75)	1.43(1.22)	1.20(1.02)	1.77(1.51)
Ph[a]	80.13				
PhCH$_2$	98.30	1.47(1.49)	1.21(1.23)	0.77(0.78)	1.09(1.11)
	98.64	1.58(1.60)	1.26(1.27)	1.05(1.07)	1.56(1.58)
Ph(CH$_2$)$_2$	116.3	2.89(2.49)	1.70(1.46)	1.22(1.05)	1.75(1.50)
	116.33	1.97(1.70)	1.40(1.21)	1.00(0.86)	1.44(1.24)
PhMeCH	115.80	2.74(2.37)	1.66(1.43)	1.18(1.02)	1.70(1.47)
	119.90	2.47(2.06)	1.57(1.31)	1.12(0.94)	1.62(1.35)
PhEtCH	129.08	1.84(1.43)	1.36(1.05)	0.86(0.67)	1.22(0.94)
	131.29	2.58(1.96)	1.61(1.22)	1.15(0.87)	1.65(1.26)
t-BuO	83.91	1.30(1.55)	1.14(1.36)	0.72(0.86)	1.02(1.22)
	84.91	1.37(1.61)	1.17(1.38)	0.98(1.15)	1.45(1.71)
n-AmO	98.11	1.62(1.65)	1.27(1.30)	1.07(1.09)	1.58(1.61)
	100.20	1.54(1.54)	1.24(1.24)	1.39(1.39)	2.04(2.04)
H[a]	7.24				
F	13.27	0.01(0.06)	0.09(0.68)	0.06(0.49)	0.09(0.70)
Cl	22.42	0.08(0.37)	0.13(0.59)	0.11(0.49)	0.16(0.73)
Br	26.52	0.02(0.06)	0.13(0.49)	0.09(0.35)	0.13(0.50)
I	32.48	0.01(0.05)	0.12(0.37)	0.10(0.31)	0.15(0.46)
FCH$_2$	31.37	0.25(0.81)	0.50(1.61)	0.32(1.02)	0.45(1.44)
ClCH$_2$	40.36	0.29(0.72)	0.54(1.33)	0.45(1.12)	0.67(1.65)
BrCH$_2$	44.97	0.36(0.81)	0.60(1.34)	0.43(0.96)	0.62(1.38)
ICH$_2$	50.81	0.22(0.44)	0.47(0.93)	0.30(0.59)	0.42(0.84)
F$_2$CH	36.12	0.10(0.27)	0.31(0.86)	0.22(0.61)	0.32(0.88)
Cl$_2$CH	54.30	0.16(0.29)	0.39(0.73)	0.25(0.46)	0.35(0.65)
Br$_2$CH	62.95	0.19(0.31)	0.44(0.70)	0.37(0.58)	0.54(0.86)
I$_2$CH	76.16	0.16(0.21)	0.40(0.53)	0.45(0.60)	0.66(0.87)
F$_3$C	40.36	0.19(0.48)	0.44(1.09)	0.28(0.69)	0.40(1.00)
Cl$_3$C	67.88	0.80(0.44)	0.55(0.81)	0.35(0.51)	0.49(0.73)
Br$_3$C	81.05	0.37(0.46)	0.61(0.75)	0.44(0.54)	0.63(0.77)

TABLE 7 (continued)
The van der Waals Volumes of the Substituents (X) Calculated by Means of the Program MON-CAVE-1 (in Å^3)

X	V^wm/M	var(%V)	SD(%V)	I_{95}(%V)	I_{99}(%V)
I_3C	99.72	0.38(0.38)	0.61(0.62)	0.51(0.52)	0.76(0.76)
$Cl(CH_2)_2$	57.63	0.37(0.64)	0.61(1.06)	0.44(0.76)	0.63(1.09)
$Br(CH_2)_2$	62.09	0.26(0.42)	0.51(0.82)	0.43(0.69)	0.63(1.02)
$I(CH_2)_2$	67.92	0.47(0.69)	0.68(1.01)	0.49(0.72)	0.70(1.04)
$MeBr_2C$	79.89	0.37(0.46)	0.61(0.76)	0.39(0.48)	0.55(0.68)
MeBrCH	62.01	0.33(0.53)	0.57(0.92)	0.48(0.77)	0.71(1.14)
MeClCH	57.35	0.40(0.70)	0.64(1.11)	0.45(0.79)	0.65(1.14)
MeNH	37.96	0.26(0.69)	0.51(1.35)	0.43(1.13)	0.64(1.67)
EtNH	38.19	0.26(0.67)	0.51(1.32)	0.36(0.95)	0.52(1.37)
EtNH	54.85	0.13(0.23)	0.35(0.65)	0.40(0.73)	0.58(1.06)
	55.30	0.09(0.16)	0.30(0.54)	0.21(0.39)	0.31(0.55)
n-PrNH	72.01	0.18(0.25)	0.42(0.59)	0.67(0.93)	1.23(1.71)
n-BuNH	85.34	0.98(1.14)	0.99(1.16)	0.83(0.97)	1.22(1.43)
	88.33	1.01(1.14)	1.00(1.14)	0.84(0.95)	1.24(1.40)
n-AmNH	105.24	1.45(1.38)	1.21(1.15)	1.01(0.96)	1.49(1.42)
H_2N	20.45	0.03(0.16)	0.18(0.88)	0.13(0.63)	0.19(0.91)
O_2N	32.16	0.08(0.24)	0.28(0.87)	0.18(0.55)	0.25(0.78)
$PhOCH_2$	107.17	1.45(1.36)	1.21(1.13)	1.01(0.94)	1.49(1.39)
	109.09	0.95(0.87)	0.98(0.89)	0.70(0.64)	1.00(0.92)
$MeOCH_2$	52.10	0.16(0.30)	0.39(0.76)	0.33(0.63)	0.49(0.94)
$HOCH_2$[a]	34.20				
H_2NCH_2[a]	38.61				
MeO	34.78	0.31(0.88)	0.55(1.59)	0.35(1.01)	0.50(1.42)
EtO	51.14	0.39(0.77)	0.63(1.23)	0.40(0.78)	0.56(1.10)
	51.63	0.31(0.60)	0.56(1.08)	0.40(0.77)	0.57(1.11)
PrO	68.07	1.28(1.88)	1.13(1.66)	0.72(1.06)	1.02(1.49)
	68.91	1.17(1.71)	1.08(1.57)	0.69(1.00)	0.97(1.41)
i-PrO	68.05	0.80(1.18)	0.90(1.32)	0.64(0.94)	0.92(1.35)
	68.31	0.74(1.09)	0.86(1.26)	0.62(0.90)	0.89(1.30)
n-BuO	83.37	1.19(1.42)	1.09(1.31)	0.78(0.93)	1.12(1.34)
	85.73	1.14(1.33)	1.07(1.24)	0.68(0.79)	0.96(1.12)
i-BuO	84.33	1.21(1.43)	1.10(1.30)	0.92(1.09)	1.36(1.61)
	85.17	0.90(1.05)	0.95(1.11)	0.60(0.71)	0.85(1.00)
s-BuO	82.07	1.23(1.50)	1.11(1.35)	0.79(0.97)	1.14(1.39)
	87.87	1.00(1.14)	1.00(1.14)	0.64(0.72)	0.90(1.02)

Note: var = variance, SD = standard deviation, I_{95} = confidence interval 95%, I_{99} = confidence interval 99%, %V(SD) = variation coefficient; m/M = minimum volume/ maximum volume, corresponding to the compact and extended conformation, respectively.

[a] = unique volumes.

From the data summarized in Table 7 it follows that the method developed for the calculation of the molecular van der Waals volumes has a very good accuracy (as compared to experimental data), a slow decrease of precision paralleling the increasing number of atoms in the molecule is noted and, for the same number of atoms, paralleling the ramification degree.

By means of Student-t test, the 95 and 99% confidence intervals were calculated. Table 7 shows that the size of the 95% confidence interval is below 4% from the calculated average value of the volume, and is of maximum 5% for the 99% trust interval. The variance of the calculated volumes is below 3% from the average value.

To check the validity of the results obtained for N = 10,000, the volume of the methyl group was calculated using a large number of aleatory points (Table 8). As expected, the

TABLE 8
Volumes Calculated for the Methyl Group Using
Various Amounts of Aleatory Points (N)

	a	b	c	d
Sequence	N = 100,000	200,000	500,000	1,000,000
V_i	26.62544	26.55897	26.56268	26.53472
	26.51204	26.66211	26.50715	26.53746
	26.38495	26.63131	26.50464	26.63131
	26.67530			
	26.63229			
V^a	26.57	26.55	26.525	26.61
var	0.0139	0.000118	0.00108	0.0044
SD	0.1179	0.010847	0.0328	0.0665

[a] Average volume.

accuracy of the calculation improves with increasing number of aleatory points, the dispersion of the results around the average value decreasing with increasing N.

However, for $N = 10^6$ points the computation time becomes restrictive, so that a compromise between accuracy and computation time has to be found. The van der Waals volume truly reflect the dimensions of the substituents (Table 7), being in this respect a valuable parameter for QSAR studies. Used in connection with other indicator variables, they may afford information concerning the nature of the biological receptor, as well as the positions and sizes of the substituents which modulate the reactivity of the effector molecule. If the biological receptor is sensitive to the effects of the van der Waals volumes of the effector, then the optimal volume of the substituent can be easily computed. Its use in the MTD-R-MC* method affords new possibilities, transposing the method from a topological space into a geometrical one, with physical significance.

b. Van der Waals Surface

In the "hard spheres" approximation (see the previous paragraph) for the structure of molecule M, a molecular van der Waals envelope (Γ) may be uniquely defined as the external surface resulted by the intersection of van der Waals spheres associated to all of the atoms composing the molecule M. Undoubtedly, the surface of the molecular van der Waals envelope (van der Waals, surface, S^w) can code very useful information for the QSAR analysis.

Recently, a series of methods were developed[100-103] for the calculation of this surface area. These methods are quite sophisticated and require powerful computers. Such studies are mainly focused toward: (1) the visualization of such surfaces;[104] (2) the understanding of the contiguity of molecules[105,106] and (3) the analysis of the similarity between molecules with related structures.[107] A more efficient and simple procedure for the calculation of such molecular van der Waals surfaces was developed by us by means of the same Monte Carlo technique. The studies we carried out[17] allowed the development of rapid and efficient algorithms for the calculation of molecular surfaces. The concept underlying the calculation is the following (see also Section III.D.3.a): on the surfaces of the atomic spheres there are generated networks of aleatory, uniformly distributed points, and from these only those belonging to the molecular van der Waals surface are detected.

Three algorithms were developed for the calculation of the molecular van der Waals surface, which differ only by the construction of the point network distributed on the surfaces of the atomic spheres: (1) aleatory generation of φ and θ angles (see Figure 8); (2) aleatory

---

* MTD-R-MC = Minimal Topological Differences — optimization based upon η values — multiple conformations.

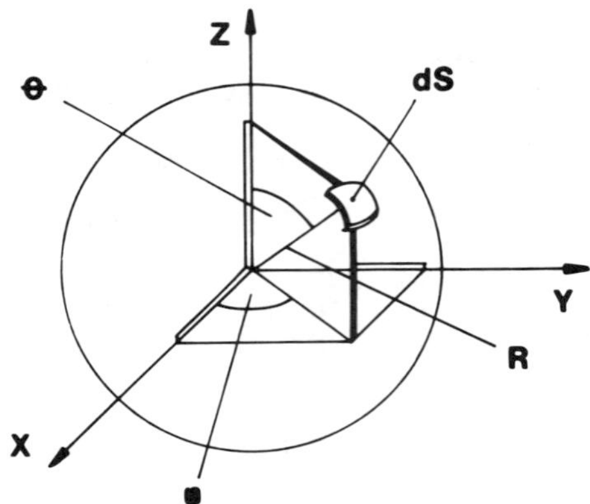

FIGURE 8.   Generation of φ and Θ angles.

TABLE 9
Comparative Study of Algorithms b and c

Network step[c]	Algorithm b (Monte Carlo)		Algorithm c (determinist)	
	Time (min)	Surface (nm²)	Time (min)	Surface (nm²)
0.02	0.33	0.5168	2.13	0.5796
0.01	1.4	0.5144	12.5	0.5566
0.0075	2.52	0.5100	28.23	0.5395
0.005	5.62	0.5120	120.0	0.5210[a]
0.004	8.78	0.5114	—	—
0.003	15.58	0.5109	—	—
0.002	35.06	0.5101	—	[b]

[a]   0.5259 (calculated according to Reference 97).
[b]   0.5139 (calculated according to Reference 97).
[c]   In nm.

generation of φ angles and Z coordinate and (3) construction of a similar point network by determinist methods, which simulate the stochastic approaches (1) and (2). This algorithm was developed in order to compare our results with those of Meyer[93,101] (see Table 9).

The performed studies[17,98] led to the conclusion that the use of the Monte Carlo method (algorithms 1 and 2) is more efficient and less time consuming than the determinist integration method.

The calculated van der Waals surfaces for various substituents are summarized in Table 10. The calculations were carried out on a Sinclair-QL personal computer.

For the substituents having a flexible conformation, van der Waals surfaces were calculated for the sterically most crowded (S_{min}) and most extended conformers (S_{max}), respectively. Usually, the *anti* (most extended) conformers have a larger van der Waals envelope. There is only one exception (marked in Table 10). Mention should be made that the same exception was also noticed by Meyer[102] (eclipsed ethane S^w = 67.79 Å², intercalated ethane S^w = 67.50 Å²). For alkyl groups with an equal number of carbon atoms, the molecular van der Waals surface increases with the degree of branching (see substituents C_3 and C_4 in Table 10), this increase being more marked for eclipsed conformers.

The same limitations for van der Waals volumes emerge in the use of S^w for different substituents in QSAR analysis. In fact, as expected, S^w and V^w are linearly related, (at least for C_1-C_{10} alkanes in extended conformations):

TABLE 10
Average van der Waals Surfaces (in Å²) of Several Substituents Calculated by the Program MOL-SURF

Substituent	S^w	Substituent	S^w	Substituent	S^w
Me	44.92	I	49.27	$H_2NCH_2CH_2$[b]	83.83
Et	67.21	FCH_2	52.63	$Me(NH_2)CH$	83.52
n-Pr	88.73	$ClCH_2$	63.50	HO	32.38
i-Pr	89.24	$BrCH_2$	68.17	CN	45.09
n-Bu	107.03	ICH_2	74.53	MeCONH	83.65
i-Bu	108.23	F_2CH	58.60	MeS	67.50
t-Bu	109.90	Br_2CH	88.44	HS	44.40
s-Bu	108.78	Cl_2CH	79.23	NO	41.27
n-Am	128.46	I_2CH	101.01	CHO	48.37
$s\text{-}BuCH_2$	127.76	F_3C	63.77	COOH	58.59
$i\text{-}PrCH_2CH_2$	123.47	Cl_3C	94.72	CH_3CO	70.71
Et_2CH	127.55	Br_3C	108.48	CH_2CN	66.11
$c\text{-}C_6H_{11}$	131.17	I_3C	126.86	H_2NCO	61.82
$c\text{-}C_6H_{11}CH_2$	151.71	$Cl(CH_2)_2$[a]	85.05	H_2NCONH	78.29
Ph	105.30	$Br(CH_2)_2$	89.62	H_2NSO_2	77.24
$PhCH_2$	128.37	$I(CH_2)_2$[b]	95.95	SO_2F	71.36
Ph(Me)CH	152.68	$MeBrCH$[a]	89.46	$HOCH_2$[b]	55.68
Ph(Et)CH	163.72	MeClCH	84.88	$Me(OH)CH$[b]	79.32
MeO	55.98	MeNH	61.01	$OH(CH_2)_2$[b]	79.05
EtO	78.02	EtNH	83.20	H_2NCH_2[b]	62.35
PrO	98.72	PrNH[a]	102.45	H	18.10
i-PrO	99.06	n-BuNH	121.71	F	27.15
n-BuO	117.81	n-AmNH[a]	146.53	Cl	38.48
i-BuO	118.22	NH_2	37.62	Br	43.01
s-BuO	116.03	t-BuO	117.90	n-AmO	134.40
PhOCH	141.50	MeOCH	77.78	NO	53.31

[a] Minimal

[b] Maximal.

$$S^w = 10.7935 \, V^w + 0.1914 \quad (S \text{ in } nm^2; \ V \text{ in } nm^3)$$

$$n = 44 \qquad n = 0.991 \tag{41}$$

c. Synthetic Indicators of Form

The shape of the effector molecules is doubtlessly the main element of most chemical interactions. It is very difficult to quantify this form, i.e., to find appropriate molecular descriptors able to express it. Most procedures are based either on comparing molecules with reference structures, or on sectorizing them and defining the sectors by means of geometric distances between certain atoms or by means of Cartesian coordinates.[102]

Using the "hard spheres" model, a series of van der Waals indicators of the shape of substituents were developed which are applicable in QSAR analysis as steric parameters. This model allows the introduction of several synthetic descriptors of form.

A first set of indicators were developed starting from the fact that a substituent may be characterized by the surface of the van der Waals envelope defined according to Equation 30. It is known that the relationship:

$$\frac{x^2}{a^2} + \frac{y^2}{b^2} + \frac{z^2}{c^2} = 1 \tag{42}$$

represents an ellipsoid. The "hard sphere" model of the considered molecule (see Figure

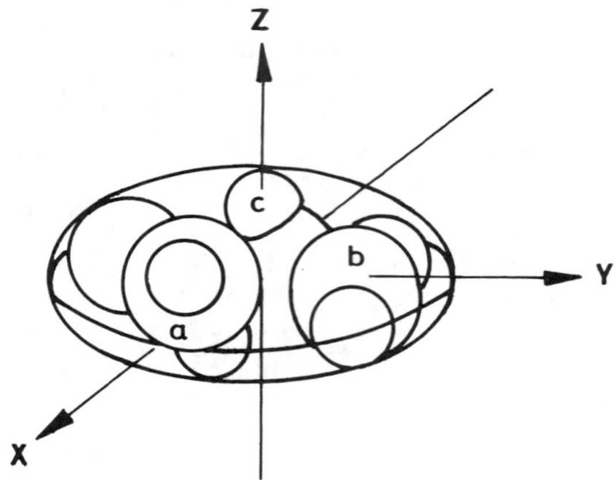

FIGURE 9.   Triaxial ellipsoid.

7) is embedded in this triaxial ellipsoid*. The semi-axes of this ellipsoid, noted a, b, c are the first set of indicators describing the substituent shape (Figure 9).

The molecular descriptors of the substituent form, given in Table 11, were calculated by the program ELLIPSOID.

It can be noticed that the linear alkyl radicals and other substituents such as NO, CHO, COOH, SO_2NH_2 etc., may be pictured as elongated ellipsoids, whereas the branched radicals (including CX_2, CHX_2 and CH_2X) resemble a flattened ellipsoid. The possibility to assimilate the substituents to spheres decreases from CF_3 to CI_3.

Starting from the concept of "packaging density" and from the fact that the determination of the transversal section area of a molecule is performed by assimilating it to a sphere, one may consider as a quantitative measure of the steric effect of the substituent the parameters u'_v and u'_s defined as follows:

$$u'_v = r(V) - 1.2; \quad r(V) = (3V^w/4\pi)^{1/3} \tag{43}$$

$$u'_s = r(S) - 1.2; \quad r(S) = (S^w/4\pi)^{1/2} \tag{44}$$

where r(V) and r(S) represent the van der Waals radii equivalent to the calculated volume (V^w) and estimated surface (S^w), respectively (see Section III.D.3.b) and 1.2 Å represents the van der Waals radius of the hydrogen atom. The values calculated with the formulae 43 and 44 are summarized in Table 11.

The ratio V^w/S^w or $(V/S)^w$ could also be a measure of the substituent form, its relative value expressing the more or less "globular" character of the substituent. Because the stereochemical variations affect the volume less than the surface of the substituent envelope, the decrease of V/S value is expected to express the increase of the substituent "globularity" (i.e., for staggered skew n-Bu, V^w/S^w is 0.716, whereas for the staggered transoid conformer, the value of this ratio is 0.705).

Mention must be made of the fact that these steric parameters have the dimensions of a radius, as Charton's γ parameter. Some values of this parameter for a series of substituents are given in Table 11.

d. STERIMOL-Type Parameters

The STERIMOL parameters were developed by Verloop et al.[109] in order to obtain more

---

*   For a = b = c, the ellipsoid is a sphere. If only two axes are equal, the equation represents a rotation (bi-axial) ellipsoid.

TABLE 11
Synthetic Descriptors of the Substituents X[a] Form

X	a	b	c	μ_v'	μ_s'	$(V/S)^w$
Me	1.700	1.983	2.104	0.651	0.691	0.591
Et	2.301	2.459	2.104	0.983	1.113	0.648
n-Pr	2.763	2.705	2.104	1.229	1.457	0.676
i-Pr	2.606	3.104	2.729	1.235	1.465	0.678
n-Bu	3.363	3.166	2.104	1.428	1.718	0.710
i-Bu	2.521	3.104	3.355	1.438	1.735	0.811
s-Bu	2.519	3.735	2.743	1.438	1.742	0.703
t-Bu	2.301	3.110	3.353	1.443	1.757	0.699
n-Am	3.825	3.412	2.104	1.609	1.997	0.723
s-BuCH$_2$	2.520	3.100	3.979	1.618	1.989	0.733
iPrCH$_2$CH$_2$	3.363	2.705	3.355	1.593	1.935	0.739
Et$_2$CH	2.689	4.216	3.355	1.599	1.986	0.720
c-C$_6$H$_{11}$	3.283	3.328	2.735	1.677	2.031	0.760
c-C$_6$H$_{11}$CH$_2$	3.246	3.675	3.365	1.833	2.275	0.770
PhCH$_2$	2.755	3.978	3.075	1.665	1.996	0.767
PhCH$_2$CH$_2$	4.458	2.736	3.075	1.828	2.251	0.777
Ph(Me)CH	3.680	4.618	2.730	1.842	2.286	0.772
Ph(Et)CH	3.680	4.618	2.763	1.944	2.409	0.795
MeO	2.321	1.983	2.104	0.825	0.911	0.621
EtO	2.921	2.459	2.104	1.107	1.292	0.659
PrO	2.681	3.048	2.104	1.338	1.603	0.694
i-PrO	2.921	3.099	2.730	1.335	1.608	0.688
n-BuO	3.984	3.151	2.104	1.523	1.862	0.718
t-BuO	2.921	3.066	3.355	1.525	1.867	0.716
H	1.200	1.200	1.200	0.000	0.000	0.400
F	1.470	1.470	1.470	0.270	0.270	0.489
Cl	1.750	1.750	1.750	0.550	0.550	0.583
Br	1.850	1.850	1.850	0.650	0.650	0.640
I	1.980	1.980	1.980	0.780	0.780	0.659
FCH$_2$	2.115	1.918	2.350	0.756	0.847	0.596
ClCH$_2$	2.299	2.188	2.637	0.932	1.048	0.640
BrCH$_2$	2.372	2.278	2.749	1.006	1.129	0.660
ICH$_2$	2.467	2.395	2.894	1.098	1.235	0.682
F$_2$CH	2.095	1.938	2.554	0.851	0.959	0.616
Cl$_2$CH	2.296	2.184	3.159	1.149	1.311	0.685
Br$_2$CH	2.371	2.276	3.388	1.268	1.453	0.712
I$_2$CH	2.467	2.395	3.684	1.430	1.635	0.754
F$_3$C	2.336	1.932	2.534	0.938	1.053	0.633
Cl$_3$C	2.893	2.182	3.155	1.331	1.545	0.717
Br$_3$C	3.101	2.306	3.387	1.485	1.738	0.747
I$_3$C	3.367	2.485	3.684	1.677	1.977	0.786
MeNH	2.379	1.973	2.092	0.887	1.003	0.624
EtNH	3.006	2.577	2.104	1.160	1.373	0.662
H$_2$N	1.567	1.902	1.780	0.496	0.530	0.544
O$_2$N	1.823	2.624	1.550	0.773	0.860	0.603
HO	1.520	1.814	1.520	0.396	0.405	0.526
NC	2.205	1.700	1.700	0.672	0.694	0.609
MeCONH	2.757	2.718	2.087	1.173	1.380	0.569
MeS	2.139	2.654	2.098	0.995	1.118	0.657
HS	1.800	2.166	1.800	0.661	0.680	0.608
OHC	1.950	2.358	1.700	0.714	0.762	0.607
HOOC	2.242	2.628	1.700	0.868	0.959	0.632
NCCH$_2$	2.073	2.867	2.098	0.986	1.094	0.662
H$_2$NCO	1.995	2.658	1.932	0.909	1.018	0.636
H$_2$NO$_2$S	2.294	2.448	2.675	1.115	1.279	0.673
FO$_2$S	2.529	1.985	2.692	1.029	1.183	0.650

[a] For the alkyl groups the a, b, c figures correspond to the intercalated conformations.

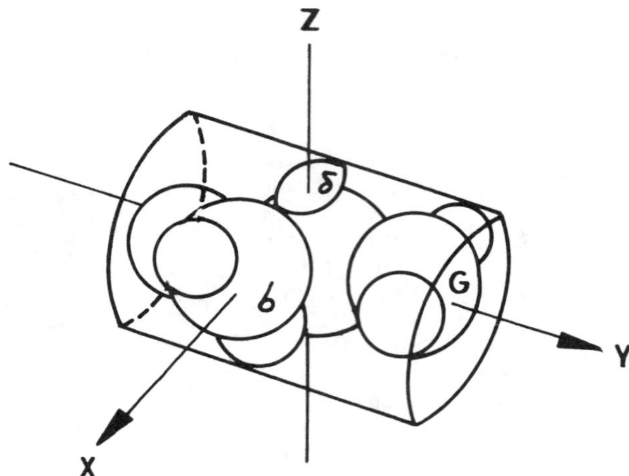

FIGURE 10.   Model for σ_i and G_i indices calculation.

appropriate descriptors of the substituents shape. According to the STERIMOL procedure a set of five parameters (L, B_1-B_4) (expressed in Å) computed for each substituent are enough to describe its shape. The index L represents the substituent length, whereas the B_1-B_4 indices characterize the "thickness" of the substituents on two orthogonal directions. These parameters represent a powerful tool in describing steric effects and were used in QSAR approaches describing the 3D-character of the substrate-effector interaction.

A new parameter of the same type was developed by one of us based on the following assumptions:

1.   The substituents are treated according to the hard spheres model (see Section III.D.3.a).
2.   The steric behavior of the substituent is due exclusively to the homogenous and isotropic molecular van der Waals space delimited by the envelope.
3.   The steric effect is of a vectorial nature. It is due to the fact that a substituent occupies a certain volume in the tridimensional space ("space filling"), relatively impenetrable to external influences.
4.   The substituents show a rotation symmetry axis linking the contact point of the substituent and the reference structure with the van der Waals weight center of the substituent (see Figure 10).

In this case, the steric anisotropy of the molecular van der Waals space is effective in two directions: (1) the direction of the rotation axis (G) and (2) the direction perpendicular to it (δ).

Values of the δ and G descriptors for a series of substituents are summarized in Table 12.

Values (δ_i, G_i) given in Table 12 concern the staggered transoid rotamer, and (δ_e, G_e) the skew one. Analysis of the parameter δ for alkyl substituents suggests its possible utility in the quantification of steric effects in organic reactions. On the other hand, parameter G representing the length of the substituent (in the direction of the rotation axis) could be very useful in QSAR studies. Therefore, the quantification of a steric receptor-effector interaction by a set of only two parameters (δ and G) (instead of five with STERIMOL procedure) may be achieved.

4. The MTD-Method

The MTD-method was described in detail elsewhere.[9] We give here only an outline of

TABLE 12
Values of the van der Waals Descriptors (δ, G)

Substituent	δ_i	G_i	δ_e	G_e	Substituent	δ	G
Et	1.420	4.876	1.625	4.276	CH_3	1.244	3.400
Pr	1.628	5.799	2.187	4.418	FCH^2	1.437	3.474
i-Pr	2.332	4.123	2.748	3.506	$ClCH_2$	1.473	4.387
n-Bu	1.656	7.409	2.121	5.622	$BrCH_2$	1.527	4.688
i-Bu	2.786	4.416	2.234	5.453	ICH_2	1.598	5.059
s-Bu	3.133	3.918	2.689	4.585	F_2CH	1.701	3.379
t-Bu	3.605	3.399	3.593	3.399	Cl_2CH	2.453	3.523
n-Am	1.811	8.318	2.640	5.492	Br_2CH	2.776	3.609
$s\text{-}BuCH_2$	3.267	4.589	2.570	5.772	I_2CH	3.265	3.712
$i\text{-}PrCH_2CH_2$	2.627	5.667	2.113	6.703	F_3C	1.889	3.400
Et_2CH	3.617	4.059	3.798	3.835	Cl_3C	3.177	3.400
$c\text{-}C_6H_{11}CH_2$	2.553	7.279	2.687	6.928	Br_3C	3.794	3.400
$PhCH_2$	2.334	6.727	2.311	6.771	I_3C	4.668	3.400
$PhCH_2CH_2$	2.106	8.787	2.353	7.868	H_2N	1.055	3.083
$Ph(Me)CH$	2.600	7.088	2.631	7.252	O_2N	1.604	3.190
$Ph(Et)CH$	2.991	6.985	3.088	6.653	HO	0.898	3.017
MeO	1.209	4.558	1.303	4.148	CN	0.991	4.410
EtO	1.455	5.608	1.900	4.160	COOH	1.409	4.184

Note: The subscript i refers to the intercalated (trans) conformer, and e to the eclipsed conformer.

this procedure. More attention will be given to recent developments and to specific difficulties of this method.

As a preliminary step, a congeneric database is constructed by listing the investigated series of molecules according to the decreasing or increasing order of their biological activities. The successive steps are *superposition of molecules, construction of the hypermolecule and description of the spatial structure of molecules.*

Consider a series of N structurally related molecules i = 1, . . . N, with known biological activities. The orientation of the molecules to be compared is performed by superimposing the atoms of the "pharmacophore constellation". Other atoms are also superimposed by respecting van der Waals contact distances. Hydrogen atoms are neglected. The superposition procedure of N molecules produce a topological network with vertices j = 1 . . . M corresponding to the approximate positions of the superimposed atoms (a tolerance of about 0.5 Å being admitted), and with edges corresponding to covalent bond between atoms.

The constitution of each molecule i is described by an occupancy vector $x_{i,j}$ (Kronecker delta) with $x_{i,j} = 1$ if the vertex is occupied by an atom of the molecule, or $x_{i,j} = 0$ if not.

Selection of a start receptor map, S_o, describing three categories of vertices: receptor cavity (beneficial) vertices with $\epsilon_j = -1$; the wall (detrimental) vertices with $\epsilon_j = +1$; and the exterior (irrelevant) vertices with $\epsilon_j = 0$. The steric misfit of molecule i is measured by MTD_i, the minimal steric (or topologic) difference, defined as:

$$MTD_i = s + \sum_{j=1}^{n} \epsilon_j x_{ij} \tag{45}$$

which gives for molecule i the number of unoccupied receptor vertices plus the number of occupied wall vertices; s is the total number of cavity vertices in the hypermolecule. The calculated biological activity A_i is given by:

$$A_i = a_0 + a_1\sigma_i + \ldots - \beta MTD_i \tag{46}$$

where a_o, a_1 . . . β are regressional coefficients. The start map can be inspired by the form of the most active molecule.

Optimization of the receptor map: in the optimization procedure, one starts from the initial set, S^o, of ϵ_i assignments and changes them, one by one, aiming at minimizing the sum Y of squares of differences between experimental activities, $\hat{A}_i$, and calculated activities A_i

$$Y = \sum_{i=1}^{N} (A_i - \hat{A}_i)^2 \tag{47}$$

The receptor map is considered to be optimized (S^*) if other, singular ϵ_j changes do not further reduce Y. This optimized receptor map, S^*, is a model of the receptor site, the main result of the MTD method.

The following specific difficulties appear with the MTD-method: (1) Construction of the hypermolecule; (2) molecules with several low energy conformations (3) the optimization method. If molecules with condensed cycles are to be superimposed (for instance: steroid-type molecules with different ring sizes or systems of double bonds in the nucleus), it is not clear how far some of the corresponding atoms fall apart if simple superposition based upon comparison of structural models is achieved. One cannot say if these corresponding atoms (of different cycles) can be ''contracted'' into single vertices or if new vertices are to be introduced in the hypermolecule. If there are several low energy conformations for one molecule we adopt the conformation which allows the best superposition with the standard molecule. In principle, one must consider the conformation which gives the lowest misfit, the lowest MTD_i value. One should check (by molecular mechanics calculations) the energy of this conformation. If no special care is taken, optimized maps with interspersed wall, cavity and exterior-vertices may result, producing complicated, unrealistic receptor site structures. The vertex attribution may also depend on other structural variables considered.

Let us consider all these problems separately. The construction of the hypermolecule can be solved on a more rigorous basis by minimizing the mean square root (MSR) deviation between the corresponding atoms, (either all of them, or selected atoms in two molecules, one of which is considered as ''standard''), yielding an initial set of vertices. New vertices are to be added for corresponding atoms which fall apart more than one standard distance (by respect to its counterpart in the ''standard'' molecule).

This procedure was applied in MTD-studies on progestational steroids by Bohl, Simon et al.[110-112] On this basis progesterone, 5α-H-androstan-3,20-dione and 9,10-dehydro-progesterone derivatives could be superimposed — with progesterone as ''standard'' — and only three new vertices had to be introduced. The standard distance of 0.5 Å was considered hereby. The C_1 and C_2 atoms of 5-H-androstane and 9,10-dehydroprogesterone fall rather far apart from C_1 and C_2 of progesterone because of a different low energy conformation of the A-ring.[34] Table 13 lists some distances between equivalent ring atoms for superposition upon the progesterone cycle. For the progesterone-testosterone superposition, several corresponding atoms fall more than 0.5 Å apart, several new vertices are to be introduced (for these atoms and the substituents bond to them) if testosterone and progesterone derivatives are to be treated in a unique series for QSAR; in the above mentioned papers,[110,111] progesterone and testosterone series were treated in separate series. X-ray crystallographic coordinates[112] were used. Table 13 presents the 17 β-OH-5H-α-androstane-3-one ring system as a model for the 5-H-androstane-3,20-dione system, and the 9,10-dehydrotestosterone system as model for the 9,10-dehydrotestosterone system. Atoms C_1, C_2 and O_{17} were not considered for the MSR procedure. For the testosterone-progesterone superposition, $O_{17-\beta}$ and O_{20} were considered also as equivalent atoms.

The hypermolecule thus contains three supplementary vertices, compared to the pro-

TABLE 13
Distances Between Equivalent Atoms for Superposition of Steroids Upon the Progesterone Molecule

Atom no.	5 AHT	4,9.T	T
C_1	—	—	0.419
C_2	—	—	0.414
C_3	0.193	0.282	0.339
C_4	0.551	0.140	0.297
C_5	0.323	0.041	0.311
C_6	0.204	0.081	0.269
C_7	0.059	0.096	0.335
C_8	0.074	0.143	0.383
C_9	0.127	0.402	0.417
C_{10}	0.098	0.369	0.376
C_{11}	0.185	0.237	0.476
C_{12}	0.146	0.120	0.557
C_{13}	0.041	0.105	0.559
C_{14}	0.029	0.060	0.495
C_{15}	0.128	0.055	0.514
C_{16}	0.324	0.048	0.658
C_{17}	0.052	0.226	0.651
C_{18}	0.111	0.151	0.500
C_{19}	0.231	—	0.328
O_3	0.279	0.159	0.320
$O_{20}(O_{17})$	—	—	0.728

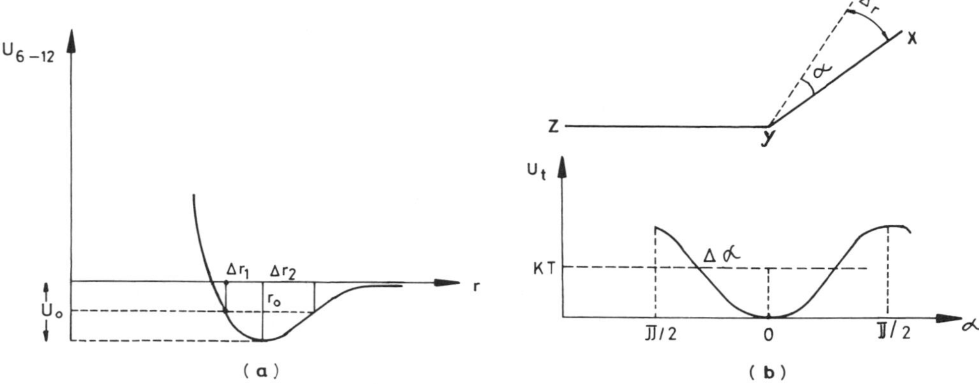

FIGURE 11. Sensitivity of some interaction potentials to distance distortion.

gesterone atoms: C_1 and C_2 in the 5Hα- and 4,9-di-Δ-rings (different A-ring conformations) and C_4 in the 5Hα-ring.

The justification of the distance limit of 0.5 Å is of interest.[111] In fact, how exact must be the steric fit, i.e., what tolerance for the positioning of an atom (of the drug molecule) in the receptor site is admissable (i.e., produces only a small difference in the interaction energy)? Such an atom displacement will affect van der Waals energies or, if steric crowding is circumvented by distortion of torsional angles, the sinusoidal potential energy for torsion (Figure 11a and b).

Consider the 6,12 van der Waals potential introduced by Lennard-Jones (Figure 11a):

$$U(r) = -A/r^6 + B/r^{12} \qquad (48)$$

The energy minimum, $U_o = -A^2/4B$ is obtained for $r_o = (2B/A)^{1/6}$. One may ask for which $r = r_o + \Delta r$ the van der Waals interaction energy U_o (corresponding to the interaction with an atom in a "cavity" vertex) is reduced to half:

$$U(r_0 + \Delta r) = \frac{1}{2} U_0 = - \frac{A^2}{8B} \tag{49}$$

The equation can be brought to a quadratic form, and one obtains two solutions:

$$r_0 + \Delta r = 1.227 \, r_0 \text{ or } 0.916 \, r_0 \tag{50}$$

With $r_o = 3.5$ Å for van der Waals contact distances:

$$\Delta r = +0.79 \text{ Å or } -0.33 \text{ Å} \tag{50a}$$

For the distortion of a torsional angle (Figure 11b), the potential is:

$$U(\alpha) = \frac{1}{2} U_0 (1 - \cos n\alpha) \quad n = 2,3 \tag{51}$$

$$\Delta U(\alpha) = U(\alpha) - U(o) = \frac{1}{2} U_0 (1 - \cos n\alpha) \tag{52}$$

The shift of atom X produced by a torsion of α-radians will be:

$$\Delta r = d_{xy} \cdot \sin_{xyz} \tag{53}$$

One can adopt as tolerable $U = kT = 4.10^{-12}$ j (for 300°K). With $d_{xy} = 1.5$ Å, $xyz = 108°30'$ (sp³ hybridization for y), and with three values for U_o of 3, 10 and 40 kcal/mol, respectively, one obtains for Δr, 0.64, 0.34 and 0.17 Å, respectively. The guess of 0.5 Å for distance tolerance is thus acceptable.

Consideration of several low energy conformations for each molecule was discussed at length in a MTD paper about substituted acetic acid derivatives with auxinic activity.[113] Low energy conformations can be considered to be those whose energy difference with respect to the one of lowest energy is not large in comparison to the mean thermal energy, kT. In principle, if there are several low-energy conformations to be considered for each molecule, a third subscript, k, must be considered and conformation k of molecule i is described by an (x_{ijk}) vector, with $x = 1$ if vertex j is occupied in the conformation k of molecule i and $x_{ijk} = 0$ if this vertex is not occupied. In the complex with the receptor, the molecule will adopt the conformation which fits best into the receptor site, i.e., has the minimal MTD value. Thus, if several conformations are considered:

$$MTD_i = Min(s + \sum_{j'=1}^{M} \epsilon_j x_{ijk}) \tag{54}$$

In most of the published MTD-works, if several low-energy conformations are possible for some molecules of the considered series, the MTD-value considered for each molecule was checked for being the lowest among those corresponding to the low energy conformations. If necessary, corrections were performed, which generally somewhat decreased the r value obtained for the optimized map. Generally, all conformations of a molecule with no obvious steric hindrance or interruption of π-electron conjugation were considered as low-energy conformations in this type of work.

A computer program for QSAR with the MTD-method with multiple conformations (with Equation 54 instead of Equation 45 for definition of MTD) was written by Ciubotariu et al.[17,114] and was used to develop a QSAR for a series of alpha-adrenergic agonists.[115]

The tendency of the MTD-optimization method to yield different optimized receptor maps (local minima) when beginning with different star-maps ($S°$) and also to yield maps with interspersed cavity, wall and exterior vertices, can be limited by imposing different restrictions on the optimization strategy. Motoc, in his SIBIS-variant of the MTD-method, considers (during the optimization procedure and for the optimized map) only maps in which all cavity vertices and all wall vertices form a unique connected set (within the hypermolecule considered as a topological network).[116] Experience with MTD-QSARs, especially the results obtained for test series, suggest that this limitation is too stringent and that the restriction of a unique connected network, applied only to the cavity vertices, gives better results.[9,64,117]

A unique connected network for wall vertices is not to be used if attractive receptor-molecule interactions are described mainly by another parameter such as hyhdrophobicity or, perhaps, polarizability parameters (molecular refraction group).[65] Actually, in the SIBIS-method of Motoc,[116] attractive interactions are described by the OV-parameter (the overlapping volume of receptor cavity and drug molecule), repulsive interactions by the NOV-parameter (overlapping volume of receptor walls and drug molecule. In the SIBIS-variant[118] one tries to describe attractive interactions by the hydrophobicity of the part of the drug molecule which overlaps with the receptor cavity (or lies within the receptor cavity). A similar idea was used in MTD-work upon progestogenic steroids.[110-112] Along with MTD, relative hydrophobicities (f) of progesterone and testosterone analogs were considered as a second structural parameter. These hydrophobicities (calculated as sums of fragmental contributions) were corrected by neglecting the contribution of the 3- and 17β-substituents which correspond to groups giving strong polar interactions (hydrogen bonding) with the progesteronic receptor. The QSARs obtained for progesterone and testosterone derivatives, respectively, are the following:[111]

$$A_{prog} = 5.493 - 0.760 \text{ MTD} + 0.698 \text{ f; n} = 55, \text{ r} = 0.934 \tag{55}$$

$$A_{testo} = 5.000 - 0.966 \text{ MTD} + 0.538 \text{ f; n} = 39, \text{ r} = 0.932 \tag{56}$$

have fairly similar regressional coefficients for MTD and f. The optimized maps also have identical attributions for substituents at the A and B ring atoms which overlap well if progesterone and testosterone are superimposed (see Table 13). When these results are compared with those for smaller series (n $=$ 34 and n $=$ 25, respectively)[110] the regressional coefficients present sufficient stability, and attributions to common vertices (in the extended and reduced series) are not changed. Only a few vertices are attributed as beneficial ($\epsilon =$ -1) in this case. As attractive interactions are described successfully by the hydrophobicity f, the irrelevant ($\epsilon_j = 0$) vertices should not correspond to parts of molecules placed in the exterior, aqueous solution. The $\epsilon_j = -1$ (beneficial) atoms also present some supplementary interactions. As a conclusion, the MTD-method is one of the first 3D-QSAR methods at a low level of sophistication (not very mugh higher than the simple, Hansch-type QSAR). As judged from results with test series[65] and stability of equations,[112] it worked satisfactory for several series of molecules up to the size of steroids. Molecules with fairly different stereochemistries can be considered within a unique QSAR.

Certainly, one should not expect correlation coefficients much higher than r $=$ 0.9 with such a simple method. Actually, an explained variance of about 75% is its predictive power, as given by results with test series.[18] Outliers are to be expected if interactions with rigid zones of the receptor site interfere, requiring a more stringent positioning of the interaction atoms of the molecule. The MTD method can be considered to have a significant predictive capacity and can certainly be recommended if some steric peculiarities of a receptor (not yet studied by X-ray crystallography) are required as an onset for a less approximate 3D-QSAR-study.

5. Molecular Shape Analysis

A somewhat similar method was developed by Hopfinger and Potenzone.[119] It is based on the volume differences between the most stable conformation of the most active compound in the congeneric database and the compound to be investigated. The most stable (probable) conformations are determined by molecular mechanics calculations.[120]

6. Topological Indices

Topological models, using the powerful generalizations of the graphs theory (a field related to combinatorics), were included in attempts to numerically express the molecular structure.[121]

Molecular topology is based on the notion of covalent chemical bond, considered as the internal connection between two atoms in the molecule. Constitutional isomerism follows directly. Therefore, in molecular topology, structural information (i.e., regarding the molecular shape and size) is implicit. A series of topological indices were developed on this basis, containing more or less structural information; they are suitable to be used as steric parameters in QSAR analysis. The molecular connectivity indices described by Randić, Kier and Hall[122,123] belong to this category. Toplogical indices as well as their applications in carcinogenesis are discussed in detail in Chapter 4.

7. Descriptors for the Connectivity Methods

Connectivity methods and those using pattern recognition techniques employ a series of specific descriptors which code in some way the information concerning the ground-state positions of atoms composing a molecule, the connections of each atom, data on the structure of the molecule, indications regarding the molecular shape, thickness, etc. Some of the new computer-assisted connectivity methods (as for instance SIMCA) also employ additional "classical parameters" such as hydrophobicity and especially electronic indices.

The descriptors briefly discussed in this section can be classified into two large distinct categories, namely topological descriptors and geometrical ones. Whereas the latter have a concrete physical significance, the former usually lack such a content.

a. Geometrical Descriptors

In contrast with steric parameters previously discussed which express the sterical features of substituents, these descriptors were developed, in order to describe the stereochemistry of the entire molecule. They include molecular volumes, molecular surfaces and the main axis of the molecule or various combinations of these data.

b. Fragment Descriptors

These are the most simple descriptors including atom types, bond types, molecular weights, some specific structural elements (e.g., number and type of saturated, nonsaturated, aromatic rings, etc.).

c. Substructure Indices

Each structure from a set of compounds is searched for the presence of substructures of interest. The number of their occurences in a given structure is taken into account. If the descriptor is not present, it is given the value zero.

Substructure indices are usually connectivity indices[124] or topological ones (see Section

D.6 in this chapter), but they can belong to other categories as well. They depend mainly on the methodology employed for the QSAR analysis. For instance, the SAR procedure developed by Einslein[121] uses a dictionary containing 148 substructures. This dictionary — named CROSSBOW — was developed by Eakin.[125] It was further expanded to 350 substructures and more recently replaced by the improved system MOLSTAC.

d. *Environment Descriptors*

The information present in the fragment and substructure descriptors indicates the components of the molecular structure. Environment descriptors supply information about their interconnection by coding the vicinities of these substructures. If a searched substructure is found, then the environment descriptor is computed by performing a path one molecular connectivity computation of the substructure atoms as embedded within the structure, and in addition of the first nearest-neighbor atoms.

This type of descriptor is often employed in ADAPT and CASE techniques. Most of them are calculated by means of specific programs packages.

IV. QSAR ANALYSIS OF MUTAGENIC AND CARCINOGENIC PROPERTIES OF CHEMICAL COMPOUNDS

There are many QSAR studies of mutagenesis and carcinogenesis. Their usefulness is obvious nowadays, as they may afford valuable and accessible prediction models concerning the apparition of this type of biological property in structurally related (congeners) or unrelated chemicals. Because only a very limited number of compounds from the enormous amount of chemicals existing in the environment have been experimentally tested for their biological properties, the development of predictive screening becomes of prime importance.

Besides, these models also afford a theoretical basis for validation and, hence, selection among various possible mechanisms of action by which compounds of a certain type exert their carcinogenic or mutagenic properties. A relevant example of a typical strategy for such an approach when dealing with a large noncongeneric database (the most general situation) was recently proposed by Loew[127] and comprises the following steps:

1. Division of the chemicals into subgroups according to structure and functional groups
2. Development of an accurate and reproducible biological database, specific for the problem approached; for carcinogenesis, this aspect was discussed in Chapter 3 and for assaying mutagenic activity, there are, nowadays, a number of tests fulfilling this requirement
3. Development of models concerning the mechanisms of action of several representative compounds in each subgroup both on an experimental basis and also by means of theoretical chemistry (quantum chemical calculations of electronic properties, chemical reactivities, etc.)
4. Selection of appropriate descriptors for evaluation of the activity; they are chosen differently when dealing with classical QSAR models, or with so called ''causal approaches''*
5. Evaluation of the selected descriptors, by correlating them to the biological properties: this evaluation can also be done experimentally as well as by theoretical methods; the descriptors proven to be useful are further employed in large-scale predictive screenings

This methodology affords a rational basis for reaching the above discussed goals.

We shall discuss briefly a part of the results obtained both by classical methods of QSAR analysis (extrathermodynamic approaches) and by connectivity methods, more recently de-

---

* ''Causal approaches'' are those studies based on methods related to connectivity, pattern recognition, etc.

TABLE 14
Qualitative SAR Studies

No.	Class of compounds	Physico-chemical parameter discussed in relation with carcinogenicity	Ref.
1.	Acetylaminofluorenes	$-CH_2$-group from fluorene moiety (isosteres: -S-, -O-, $-SO_2$-, etc.)	127
2.	Amino-stilbenes	Planarity and uninterrupted conjugation	128, 129
3.	PAHs	Planarity	130, 131
4.	PAHs	Stability (melting points) of the picrates	132
5.	PAHs	Presence of a phenanthrene skeleton	133
6.	Methylated-PAHs	Site of methylation and ultraviolet absorption (bathocromic shift)	134, 135
7.	PAHs	Reaction rate and extend for oxidation with perbenzoic acid osmium tetroxide, etc.	136, 138

veloped. An excellent review of both such methods belongs to Frierson, Klopman and Rosenkranz.[6]

A. CLASSICAL QSAR METHODS FOR THE STUDY OF MUTAGENICITY AND CARCINOGENICITY

The first studies concerning structure-activity relationships obviously had an empirical (and usually not quantitative) character. However, even these qualitative conclusions contributed to a deeper understanding of the molecular basis for chemical mutagenesis and carcinogenesis, and to the connections between these closely related areas. A series of such correlations is summarized in Table 14.

An obvious progress has been made by using Hansch's extrathermodynamic approach in the development of quantitative models, the only ones which are able to afford a real basis for predicting carcinogenic and mutagenic activities. One of the first papers is concerned with the correlation between the carcinogenic properties of a series of aromatic amines (*p*-dimethylamino-azobenzenes) (**5**) and their structure.[127] Separate regression equations were computed for two subgroups of amines containing the substituents on ring a or on ring b:

a—N=N—b—$N(CH_3)_2$

5

$$\log A_a = -2.06\pi^2 + 0.94\pi - 0.12\sigma + 0.83 \tag{57}$$
$$r = 0.710 \qquad s = 0.210$$

$$\log A_b = -2.02\pi^2 + 0.93\pi + 0.81 \tag{58}$$
$$r = 0.699 \qquad s = 0.241$$

The main conclusion of this study is that the substituents located on ring b of the aromatic system do not affect carcinogenicity through electronic effects (because the term σ does not appear in Equation 58). However, they indirectly influence the activity through their own lipophilicity.

A class of compounds extensively investigated by quantitative approaches is the class of polycyclic aromatic hydrocarbons (PAHs). In this case one cannot discuss linear free-energy equations because of the mode in which carcinogenic activity (independent variable) is often expressed. In PAH activity quantification, QSAR analysis appears as a multiparametric model (see Chapter 5, Section II.A), and the parameters of choice for the independent variables are quantum-mechanical indices.

Among the first attempts for quantitative correlations, we mention those of Smith et al.[139] Various quantum mechanical indices calculated for "key"-bonds or -regions of the PAH molecule (i.e., I_A, I_B, I_K*) were computed and correlated with delocalization energy (ΔE_{deloc}), supposed to be a valuable indicator of the PAH carcinogenic potency (according to the bay-region theory). This approach finally led to a first selection of appropriate quantum mechanical descriptors, expressing the carcinogenicity of these molecules.

The carcinogenic activity quantification actually represents the critical difficulty in correlational calculations for any type of carcinogens. First, the experimental imprecision of these determinations has to be taken into account because it will heavily influence the quality of the correlation. The situation is even more critical when a discontinuous (conventional) mode of expression is used.

Iball's indices (as well as Badger's, etc.),[141] the most frequently used as carcinogenicity indices, express this property as a function of the percent of animals with tumors and the latency period of their apparition (against controls). Employing these indices for PAH carcinogenicity quantification, the following relationship was obtained:

$$\text{Iball} = 267.4I_A + 414.9\Delta E_\pi - 830.6$$
$$r = 0.853 \qquad p < 0.0001 \tag{59}$$

where ΔE_π represents the difference of π electron energy between the ultimate carcinogen diol-epoxide and the corresponding carbocation.[142]

A similar regression equation is also obtained for a sample of eleven PAHs containing methylated derivatives, namely:

$$\text{Iball} = -333.2Q_b + 506.1I_A - 780.0$$
$$n = 11 \qquad r = 0.942 \qquad p < 0.0014 \tag{60}$$

where Q_b is the π charge density at the benzylic carbon of the carbocation. Both equations suggest that: (a) the sensibility of the distal bay-region (A zone) to oxidation by the enzymatic activation systems has an important contribution in determining the carcinogenic properties of the PAH and (b) the ease of benzylic carbocation formation has a similar effect (see Chapter 3).

A more complex predictive model was developed by Szentpaly[140] for 25 PAHs:

$$I = -(80.47 \pm 9.46)M + (8.244 + 5.10)(E_D + E_C) - (0.0739 \pm 0.0107)\Delta - (331.7 \pm 21.6)$$
$$n = 25 \qquad r = 0.961 \qquad s = 6.8 \qquad F = 87.455 \tag{61}$$

where M is a metabolic parameter describing the balance between the primary epoxidation (at the distal bay-region) and the detoxication reactions, Δ is a parameter describing the size of the molecule, E_D is the delocalization energy, and E_C is the charge dispersal energy.**)

Equation 61 was complemented by the same group[144] with a set of 14 PAHs also containing heterocyclic and methylated congeners. A similar equation was obtained:

* The definition of I_A, I_B and I_K indices is given in Chapter 3.
** A more detailed discussion of this model is given in Chapter 3.

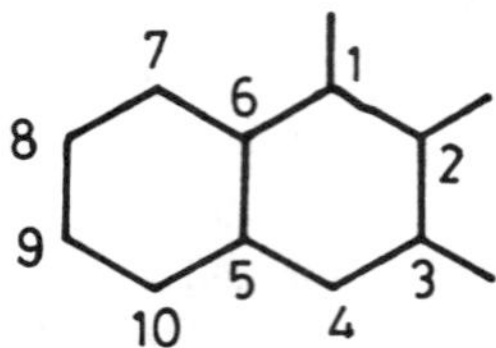

FIGURE 12.   Numbering of atoms in the PAH used in Equations 64 to 66.

$$I = (131.59 \pm 16.27)C - (54.25 \pm 11.98)M_r - (0.632 \pm 0.212)\Delta - 38.1$$

$$n = 14 \qquad r = 0.940 \qquad s = 10.4 \qquad F = 22.65 \tag{62}$$

where C measures the ease of the bay-region carbocation formation, M and Δ have the same meanings as in Equation 61. Mention must be made that this equation, through the inclusion of the M parameter, affords suggestions regarding the metabolic pathways and activation mechanism of these compounds.

More recently, structure-activity relationships in this field were described using quantum mechanical parameters and lipophilicity constants, wherein carcinogenicity (the dependent variable) was replaced by a series of other measurable biological properties (supposed to be linearly related with this parameter). These properties[143] namely: the constant of the binding to human seric albumin (K),[145] inhibition of dimethylnitrosoamine demethylase (A),[146] the formation rate of 3-hydroxybenzo(a)pyrene (R),[147] etc. could be measured without difficulty and are more accurate than for carcinogenicity determinations. The best correlations were:

$$\log A = 5.229Q(8)_{HOMO} + 0.477S_N(9) - 0.500$$

$$n = 7 \qquad r = 0.959 \qquad s = 0.219 \qquad F = 22.67 \tag{63}$$

$$\log K = 52.130S_E(7) + 0.030H_f + 16.623$$

$$n = 7 \qquad r = 0.999 \qquad s = 0.035 \qquad F = 1565.5 \tag{64}$$

$$\log M = 13.016Q(8)_{LEMO} + 1.085S_N(9) - 3.738$$

$$n = 7 \qquad r = 0.968 \qquad s = 0.44 \qquad F = 30.01 \tag{65}$$

where: $Q(a)_{HOMO}$ refers to the electron population in the highest occupied molecular orbital in the atom a, $Q(a)_{LEMO}$, idem for the lowest empty MO, $S_N(a)$, $S_E(a)$ nucleophilic and electrophilic superdelocalizability,[148] respectively, in atom a.* The numbers in brackets concern the numbering of atoms in the PAH according to Figure 12.

For a number of nine PAHs, a parallelism between total electrophilic superdelocalizability (S_E) and the hydrophobicity parameter was found:

$$\log P = 0.974S_E + 0.102$$

$$n = 9 \qquad r = 0.999 \qquad s = 0.086 \qquad F = 2147.9 \tag{66}$$

---

* A more detailed discussion of this model is given in Chapter 3.

This relationship agrees with the equations developed by Roger and Camarata. The correlations obtained are excellent, although the number of compounds analyzed is relatively small; however, the degree in which the biological parameters A and K reflect the actual carcinogenicity of this PAH raises some questions.

Finally, a conventional expression of carcinogenicity, by using an arbitrary scale (J), with discrete values of 0, 1, 2, 3 and 4 for for inactive $(-)$, slightly active $(+)$, moderately active $(+ +)$, active $(+ + +)$ and very active $(+ + + +)$ was proposed.[149] This scale was used for the estimation of carcinogenicity in the bay-region theory. More recently, Miyashita et al.[150] used the same expression of carcinogenicity in attempts to correlate this property with a series of quantum mechanical parameters for a set of 21 PAHs (among which 15 were carcinogenic and 6 noncarcinogenic) using a multiparametric approach. The following equation was obtained:

$$J = 8.64\Delta E_\pi + 12.43\Delta E_{deloc} - 0.34I_L + 21.61$$

$$n = 21 \qquad r = 0.91 \qquad s = 0.62 \qquad F = 26.45 \tag{67}$$

where ΔE_π is the energy modification (expressed in β units*) during the A-region (distal bay-region) dihydrodiol formation, from the parent PAH,** ΔE_{deloc} is the delocalization energy calculated by HMO, and I_L is the sum of the two atomic superdelocalizabilities involved in L-region.

The predicted carcinogenicities satisfactorily agree with experimental data, thus showing the validity of the proposed model and justifying this type of approach.

The same way of expressing carcinogenicity was employed by Loew's group in order to calculate, for instance, a simple molecular descriptor rationalizing the carcinogenic potency of 44 PAHs (also containing methylated and fluorinated congeners). This descriptor is actually the relative delocalization energy, ΔE_{rel}, expressing the formation easiness of the bay-region carbocation, and is calculated with respect to a strong carcinogen taken as standard compound (6,12-dimethylbenzen(a)anthracene), according to the relationship:

$$\Delta E_{rel} = \Delta E_{deloc, standard} - \Delta E_{deloc, X} \tag{68}$$

where $\Delta E_{deloc,X}$ is calculated for hydrocarbon X. Calculated ΔE_{rel} values greater than 15 kcal/mol indicate low or no carcinogenic activity.[126]

Considering that the relative carcinogenic activity may be expressed by any value between 0 and 1 so that A is 1 for PAH inducing tumors in all experimental animals and A = O for the inactive ones, Simon et al.[151] obtained a satisfactory regression equation using the delocalization energy (ΔE_{deloc}) and the MTD parameter as independent variables:

$$A = -6.397 + 9.597\Delta E_{deloc} - 0.303MTD$$

$$n = 29 \qquad r = 0.860 \qquad a = 0.222 \qquad F = 26.0 \tag{69}$$

Despite the correlation found between the mutagenicity and the carcinogenicity of a broad spectrum of chemicals, the ultimate values of bacterial tests for predictive screening raise some doubts.

In order to compare the structural requirements for these two types of biological activity, the MTD technique was used to formulate QSAR[152] for a series of 43 structurally related heterocyclic PAHs belonging to two series of congeners: (a) benzo(thio)pyranoquinolines **6(a,b)** and (b) benzo(thio)pyranoindoles **7(a,b)** for: (1) their mutagenicity against S. *thy-*

---

* 1 β unit $\cong$ 20 kcal/mol.

** For definition and discussion of all these parameters see Chapter 3.

phimurium his⁻ strains TA 98, TA 100 and TA 1537 expressed as the numbers of revertants per nmol of test compounds[153] and (2) the carcinogenic activity (Ca) of the same compounds determined in mice by a standard procedure.[153]

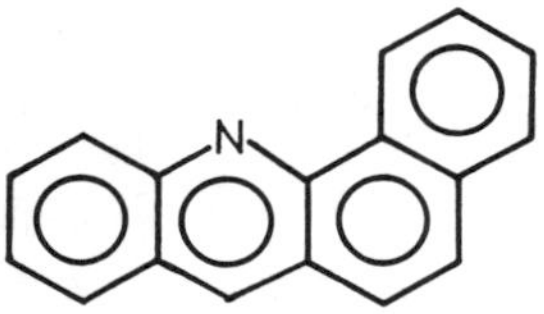

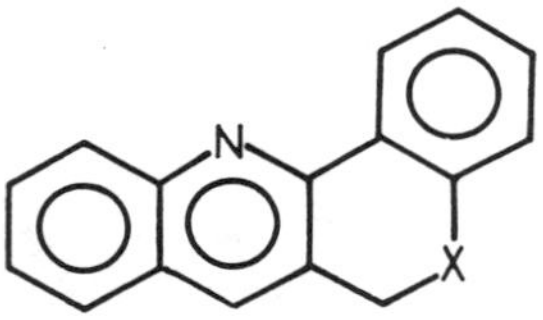

X = O, S

6a   **6b**

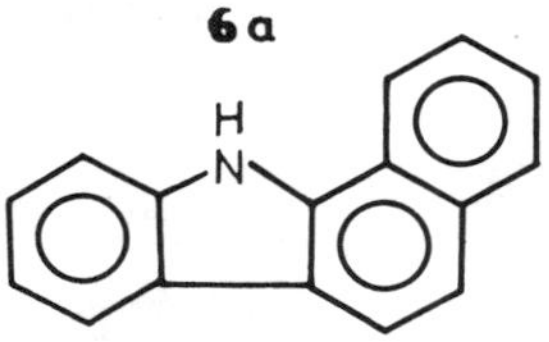

7a 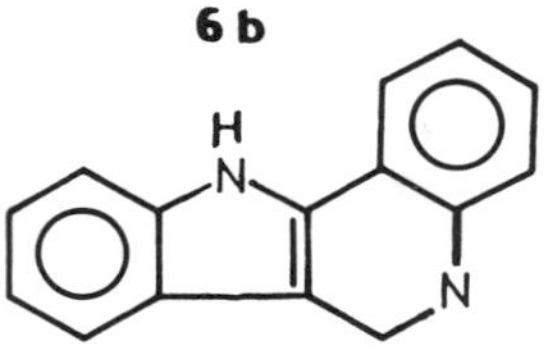   **7b**

The MTD indices (see this chapter, D.4) and the lipophilicity indices were considered for this approach. Mention should be made that only relative log P values were used; log P_{rel} = 0.0 was assigned to the simplest congeners of each series (unsubstituted hydrocarbon). The best equations obtained for each series and each type of activity were:

Series (a): (6H-1-benzothiopyrano(4,3,b)quinolines; **6a**, **6b**)

$$\log Ca = 17.16(\pm 3.39) - 2.57(\pm 0.50)MTD + 0.07(\pm 0.04)\pi$$

$$n = 15 \qquad r = 0.830 \qquad s = 0.77 \qquad F = 13.26 \qquad (70)$$

$$\log TA = 1.14(\pm 0.30) - 0.27(\pm 0.06)MTD - 0.21(\pm 0.14)\pi$$

$$n = 15 \qquad r = 0.860 \qquad s = 0.28 \qquad F = 17.03 \qquad (71)$$

Series (b): (benzothiopyrano(4,3,b)indoles; **7a**, **7b**)

$$\log Ca = 3.68(\pm 0.74) - 0.53(\pm 0.11)MTD - 0.01(\pm 0.22)\pi$$

$$n = 28 \qquad r = 0.700 \qquad s = 0.90 \qquad F = 12.02 \qquad (72)$$

$$\log TA = 1.71(\pm 0.33) - 0.34(\pm 0.05)MTD - 0.35(\pm 0.25)\pi + 0.18(\pm 0.13)\pi^2$$

$$n = 28 \qquad r = 0.904 \qquad s = 0.21 \qquad F = 35.61 \qquad (73)$$

The analysis of (1) MTD indices and (2) the vertices distribution in the calculated hypermolecules for both regression equations allow us to stress that the structural requirements for carcinogenic activity seem to be different from those for mutagenic activity. In this respect, the requirements for mutagenicity against TA 100 strain parallels to a great extent those required by carcinogenicity against XVII ne/Z mice.

A similar study on a number of 30 PAHs was recently carried out by Hopfinger.[154] In this study the mutagenic potency of each compound has been reported in terms of the lowest concentration, C, of PAH required to produce an induced mutation.

As independent variables were used:

$$\Delta E = E_{LEMO} - E_{HOMO} \qquad (74)$$

(E_{LEMO}, E_{HOMO} being the energy in β units of the lowest empty and highest occupied molecular orbital, respectively) and V_o serves as a quantitative measure of shape similarity according to MSA procedure (see this chapter, D.5). The best equation obtained was the following:

$$\log (1/C) = -0.62\Delta(\pm 0.09)E + 4.1 \cdot 10^{-5}(\pm 0.7 \cdot 10^{-5})(\Delta V_0)^2 + 7.6(\pm 0.08)$$

$$n = 30 \qquad r = 0.876 \qquad s = 0.37 \qquad F = 44.42 \tag{75}$$

The most important contribution to the mutagenicity belongs to the shape term (which exhibits a maximal explained variance of 49%), but it is difficult to assign a definitive geometric meaning to this parameter. An important contribution also belongs to the ΔE parameter (explaining approximately 43% from the variance), the mutagenicity being inversely proportional to its value. In other words, the more stable a PAH, the less prone it will be to metabolic activation.

More recently, Lewis[143] obtained the following equation using a set of seven PAHs, their mutagenicity being expressed at the logarithm of revertants per nanomole of PAH on *S. thyphimurium* TA 100 (log M):

$$\log M = 13.016Q(8)_{LEMO} + 1.085S_N(9) - 3.738$$

$$n = 7 \qquad r = 0.968 \qquad s = 0.44 \qquad F = 30.01 \tag{76}$$

where $Q(8)_{LEMO}$ AND $S_N(9)$ have the meaning given in Equations 63 to 65. This very good correlation (although n is small) confirms the important contribution of electronic factors to PAH mutagenicity.

Triazenes were another class of compound studies in order to identify the structural and physicochemical features responsible for their mutagenic and antitumor effectiveness in an attempt to optimize their antitumor activity by limiting their mutagenicity. The equation developed for the mutagenicity of 1-(X-phenyl)-3,3-dialkyltriazenes was:[155]

$$\log (1/C) = 1.09 \log P - 1.63\sigma^+ + 5.58$$

$$n = 17 \qquad r = 0.974 \qquad s = 0.316 \tag{77}$$

where C is the concentration which induces 30 mutations/10^8 bacteria. This equation suggests that an increase in the lipophilicity of triazenes and an increase of electron release via through-resonance enhance mutagenicity. The use of σ^+ indices (instead of σ) leads to a better correlation suggesting that the activation of triazenes occurs by a mechanism in which the first step consists in the oxidation of an *N*-alkyl group:

$$X\text{–}C_6H_4N = N - N(CH_3)_2 \xrightarrow[\text{microsomes}]{[O]} X\text{–}C_6H_5N = N - N(CH_3)CH_2OH$$

8   **9**

A second argument favoring this assumption is represented by the important contribution of lipophilicity to Equation 77, which is in good agreement with the correlation found between the Michaelis constant K_M of the microsomal oxidation of organic compounds and log P:

$$-\log K_M = 0.69 \log P + 2.90$$

$$n = 14 \qquad r = 0.920 \qquad s = 0.330 \tag{78}$$

Regarding the antitumor activity (against L 1210) of a much larger set of triazenes, the following equation was computed by the same group:

$$\log 1/C = 0.10 \log P - 0.042(\log P)^2 - 0.315\sigma + -0.18MR_{2,6} + 0.39E_{s-R} + 4.12$$

$$n = 61 \qquad r = 0.836 \qquad s = 0.191 \tag{79}$$

where the $MR_{2,6}$ parameter indicates the deleteriour effect produced by *ortho*-substitution of some congeners, and E_{s-R} represents the steric constants (see this chapter, D.2) of the nitrogen alkyl substituent.

On comparing Equation 77 and Equation 79, Hansch concluded that: by manipulating the electronic and lipophilic character of substituents much can be done to decrease mutagenicity without affecting the pharmaceutical properties of a drug.[156]

A study of the same class of substances using Hansch's and steric parameters MSA was reported by Hopfinger and Potenzone.[119]

An interesting attempt to compare by QSAR analysis the carcinogenicity (measured by the number of tumors induced in A mice) with the mutagenicity (determined on *S. typhimurium* TA 100 and TA 1535 lines, by activation of carcinogens with S_9 fraction) of several aromatic nitrogen mustards was carried out by Leo et al.[157] The equation thus obtained:

$$\log 1/C_M = 0.35(\pm 0.10)\pi - 0.087(\pm 0.059)\pi^2 + 1.64$$

$$n = 13 \qquad r = 0.941 \qquad s = 0.225 \qquad F = 38.34 \tag{80}$$

suggests that mutagenicity, expressed as the concentration which induces 200 revertants above the threshold concentration (concentration — at which the mutagenic activity rises rapidly with dose), depends only on lipophilicity and not on electronic factors (optimal lipophilicity, $\pi_o = 2.16$).

The equation proposed for carcinogenic activity is:

$$\log 1/C_c = -1.68(\pm 0.91)I_4 + 2.65(\pm 2.5)\sigma^2 - 1.30(\pm 1.09)\sigma + 3.75(\pm 0.75)$$

$$n = 11 \qquad r = 0.889 \qquad s = 0.530 \qquad F = 8.83 \tag{81}$$

where C_c is the concentration which induces a single tumor in mice, and I_4 is an indicator variable having the value 1 for congeners possessing a substituent in position 4, and 0 for the others.

Equation 81 reflects the fact that a substituent in position 4 considerably decreases (by a factor of more than 10) the carcinogenicity of aromatic nitrogen mustards. Unusually, Equation 81 has a σ^2 term, suggesting a change in the mechanism of tumor induction vs. the increasing value of the electronic parameters σ ($\sigma_{optimal} = 0.19$). Direct comparison between carcinogenicity and mutagenicity leads to the expression:

$$\log 1/C_c = -0.64(\pm 0.92)\log 1/C_M + 3.82(\pm 1.36)$$

$$n = 11 \qquad r = 0.47 \qquad s = 0.90 \qquad F = 2.5 \tag{82}$$

Surprisingly, this relationship indicates a lack of correlation between carcinogenic and mutagenic activity for aromatic nitrogen mustards. There are some tentative explanations of this unexpected conclusion. One of them could be that different mechanisms are involved in mutagenicity and carcinogenicity of nitrogen mustards. Thus, if direct alkylation (via aziridinium intermediates) and activated alklyation (via a possible arene oxide metabolite) could be postulated as possible activation paths, the latter appears to be preponderant in

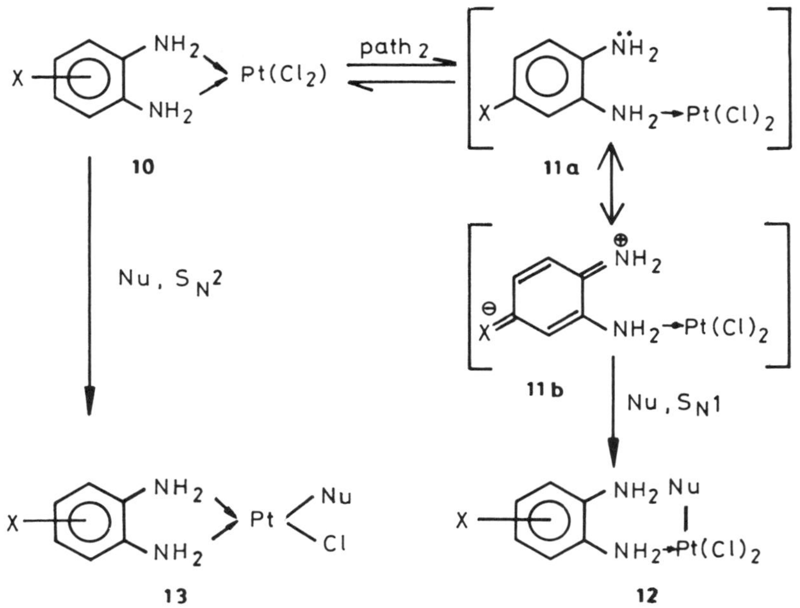

SCHEME 2. The two possible paths of nucleophilic substitution of an organic platinum derivative.

mutagenesis. In contrast, it is possible that only direct alkylation (via aziridium intermediates) leads to promutagenic lesions responsible for the cancerogenic properties of nitrogen mustards.

The organo-platinum derivatives were also submitted by Hansch[156] to a QSAR analysis of their mutagenicity (on *S. typhimurium* TA 92 with S_9 activation). The following correlation was obtained:

$$\log 1/C = 2.23 \sum_i (\sigma_i^-) + 5.78$$

$$n = 13 \qquad r = 0.98 \qquad s = 0.26 \qquad (83)$$

where C is the molar concentration which produces 30 mutations/10^8 surviving bacteria and σ^- is the nucleophilic Hammett constant. The strong dependence on the σ^- constant (characterizing the reactions in which a negative charge is developed at the reaction center and the π-electrons delocalization occurs by through-resonance) suggests that, among the two possible paths of nucleophilic substitution (see Scheme 2), the most probable is pathway II exhibiting an S_N1-like mechanism. If the nucleophilic attack occurs directly on the platinum atom, then in Equation 83, it is expected that σ will be more relevant than σ^-. As this is not the case, it appears reasonable that breaking of the bonds in the platinum complex occurs with the amino ligand acting as leaving group rather than the chlorine atom. The hydrophobic effects do not appear as significant for the mutagenicity of these compounds.

A very similar relationship was proposed by Sugiura[158] for the rationalization of the mutagenicity of substituted styrene oxides (estimated on *S. typhimurium* TA 100):

$$\log 1/C = -1.56(\pm 1.2)\sigma + 6.18(\pm 0.27)$$

$$n = 4 \qquad r = 0.971 \qquad s = 0.113 \qquad (84)$$

where C is the molar concentration of the compounds which produces 200 mutants/10^9 survivors. However, Equation 84 does not contain enough points to be significant.

Nitroso-derivatives are another important class of carcinogens extensively studied concerning their possible activation pathways, as well as the possible correlations between their carcinogenic and mutagenic activity and a series of physicochemical and structural parameters.

The first correlation attempts belong to Wisnok et al.,[159] but the results obtained when expressing the carcinogenic activity as a function of the lipophilicity constant determined in hexane (N) were poor:

$$\log 1/C_{50} = 2.94 - 0.2N$$

$$n = 47 \qquad r = 0.64 \tag{85}$$

where C_{50} is the carcinogen concentration (expressed in moles/kg b.w.) which induces tumors in 50% of the animals.

In a subsequent stage, a much better correlation was obtained on a restricted set using a series of indicator variables in Hansch's equation:[160]

$$\log 1/C_{50} = 4.08 - 0.23\pi^2 + 0.64 - 0.25A - 0.72B - 0.70C$$

$$n = 24 \qquad r = 0.94 \qquad s = 0.29 \tag{86}$$

C_{50} has the same meaning as above, and the indicator variables express the following properties:

1.   A — cyclic nitrosoamines with the amino-nitrogen in the ring and acyclic nitrosoamines
2.   B — presence and location of OH, aromaticity and double bonds
3.   C — the number of hydrogens located in α to the nitroso-function and the number of nitroso groups

Another study, carried out on a restricted number of N-nitrosoamines[161] suggests that lipophilicity alone can account for their carcinogenic potency expressed as the relative number of tumor bearing animals (RTBA):

$$\log (RTBA) = -0.0813 \log P + 0.09$$

$$n = 6 \qquad r = 0.97 \qquad s = 0.019 \tag{87}$$

This relationship proved to be valid only for acyclic N-nitrosoamines.

Very recently, in his attempts to elucidate the mechanisms involved in N-nitrosourea activation, Frecer[162] proposes (for a restricted set of N-nitrosoureas) an equation correlating their carcinogenic activity to quantum mechanical parameters:

$$\log (1/C_{50}) = -0.06 \, S_{01}^{E} - 0.46 \, S_{N2}^{E} - 2.02$$

$$n = 6 \qquad r = 0.998 \qquad F = 235.5 \tag{88}$$

where C_{50} has the meaning from Equation 85, and S^{E} are indices of electrophilic superdelocalizability calculated by MINDO/3 method for O^1 and N^2 atoms, respectively (see formula **14**)

$$N$$
$$|$$
$$R_3 - \overset{|}{\underset{|}{C_7}} - H$$
$$R_1 R_2 N_6 - \overset{\|}{C_4} - N_3 - N_2 = O_1$$
$$O_5$$
$$R_1, R_2, R_3 = H, CH_3$$

14

If the most significant correlations between the reactivity indices of the solvated nitro-soureas and their relative carcinogenic potencies are also considered:

$$\log (1/C_{50}) = -0.35\ S_{N^3}^{E} + 0.57\ S_{C^7}^{E} + 2.65$$

$$n = 6 \qquad r = 0.911 \qquad F = 56.75 \tag{89}$$

then the key function of the nitroso group (N^2 and O^1) and of the N^3-C^7 fragment in the decomposition studied, becomes obvious.

Besides the above approaches a series of similar studies reviewed QSARs for aromatic amines,[163,164] chloroethanes and chloroethylenes,[126] unsaturated dialdehydes,[166] etc.

B. MUTAGENIC-CARCINOGENIC STUDIES USING CONNECTIVITY METHODS

As previously discussed (see this chapter, Section II.B), the methods based on connectivity and pattern recognition techniques are usually classification procedures which are extremely useful for predictive screening of mutagens and carcinogens, especially when noncongeneric databases are available. However, their contribution in mechanistic studies of carcinogenesis and mutagenesis is quite restricted.

1. SIMCA Method

This computer-assisted method using as molecular descriptors the parameters usually employed in Hansch's equation has been little employed in the classification of carcinogens and mutagens.

Among the first studies carried out by means of this method we can recall the study of Norden et al.[165] aiming at the classification of 32 PAHs. Quantum mechanical indices, especially for the carbons contributing to the K- and L-regions were used in the development of correlational equations.

Another typical example is the attempt of Dunn and Wold[167] to rationalize the carcinogenicity of a set of 61 N-nitroso-derivatives (50 active and 11 inactive). Constants σ^x, Taft's E_s molar refeactivity, Rekker parameters (describing lipophilicity) and several of the STERIMOL parameters were employed as independent variables. The use of this set of descriptors for the entire population does not allow separation of classes of compounds with a definite internal structure. Therefore, the active N-nitrosoderivatives were divided into direct-acting carcinogens and compounds requiring previous activation. The latter were further divided into compounds leading by activation (1) to a cation or (2) to a diazoalkane. These additional features lead to the delimitation of two classes of compounds, the first inducing esophageal, nasal and liver tumors, the second one inducing only liver tumors. An electronic parameter, σ^x, appears to be important for the first class of carcinogens, electron withdrawing or electron neutral substituents being associated to higher carcinogenic activity.

A similar methodology is also reported in the paper of Dunn and Wold,[168] which evalutes the carcinogenicity of 4-nitroquinoline-1-oxides.

2. ADAPT Method

This method was promoted by Jurs' group and was used in the QSAR analysis of the biological activity of several large series of compound including mutagens and carcinogens. Thus, the ADAPT method was applied in order to classify a database containing 200 PAHs into carcinogenic and noncarcinogenic compounds. The use of 28 descriptors was required for computing a decision surface able to classify correctly 191 compounds (from the 200, i.e., 96%). Among these descriptors we mention: substructure representing the bay-region, log P, descriptors representing the shape, the area, the volume and the number of aromatic rings in a molecule, as well as a series of electronic indices related especially to the substructure describing bay-region.[169]

A similar approach was carried out on a sample of 153 *N*-nitroso-derivatives (198 carcinogenic, 35 noncarcinogenic). Fifteen descriptors were employed for the classification, namely: six fragment descriptors (number of carbon and nitrogen atoms, bonds, aromatic rings, etc.), five molecular connectivity indices, one geometric variable, one environmental descriptor and two charge descriptors (σ). The overall predictive ability was 91%. The requirement for the two charge indicators suggests the importance of α-hydroxylation for the expression of the carcinogenic properties of *N*-nitrosoderivatives.[170] The results obtained for this type of carcinogens were re-evaluated later,[171] using 150 *N*-nitrosoderivatives (112 carcinogenic, 38 noncarcinogenic). Among the descriptors employed, of particular importance are: a symmetry descriptor of connectivity, as well as the substructures chosen on the basis of the assumption that positions α and β (by respect to the nitroso group) are involved in the activation process of these carcinogens. The overall predictive ability of the obtained correlation was evaluated at 86%, being even better if we consider the group of carcinogens alone ($\sim$90%). Mention must be made that the four substructures representing positions α and β are able to classify 97% from the data, whereas descriptors concerning the shape and size of the molecule accounted for only 20% of the separability.

Similar studies can also be cited for aromatic amines.[172] Employing a set of 157 amines and similar descriptors, a separability of 90% into carcinogens and noncarcinogens was achieved and the overall predictive ability was estimated at 85 to 95%. The molecular volume was suggested to represent a critical parameter for this series of compounds.

3. CASE Method

This program developed by Klopman proved to be useful in the analysis of the carcinogenicity and mutagenicity of a large series of compounds. Using the same database of 200 PAHs previously analyzed by the ADAPT method[169] the CASE method correctly classifies 89% of them.[6] Although the precision is slightly lower, this was achieved with half as many descriptors as for the ADAPT program. Moreover, the CASE method does not require introduction of special data regarding the mechanism of action of these compounds, such as information about bay-region, etc. which depends on the researcher's experience and imagination.

Another study, conducted in the same manner, on a set of 56 PAHs (17 carcinogenic, 33 noncarcinogenic, 6 with questionable carcinogenicity) led to the identification of three substructures having a 99% chance of being responsible for the carcinogenicity of these compounds: these are fragments representing essential features of bay-regions, L-regions and pseudo bay-regions.[34] Using a similar approach on a set of substituted PAHs, Mitchell et al.[173] arrived at the extremely interesting conclusion that the bay-region is a structural element much more important in carcinogenesis than in mutagenesis.

An interesting tentative way to classify a sample of aromatic amines according to their mutagenic activity on *S. typhimurium* TA 98 and TA 100 (S_9-activated)[174] leads to the

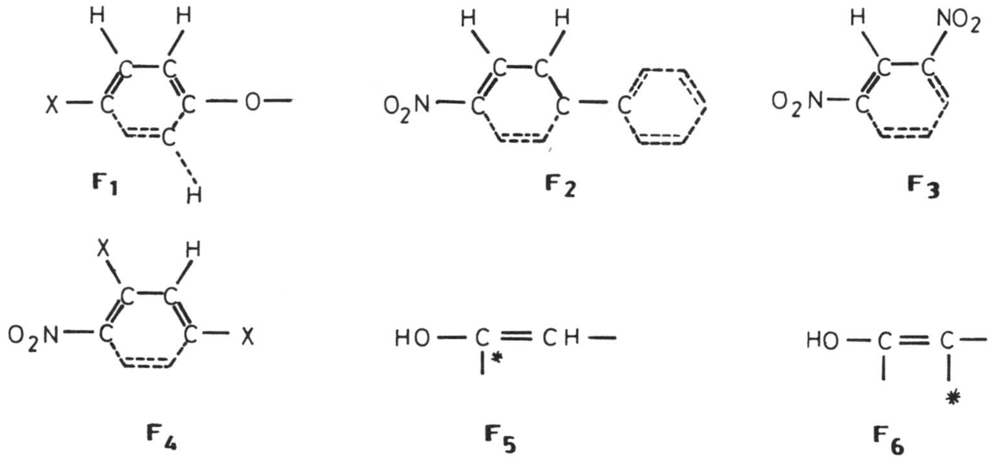

FIGURE 13. Activating and deactivating fragments selected by GST for the mutagenicity of nonfused aromatic compounds. F_5 and F_6 are deactivating fragments, whereas the others are activating ones.

following suggestions: (1) substitution of the nitrogen function by alkyl groups is an unfavorable event for mutagenicity both in TA 98 and in TA 100 strains and (2) the fragment CH_2CH_2OH has a deactivating character regardless of being attached to a nitrogen or not.

The separability of mutagens from nonmutagens is 88% for TA 98, and 84% for TA 100 database.

More recently, mutagenicity in a set of 233 nonfused ring nitroarenes and related compounds (from which 99 are mutagenic) was also investigated[175] by means of the CASE method; 18 fragments (F_1-F_{18}) (substructural descriptors) were identified, among which six (F_1-F_6) are the most important ones for the classification of these compounds. These six fragments are represented in Figure 13.

QSAR analysis of the mutagenicity of these derivatives on the basis of fragment contribution leads to the equation:

$$\text{Calcd} = 17.2 + 2.83(F_7) - 6.37(F_5) - 9.18(F_8) + 5.35(F_9) + 17.40(F_{10})$$

$$+ 6.24(F_{11}) + 7.65(F_2) + 6.21(F_1) - 13.03(F_{13}) + 10.04(F_{14}) + 5.06(F_{15})$$

$$n = 223 \qquad r = 0.848 \qquad s = 8.87 \qquad F = 41.57 \tag{90}$$

where $\text{Calcd} = 10 \times \log(\text{rev/nmol})/0.01 + 2$. Using this equation, a very good separation of active from inactive compounds is achieved (only 8 falsely positive and 15 falsely negative predictions).

The use of the CASE method for evaluating the mutagenicity of several pesticides employing a database of 54 compounds should also be cited.[176] Mention should be made that the CASE procedure can also handle noncongeneric databases.

4. Einslein's Method

Einslein's method was initially used for the classification of a noncongeneric database belonging to IARC (International Agency for Research on Cancer), which contained 343 compounds (223 carcinogenic and 120 noncarcinogenic).[36] The descriptors employed were structural fragments from the CROSSBOW-WLN codes,* molar weights, and molar refractivity.

---

* WLN is the Wiswesser Line Notation, and the CROSSBOW system is mentioned in this chapter, Section III.D.7.c.

The discriminant equation containing 79 descriptors correctly classifies 87 to 91% of the carcinogens and 78 to 80% of the noncarcinogens.

A similar study concerning carcinogenicity was recently carried out on a noncongeneric set of 343 compounds and 63 aromatic amines.[122] The same research group analyzed the mutagenicity properties of 532 compounds (301 mutagenic, 231 nonmutagenic) from a noncongeneric database. The 532 compounds were divided into 474 compounds which were used for establishing the discriminant equation, and a second group of 58 compounds, randomly chosen, which were retained as the test series.

The obtained equation is able to classify correctly 86% of these mutagenic compounds. When applied to the test series, the obtained classification proved to be 80% correct.[37]

REFERENCES

1. **Hansch, C.,** The physico-chemical approach to drug design and discovery (QSAR), *Drug Dev. Res.,* 2, 267, 1981.
2. **Martin, Y. C.,** *Quantitative Drug Design. A Critical Introduction,* Marcel Dekker, New York, 1978.
3. **Franke, R.,** *Theoretical Drug Design Methods,* Academic Verlag, Berlin, 1984.
4. **Martin, Y. C.,** A practitioner's perspective of the role of quantitative structure-activity relationships in medicinal chemistry, *J. Med. Chem.,* 24, 229, 1981.
5. **Hansch, C. and Blaney, J. M.,** The new look in QSAR, in *Drug Design: Fact or Fantasy,* Husch, C., Ed., Academic Press, London, 1984, 185.
6. **Frierson, M. R., Klopman, G., and Rosenkranz, H. S.,** Structure-activity relationships (SARs) among mutagens and carcinogens: a review, *Environ. Mutagen.,* 7, 283, 1986.
7. **Trinajstič, N., Randič, M., and Klein, D. J.,** On the QSAR in drug research, *Acta Pharm. Jugosl.,* 36, 267, 1986.
8. **Balaban, A. T., Chiriac, A., Moţoc, I., and Simon, Z.,** *Steric Fit in QSAR,* Lecture Notes in Chemistry, No. 15, Springer, Berlin, 1980.
9. **Simon, Z., Chiriac, A., Holban, S., Ciubotariu, D., and Mihalaş, G. I.,** *Minimum Steric Difference,* Research Studies Press, Letchworth, England, 1984.
10. **Crippen, G. E.,** *Distance Geometry and Conformational Calculations,* Research Studies Press, Letchworth, England, 1981.
11. **Cramer, R. D., III, Patterson, D. E., and Bruce, J. D.,** Comparative molecular field analysis (CoMFA). I. Effect of shape on binding steroids to carrier proteins, *J. Am. Chem. Soc.,* 110, 5959, 1988.
12. **Gollender, V. E. and Rosenblit, A. B.,** *Logical and Combinatorial Algorithms for Drug Design,* Research Studies Press, Letchworth, England, 1983.
13. **Ariens, E. J.,** Receptor-effector theory and structure-action relationship, *Adv. Drug Res.,* 3, 235, 1961.
14. **Mezey, P. C.,** *Chemical Applications of Topology and Graph Theory,* King, R. B., Ed., Elsevier, Amsterdam, 1983, 40.
15. **Meyer, H.,** Zur Theorie der Alcohol Narkose. Erste Mitteilung. Welche Eigenschaft der Anesthetica bedingt ihre narkotische Wirkung?, *Arch. Exp. Pathol. Pharmacol.,* 42, 110, 1899.
16. **Overton, E.,** *Studien über die Narkose,* Fischer, Jenz, 1901.
17. **Ciubotariu, D.,** Structure-Reactivity Relation in the Class of Carbonic Acids Derivative, Ph.D. thesis, Polytechnical Institute of Bucharest, 1987.
18. **Charton, M. and Moţoc, I.,** *Steric Effects in Drug Design, Topics in Current Chemistry,* Vol. 114, Springer Verlag, Berlin, 1983, 106.
19. **Hammett, L. P.,** The effect of structure upon the reaction of organic compounds. Benzene derivatives, *J. Am. Chem. Soc.,* 59, 96, 1937.
20. **Shorter, J.,** Correlation analysis, in *Organic Chemistry: An Introduction to Linear Free-Energy Relationships,* Clarendon Press, Oxford, 1973.
21. **Hansch, C. and Fujita, T.,** o-σ-π analysis. A method for the correlation of biological activity and chemical structures, *J. Am. Chem. Soc.,* 86, 1616, 1964.
22. **Trinajstič, N., Randič, M., and Klein, D. J.,** On the quantitative structure-activity relationship in drug research, *Acta Pharm. Jugos.,* 36, 267, 1986.
23. **Hansch, C.,** On the structure of medicinal chemistry, *J. Med., Chem.,* 19, 1, 1976.
24. **Lewi, P. J.,** Multivariate data-analysis in structure-activity relationships, *Drug Design,* Ariens, E. J., Ed., Academic Press, New York, 1980, 307.

25. **Rogers, K. S. and Cammarata, A.,** Superdelocalizability and charge density. A correlation with partition coefficients, *J. Med. Chem.,* 12, 692, 1969.

26. **Free, S. M. and Wilson, J. W.,** A mathematical contribution to structure-activity studies, *J. Med. Chem.,* 7, 395, 1964.

27. **Osman, R., Weinstein, H., and Green, J. P.,** Parameters and methods in quantitative structure-activity relationships, Olson, E. C. and Cristoffersen, R. E., Eds., Computer Assisted Drugs, ACS Symp, Ser. 112, ACS, Washington, D.C., 1979, 71.

28. **Stuper, A. G., Brugger, W. E., and Jurs, P. C.,** A computer system for structure-activity studies using chemical structure information handling and pattern recognition techniques, in *Chemometrics: Theory and Application,* Kowalski, B. R., Ed., ACS, Symp. Ser. 52, ACS, Washington, D.C., 1977, 165.

29. **Wold, S. and Sjostrom, M.,** SIMCA, a method for analyzing chemical data in terms of similarity and analogy, in *Chemometrics: Theory and Application,* Kowalski, B. R., Ed., ACS Symp. Ser. 52, ACS, Washington, D.C., 1977, 243.

30. **Stuper, A. J., Brugger, W. E., and Jurs, P. C.,** *Computer-Assisted Studies of Chemical Function,* John Wiley & Sons, New York, 1979.

31. **Jurs, P. C., Chov, J. T., and Yuan, M.,** Studies of chemical structure-biological activity relations using pattern recognition, in *Computer Assisted Drug Design,* Olson, E. C. and Cristofferson, R. E., Eds., ACS Symp. Ser. 112, ACS, Washington, D.C., 1978, 103.

32. **Klopman, G. and Rosenkranz, H. S.,** Structural requirements for the mutagenicity of environmental nitroarenes, *Mutat. Res.,* 126, 226, 1984.

33. **Klopman, G., Nambodiri, K., and Kalos, A.,** Computer automated evaluation and prediction of the Iball index of carcinogenicity of polycyclic aromatic hydrocarbons, in *Molecular Bases of Cancer, Part A: Macromolecular Structure, Carcinogens and Oncogenes,* Rein, R., Ed., Alan R. Liss, New York, 1985, 287.

34. **Weissberg, S.,** *Applied Linear Regression,* John Wiley & Sons, New York, 1980.

35. **Einslein, K. and Craig, P. N.,** A toxicity estimation model, *J. Environ. Pathol. Toxicol.,* 2, 215, 1978.

36. **Einslein, K. and Craig, P. N.,** Carcinogenesis: a predictive structure-activity model, *J. Toxicol. Environ. Health,* 10, 521, 1982.

37. **Einslein, K., Lanter, T. R., and Strange, J. R.,** Teratogenesis; a statistical-structure activity model, *Teratogen, Carcinogen, Mutagen,* 3, 429, 1983.

38. **Hodes, G. F., Hazard, R., Geran, I., and Richman, S.,** A statistical-heuristic method for automated selection of drugs, *J. Med. Chem.,* 20, 469, 1977.

39. **Tinker, J.,** A computerized structure-activity correlation program for relating bacterial mutagenesis, *J. Comp. Chem.,* 2, 231, 1981.

40. **Chu, K. C., Feldman, R. J., Shapiro, M. D., Hazard, G. F., and Geran, R. I.,** Pattern recognition and structure-activity relationship studies. Computer-assisted production of antitumor activity in structurally diverse drugs in an experimental mouse brain tumor system, *J. Med. Chem.,* 18, 539, 1975.

41. **Hansch, C. and Klein, T. E.,** Molecular graphics and QSAR in the study of enzyme ligand interactions. On the definition of bioreceptors, *Acc. Chem. Res.,* 19, 392, 1986.

42. **Arteca, G. A., Jammel, V. B., Mesey, P. G., et al.,** Shape group studies of molecular similarity; relative shapes of van der Waals and electrostatic potential surfaces of nicotinic agonists, *J. Mol. Graphics,* 6, 45, 1988.

43. **Arteca, G. A. and Mesey, P. G.,** A topological characterization for simple molecular surfaces, *J. Mol. Struct. (Theochem.),* 166, 11, 1988.

44. **Marshall, G. R. and Craven, P. D.,** Three dimensional structure-activity relationships, *Trends Pharmacol. Sci.,* 9, 285, 1988.

45. **Cramer, R. D., III, Peterson, D. E., and Bruce, J. D.,** Recent advances in molecular field analysis. Quantitative structure-activity relationship, in *Drug Design,* Alan R. Liss, New York, 1989, 161.

46. **Moţoc, I., Labanowski, J., and Bender, C. F.,** *Molecular Design of Bioactive Molecules: Pharmacophone Model, Bioactive Conformation and 3D-QSAR,* in Proc. Int. Course Conf. Interfaces between Math., Chem. Comput. Sci., Elsevier, Amsterdam, 1989.

47. **Moţoc, I., Dammkoehler, R. A., and Marshall, G. R.,** in *Mathematics and Computational Concepts in Chemistry,* Trinajtič, N., Ed., Ellis Horwood, Chichester, England, 1986, 20.

48. **Collander, R.,** The permeability of nitella cells to nonelectrolytes, *Physiol. Plant.,* 7, 420, 1954.

49. **Leo, A., Hansch, C., and Elkins, D.,** Partition coefficients and their uses, *Chem. Rev.,* 71, 525, 1971.

50. **Hansch, C. and Leo, A. J.,** *Substituent Constants for Correlation Analysis in Chemistry and Biology,* John Wiley & Sons, New York, 1979.

51. **Klopman, G. and Nambodiri, K.,** A simple method of computing the partition coefficient, *J. Comput. Chem.,* 28, 1985.

52. **Rekker, R. F.,** *The Hydrophobic Fragmental Constant,* Pharmacochemistry Library, Elsevier, New York, 1977.

53. **Wepster, B. M., Hoefnagel, A. J., Monshouwer, J. C., and Snorn, E.,** Substituents effects. III. Dissociation constants of β-arylpropionic acids, β-arylisovaleric acids, *N*-arylglycines, aryloxyacetic acids, *N*-aryl-β-alanines and some related systems, *J. Am. Chem. Soc.,* 95, 5350, 1973.

54. **Taft, R. W., Ehrenson, S., Lewis, I. C., and Glick, R. E.,** Evaluation of resonance effects on reactivity by application of the linear inductive energy relationship. VI. Concerning the effects of polarization and conjugation on the mesomeric order, *J. Am. Chem. Soc.,* 81, 5352, 1959.

55. **Jdanov, Yu. A. and Minkin, V. I.,** Correlational Analysis in Organic Chemistry (in Russian), Rostov University (USSR), 1966.

56. **Wells, P. R.,** *Linear Free-Energy Relationships,* Academic Press, London, 1968.

57. **Taft, R. W.,** Sigma values from reactivities, *J. Phys. Chem.,* 64, 1805, 1960.

58. **Taft, R. W.,** Linear free energy relationships from rates of esterification and hydrolysis of aliphatic and ortho substituted benzoate esters, *J. Am. Chem. Soc.,* 74, 2729, 1952.

59. **Taft, R. W.,** The general nature of the proportionality of polar effects of substituent groups in organic chemistry, *J. Am. Chem. Soc.,* 75, 4231, 1953.

60. **Johnson, C. E.,** *The Hammett Equation,* Cambridge University Press, New York, 1973.

61. **Kibuchi, O.,** Systematic QSAR procedures with quantum chemical descriptor, *Quant. Struct.-Act. Relat.,* 6, 179, 1987.

62. **Pritchard, D. C., Cerembery, D. A., and Snyden, S. H.,** Binding characteristics of radiolabeled agonists and antagonists at central nervous system alpha adrenergic receptor, *Mol. Pharmacol.,* 13, 453, 1977.

63. **Pincus, M. R.,** Protein structure and oncogenesis: a study of p21 protein, in *Computer Simulation of Carcinogenic Process,* Silverman, B. D., Ed., CRC Press, Boca Raton, FL, 1989, 37.

64. **Garnier, J. and Robson, B.,** Conformational calculations of oncogene products in *Computer Simulation of Carcinogenic Process,* Silverman, B. D., Ed., CRC Press, Boca Raton, FL, 1989, 37.

65. **Simon, Z.,** Stereochemical and informational aspects in QSAR and MTD, *Rev. Roum. Chim.,* 32, 1103, 1987.

66. **Topliss, J. G. and Costello, R. J.,** Chance correlation in structure-activity studies using multiple regression analysis, *J. Med. Chem.,* 15, 1066, 1972.

67. **Topliss, J. G. and Edwards, P. P.,** Chance factors in studies of quantitative structure-activity relationships, *J. Med. Chem.,* 22, 1238, 1979.

68. **Wold, S., Ruse, A., Wold, W., and Dunn, W. J.,** Partial least square method in multivariate analysis, SIAM, *J. Sci. Stat. Comput.,* 5, 735, 1984.

69. **Shorter, J.,** The separation of polar, steric and resonance effects by the use of linear free energy relationships, in *Advances in Linear Free Energy Relationships,* Chapman, N. B. and Shorter, J., Eds., Plenum Press, New York, 1972, 71, 2.

70. **Verloop, A., Hoogenstraten, W., and Tipker, J.,** STERIMOL parameters. Applications to drug design, in *Drug Design,* Vol. VII, Ariëns, E. J., Ed., Academic Press, New York, 1976, 1965.

71. **Charton, M.,** The prediction of chemical lability through substituent effects, in *Design of Biopharmaceutical Properties Through Pro-drugs and Analogs,* Roche, E. B., Ed., Am. Pharm. Assoc. Acad. Pharm. Sci., Washington, D.C., 1977.

72. **Kier, L. B. and Hell, L. H.,** *Molecular Connectivity in Chemistry and Drug Research,* Academic Press, New York, 1976.

73. **Ciubotariu, D., Holban, S., Mihalaş, G. I., Simon, Z., and Chiriac, A.,** Computer programs for the MTD method. 2. The MTD-program, Preprint, University of Timişoara, Ser. Chim., 1983, 2.

74. **Taft, R. W.,** Separation of polar, steric and resonance effects, *J. Am. Chem. Soc.,* 74, 3120, 1952.

75. **Taft, R. W.,** Separation of polar, steric and resonance effects in reactivity, Chapter 13, in *Steric Effects in Organic Chemistry,* Newman, M. S., Ed., John Wiley & Sons, New York, 1956, 556, 13.

76. **Gallo, R.,** Treatment of Steric Effects, *Prog. Phys. Org. Chem.,* 14, 115, 1983.

77. **Unger, S. H. and Hansch, C.,** Quantitative models of steric effects, *Prog. Phys. Org., Chem.,* 12, 91, 1976.

78. **Hansch, C.,** Drug design, in *Medicinal Chemistry,* Vol. I, Ariëns, E. J., Ed., Academic Press, New York, 1971, 271.

79. **Hansch, C. and Leo, A.,** Substituent constants for correlation analysis, in *Chemistry and Biology,* Wiley-Interscience, New York, 1980.

80. **Charton, M.,** The nature of the ortho effect. II. Composition of the Taft steric parameters, *J. Am. Chem. Soc.,* 91, 619, 1969.

81. **Fujita, T. and Iwamura, H.,** Applications of various steric constants to quantitative analysis of structure-activity relationships, in *Steric Effects in Drug Design,* Charton, M. and Moţoc, I., Eds., Topics Curr. Chem., Vol. 114, Springer-Verlag, Berlin, 1983, 76.

82. **Hancock, C. K., Meyens, E. A., and Yogen, J. B.,** Quantitative separation of hyperconjugation effects from steric substituent constants, *J. Am. Chem. Soc.,* 83, 4211, 1961.

83. **Kreevoy, M. M. and Eyning, H.,** The evaluation of inductive and resonance effects on reactivity. I. Hydrolysis rates of acetals of nonconjugated aldehydes and ketones, *J. Am. Chem. Soc.,* 77, 5590, 1955.

84. **Charton, M.,** Steric Effects. I. Esterification and acid-catalysed hydrolysis of esters, *J. Am. Chem. Soc.,* 97, 1552, 1975.

85. **Mc Phee, J. A., Panaye, A., and Dubois, J. E.,** Sterid Effects, I. A critical examination of the Taft steric parameter-E_s. Definition of a revised, broader and homogeneous scale. Extension to highly congested alkyl groups, *Tetrahedron,* 34, 3553, 1978.

86. **Talvik, J. V. and Palm, V. A.,** The effect of α-C hyperconjugation on E_s — Taft steric parameter, *Org. React. (USSR),* 2, 445, 1971.

87. **McPhee, J. A., Panaye, A., and Dubois, J. E.,** Operational definition of the Taft steric parameter. An homogeneous scale for alkyl groups. Experimental extension to highly hindered groups, *Tetrahedron Lett.,* 3293, 1978.

88. **Panaye, A., McPhee, J. A., and Dubois, J. E.,** Steric effects. II. Relationship between topology and the steric parameter. E'_s — topology as a tool for the correlation and prediction of steric effects, *Tetrahedron,* 36, 759, 1980.

89. **Lee, J. D. and Lee, T. D.,** *Statistic and Computer Methods in BASIC,* Van Nostrand and Reinhold, New York, 1982, 13.

90. **Hirschfelder, J. O.,** Intermolecular Forces, *Adv. Mol. Phys.,* Vol. 12, Interscience, New York, 1967, 5.

91. **Bondi, A.,** Van der Waals volumes and radii, *J. Phys. Chem.,* 68, 441, 1964.

92. **Bondi, A.,** Van der Waals volumes and radii of metals in covalent compounds, *J. Phys. Chem.,* 80, 3006, 1966.

93. **Meyer, A. Y.,** Molecular mechanics and molecular shape. Part 1. Van der Waals descriptors of simple molecules, *J. Chem. Soc.,* II, 1161, 1985.

94. **Allinger, N. L.,** *Pharmacology and the Future of Man,* Proc. 5th Int. Cong. Pharmacol., Maxwell, R. A., Ed., S. Karger, Basel, 57, 1972.

95. **Duchamps, D. J.,** *Computer-Assisted Drug Design,* Olson, E. D. and Christoffersen, R. E., Eds., American Chemical Society, Washington, D.C., 1979, 89.

96. **Karfunkel, H. R. and Eyrand, V.,** An algorithm for the representation and computation of supermolecular surfaces and volumes, *J. Comput. Chem.,* 10, 628, 1989.

97. **Ciubotariu, D., Gogonea, V., Holban, S., Chiriac, A., and Simon, Z.,** Two algorithms for the computation of van der Waals volume of the molecules by means of the Monte Carlo method, Preprint, University Timişoara, Ser. Chim., 1985, 10.

98. **Demidovich, B. P. and Meron, J.,** *Computational Mathematics,* Mir, Moscow, 1981, 649.

99. **Vilkov, L. V., Mastryukov, V. S., and Sadova, J. N.,** *Determination of the Geometrical Structure of Free Molecules,* Mir, Moscow, 1983.

100. **Meyer, A. Y.,** Molecular mechanics and molecular shape. Part II. Beyond the van der Waals descriptors of shape, *J. Mol. Struct. (Theochem.),* 124, 93, 1985.

101. **Meyer, A. Y.,** Molecular mechanisms and molecular shape. III. Surface area and cross-sectional areas of organic molecules, *J. Comput. Chem.,* 7, 144, 1986.

102. **Gogonea, V., Motsenigos, A., Ciubotariu, D., Deretey, E., Chiriac, A., and Simon, Z.,** Molecular mechanics and molecular shape descriptors. 2. Comparative treatments of four methods for molecular surface calculation, Preprint, University of Timişoara, Ser. Chim., 1987, 1.

103. **Pearlman, R. S.,** Molecular surface area and volumes and their use in structure-activity relationships, in *Physical Chemistry Properties of Drugs,* Yalkovsky, S. H., et al., Eds., Marcel Dekker, New York, 1980, 321.

104. **Motsenigos, A., Ciubotariu, D., Gogonea, V., Chiriac, A., and Simon, Z.,** Molecular mechanics and molecular shape descriptors. 4. Computer program for interactive generation of molecular structures. Preprint, University of Timişoara, Ser. Chim., 1987, 2.

105. **Meyer, A. Y., Farin, D., and Avnir, D.,** Cross-sectional areas of alkanoic acids. A comparative study applying fractal theory of adsorption and considerations, *J. Am. Chem. Soc.,* 108, 7897, 1986.

106. **Meyer, A. Y.,** Algorithm for calculation of van der Waals substituents surfaces, *J. Chem. Soc.,* 11, 1161, 1985.

107. **Meyer, A. Y.,** The size of molecules, *Chem. Soc. Rev.,* 15, 449, 1986.

108. **Cohen, N. C.,** Computer assisted drug design, in ACS Symp. Ser. No. 112, ACS, Washington, D.C., 1979, 371.

109. **Verloop, A., Hoogenstraten, W., and Tipker, J.,** Development and applications of new steric parameters in drug design, in *Drug Design,* Vol. 7, Ariëns, E. J., Ed., New York, Academic Press, 1976, 165.

110. **Bohl, M., Simon, Z., Vlad, A., Kaufman, G., and Ponsold, R.,** MTD calculations on quantitative structure-activity relationships of steroids binding to progesterone receptor, *Z. Naturforsch.,* 42c, 935, 1987.

111. **Gergen, I., Bohl, N., Simon, H., and Simon, Z.,** Structure-activity relations for steroids by the MTD method. Superposition procedures for molecules with different condensed cycles, *Rev. Roum. Chim.,* 34, 995, 1989.

112. **Bohl, M., Simon, Z., and Lochmann, J. R.,** Theoretical investigations on the role of steroid skeleton C_4-C_5 unsaturation in competitive aromatase inhibition, *Z. Naturforsch.,* 44c, 217, 1989.

113. **Chiriac, A., Chiriac, V., Ciubotariu, D., Holban, St., and Simon, Z.,** Minimal steric difference MTD study for the flexible molecules. Acetic acid derivatives with anxinic activity, *Eur. J. Med. Chem.,* 18, 507, 1983.

114. **Motsenigos, A.,** Chemical Structure-Biological Activity Relationships by the MTD Method Compounds with Conformational Flexibility, Ph.D. thesis, University of Timişoara, 1988.

115. **Motsenigos, A.,** QSAR analysis of clonidine derivatives by the MTD-multiconformational method, *Rev. Roum. Chim.,* in press.

116. **Moţoc, I. and Dragomir-Filimonescu, O.,** Molecular interactions in biological systems. I. Steric interactions. The SIBIS algorithm, *Math. Chem. (Weinheim),* 12, 117, 1981.

117. **Simon, Z.,** Steric fit in QSAR, the MTD and SIBIS methods, critique and perspectives, *Math. Chem. (Weinheim),* 13, 356, 1982.

118. **Moţoc, I. and Dragomir-Filimonescu, O.,** Molecular interactions in biological systems. II. Hydrophobic interactions. The HIBIS algorithm, *Math. Chem. (Weinheim),* 12, 127, 1981.

119. **Hopfinger, A. J. and Potenzone, R., Jr.,** Ames test and antitumor activity of 1-(1-phenyl)-3,3-dialkyl triazenes, *Mol. Pharmacol.,* 21, 187, 1982.

120. **Burkert, U. and Allinger, N. L.,** *Molecular Mechanics,* American Chemical Society, Washington, D.C., 1982.

121. **Balaban, A. T.,** Applications of graph theory in chemistry, *J. Chem. Inf. Comput. Sci.,* 25, 334, 1985.

122. **Einslein, K., Borgstedt, H. H., Tomb, M. E., Blake, B. W., and Hart, J. B.,** A structure-activity prediction model of carcinogenicity based on NCI/NTP assays and food additives, *Toxicol. Ind. Health,* 3, 267, 1987.

123. **Kier, L. B. and Hall, L. H.,** *Molecular Connectivity in Chemistry and Drug Research,* Academic Press, New York, 1976.

124. **Randič, M.,** On characterization of molecular bonding, *J. Am. Chem. Soc.,* 97, 6609, 1975.

125. **Eakin, D. L., Hyde, E., and Parker, G.,** The CROSSBOW-system, *Pestic. Sci.,* 5, 319, 1974.

126. **Loew, G. H., Poulsen, M., Kirkjan, E., Ferrel, J., Sudhindra, B. S., and Rebagliati, M.,** Computer assisted mechanistic structure-activity studies: application to diverse classes of chemical carcinogens, *Environ. Health Persp.,* 61, 69, 1985.

127. **Miller, E. C., Miller, J. A., Sandin, R. B., and Brown, R. K.,** The carcinogenic activities of 2-ethylaminofluorene in the rat, *Cancer Res.,* 9, 504, 1949.

128. **Haddow, A., Harris, R. J. C., Kon, G. A. R., and Roe, E. M. F.,** The growth inhibitory and carcinogenic properties of 4-aminostilbene and derivatives, *Trans. R. Soc. London,* 241A, 147, 1948.

129. **Sandin, R. B., Melby, R., Hay, A. S., Jones, R. N., Miller, E. C., and Miller, J. A.,** Ultraviolet spectra and carcinogenic activities of some fluorene and biphenyl derivatives, *J. Am. Chem. Soc.,* 74, 5073, 1952.

130. **Badger, G. M.,** The carcinogenic hydrocarbons: chemical constitution and carcinogenic activity, *Br. J. Cancer,* 2, 309, 1948.

131. **Haddow, A. and Kon, G. A.,** Chemistry of carcinogenic compounds, *Br. Med. Bull.,* 4, 314, 1947.

132. **Orchin, M.,** Steric effects in complex compound formation, *J. Org. Chem.,* 16, 1165, 1951.

133. **Robinson, R.,** Aspects of chemistry related to medicine, *Br. Med. J.,* 1, 943, 1946.

134. **Badger, G. M., Pearce, R. S., and Pettit, R.,** Substituted anthracene derivatives. Part V. The conjugating power of the substitution position in 1-2 benzanthracene, *J. Chem. Soc.,* 112, 1952.

135. **Badger, G. M. and Lynn, K. R.,** The relative reactivity of aromatic double bonds. Part II. Addition of osmium tetroxide to substituted position in 1-2 benzanthracene, *J. Chem. Soc.,* 1726, 1950.

136. **Boyland, E.,** The biochemistry of abnormalities in cell division, *Biochem. Biophys. Acta,* 4, 293, 1950.

137. **Badger, G. M.,** The relative reactivity of aromatic double bonds, *J. Chem. Soc.,* 456, 1949.

138. **Cook, J. M. and Schowenthal, R.,** Oxidation of carcinogen hydrocarbons, *J. Chem. Soc.,* 170, 1948.

139. **Smith, I. A., Berger, G. D., Seybold, P., and Serve, M. P.,** Relationships between carcinogenicity and theoretical reactivity indices in polycyclic aromatic hydrocarbons, *Cancer Res.,* 38, 2968, 1978.

140. **Szentpaly, L.,** Carcinogenesis by polycyclic aromatic hydrocarbons: a multilinear regression on new type PMO indices, *J. Am. Chem. Soc.,* 106, 6021, 1984.

141. **Badger, G. M.,** Chemical constitution and carcinogenic activity, *Adv. Cancer Res.,* 2, 73, 1954.

142. **Seybold, P. G.,** Steric and electronic determinants of carcinogenicity in polycyclic aromatic hydrocarbons: use in short time test, in *Polynuclear Aromatic Hydrocarbons: Chemistry, Characterization and Carcinogenesis,* Cooke, M. and Dennis, A. J., Eds., Battelle Press, Columbus, OH, 1986, 839.

143. **Lewis, D. F.,** Molecular orbital calculations and quantitative structure-activity relationships for some polyaromatic hydrocarbons, *Xenobiotica,* 17, 135, 1987.

144. **Szentpaly, L. and Parkanyi, C.,** The MCS model of chemical initiation of cancer: PPP calculation on methylated and N-heteroaromatic polycycles, *J. Mol. Struct.,* 151, 245, 1987.

145. **Franke, R.,** Structure-activity relationships in polycyclic aromatic hydrocarbons. Induction of microsomal arylhydrocarbon hydroxylase and its importance in chemical carcinogenesis, *Chem. Biol. Interact.,* 6, 1, 1973.

146. **Kaliszan, R., Lemparczyk, H., and Radecki, A.,** A relationship between repression of dimethyl-nitrosoamine-demethylase by polycyclic aromatic hydrocarbons and their shape, *Biochem. Pharmacol.*, 28, 123, 1979.

147. **Huberman, E. and Sachs, L.,** Mutability of different genetic loci in mammalian cells by metabolically activated carcinogenic polycyclic hydrocarbons, *Proc. N.Y. Acad. Sci. U.S.A.*, 731, 188, 1976.

148. **Fukui, K., Yonezawa, T., and Nagata, C.,** Theory of substitution in conjugated molecules, *Bull. Chem. Soc. Jpn.*, 27, 423, 1954.

149. **Jerina, D. M., Lehr, R., Schaefer-Rider, M., Yagi, H., Karle, J. M., Thakker, D. R., Wood, A. H., Lu, A. Y., Ryan, D., West, S., Levin, W., and Conney, A. H.,** Bay region epoxides of dehydrodiols: a concept explaining the mutagenic and the carcinogenic activity of benzo(a)pyrene and benzo(a)anthracene, in *Origins of Human Cancer*, Hiatt, H., Watson, J. D., and Winstin, I., Eds., Cold Spring Harbor Laboratory, Cold Spring Harbor, NY, 1977, 639.

150. **Miyashita, Y., Okuyama, T., Yamamura, K., Jinno, K., and Sasaki, S. I.,** Production of carcinogenicity of polynuclear aromatic hydrocarbons on the basis of their chemical structures, *Anal. Chim. Acta*, 202, 237, 1987.

151. **Simon, Z., Balaban, A. T., Ciubotariu, D., and Balaban, T. S.,** QSAR for carcinogenesis by polycyclic aromatic hydrocarbons and derivatives in term of delocalization energy, minimal sterical differences and topological indices, *Rev. Roum. Chim.*, 30, 985, 1985.

152. **Niculescu-Duvăz, I., Tugulea, M., Croisy, A., and Jacquignon, P. C.,** A quantitative structure-activity analysis of the mutagenic and carcinogenic action of 43 structurally related heterocyclic compounds, *Carcinogenesis*, 2, 269, 1981.

153. **Glatt, H. R., Scwind, H., Zajdela, F., Croisy, A., Jacquignon, P., and Oesch, F.,** Mutagenicity of 43 structurally related heterocyclic compounds and its relationships to their carcinogenicity, *Mutat. Res.*, 66, 307, 1979.

154. **Hopfinger, A. J.,** Intra and intermolecular modelling studies of polycyclic aromatic hydrocarbons, in *Molecular Basis of Cancer, Part A. Macromolecular Structure, Carcinogens and Oncogenes*, Alan R. Liss, New York, 1985, 277.

155. **Hansch, C., Venger, B. H., Hathaway, G. J., and Amrein, Y. U.,** Ames test of 1(x-phenyl)-3,3-dealkyltriazenes, *J. Med. Chem.*, 22, 473, 1979.

156. **Hansch, C., Venger, B., and Panthahanickal, A.,** Mutagenicity of substituted (o-phenyldiamine) platinum dichlorides in the Ames test. A quantitative structure-activity study, *J. Med. Chem.*, 23, 459, 1980.

157. **Leo, A., Panthahanickal, A., Hansch, C., Theiss, J., Shimkin, M., and Andress, A. W.,** A comparison of mutagenic and carcinogenic activities of aniline mustards, *J. Med. Chem.*, 24, 859, 1981.

158. **Sugiura, K. and Goto, M.,** Mutagenicities of styrene-oxide derivatives on bacterial test systems: relationship between mutagenic potencies and chemical reactivity, *Chem. Biol. Interact.*, 35, 71, 1981.

159. **Wishnok, J. S. and Archer, M. C.,** Structure-activity relationships in nitrosoamine carcinogenesis, *Br. J. Cancer*, 33, 307, 1976.

160. **Wishnok, J. S., Archer, M. C., Edelman, E. S., and Rand, W. M.,** Nitrosoamine carcinogenicity: a quantitative Hansch-Taft structure-activity relationship, *Chem. Biol. Interact.*, 20, 43, 1978.

161. **Singer, G. M., Taylor, H. W., and Lijinsky, W. I.,** Liposolubility as an aspect of nitrosoamine carcinogenicity. Quantitative correlations and qualitative observations, *Chem. Biol. Interact.*, 19, 133, 1977.

162. **Frecer, V. and Miertus, S.,** Theoretical study of *N*-nitrosoureas and mechanism of their carcinogenic effect, *Neoplasma*, 36, 257, 1989.

163. **Loew, G. H., Philips, G., and Pack, G.,** Quantum chemicals studies of the polycyclic aromatic amines and the stabilities and electrophylicities of their arylnitrenium ions in relation to their mutagenic-carcinogenic potencies, *Cancer Biochem. Biophys.*, 3, 101, 1979.

164. **Loew, G. H., Sudhindra, B. S., Walker, J. M., Sigman, C. C., and Johnson, H. I.,** Correlation of calculated electronic parameters of fifteen aniline derivatives with their mutagenic potencies, *J. Environ. Pathol. Toxicol.*, 2, 1069, 1979.

165. **Norden, B., Edlund, U., and Wold, S.,** Carcinogenicity of polycyclic aromatic hydrocarbons, studied by SIMCA pattern recognition, *Acta Chem. Scand.*, Series B, 32, 602, 1978.

166. **Nilson, L. M., Carter, R. E., Sterner, O., and Liljefors, T.,** Structure-activity relationships for unsaturated dialdehydes ZAPLS correlation of theoretical descriptors for six compounds with mutagenic activity in Ames Salmonella assay, *Quant. Struct. Act. Relat.*, 7, 84, 1988.

167. **Dunn, W. J. and Wold, S.,** The carcinogenicity of *N*-nitrosocompounds: a SIMCA pattern-recognition-study, *Bioorg. Chem.*, 10, 29, 1981.

168. **Dunn, W. J. and Wold, S.,** A structure-carcinogenicity study of 4-nitroquinoline-1-oxides using the SIMCA method of pattern-recognition, *J. Med. Chem.*, 21, 1001, 1978.

169. **Yuan, M. and Jurs, P. C.,** Computer assisted structure-activity studies of chemical carcinogens. A polycyclic aromatic hydrocarbon data set, *Toxicol. Appl. Pharmacol.*, 52, 294, 1980.

170. **Chou, J. T. and Jurs, P. C.,** Computer assisted studies of chemical carcinogens. An *N*-nitroso-compounds data set, *J. Med. Chem.*, 22, 792, 1979.

171. **Rose, S. L. and Jurs, P. C.,** Computer assisted studies of structure-activity relationships of *N*-nitroso-compounds using pattern recognition, *J. Med. Chem.,* 25, 769, 1982.

172. **Yuta, K. and Jurs, P. C.,** Computer assisted structure-activity studies of chemical carcinogens. Aromatic amines, *J. Med. Chem.,* 24, 241, 1981.

173. **Mitchell, C. S., Klopman, G., and Rosenkrantz, H. S.,** Computer automated evaluation of mutagenicity of selected polycyclic aromatic hydrocarbons, in *Polycyclic Aromatic Hydrocarbons,* Ninth Int. Symp., Battelle Press, Columbus, OH, 1986.

174. **Klopman, G., Frierson, M. R., and Rosenkrantz, H. S.,** Computer analysis of toxicological databases: mutagenicity of aromatic amines in Salmonella tester strains, *Environ. Mutagen.,* 7, 625, 1985.

175. **Klopman, G., Kalos, A. N., and Rosenkrantz, H. A.,** Computer automated study of the structure-mutagenicity relationships of non-fused ring nitroarenes and related compounds, *Mol. Toxicol.,* 1, 61, 1987.

176. **Klopman, G., Contreras, R., Rosenkrantz, H. S., and Waters, M. D.,** Structure genotoxic activity relationship of pesticides: comparison between the results of several short-term assays, *Mutat. Res.,* 147, 1985.

Chapter 6

QUANTITATIVE APPROACH TO CARCINOGENESIS INHIBITION: A QSAR ANALYSIS

Nicolae Voiculetz, Alexandru T. Balaban, and Ion Niculescu-Duvăz

TABLE OF CONTENTS

I. INTRODUCTION

Increasing evidence demonstrates that the concept of cancer chemoprevention, as well as its strategy, are founded on the possibility of modulating the effect of the environmental carcinogens (especially chemicals) by means of pharmacological agents able to activate, inhibit or reverse the carcinogenic process.

Although the concept of cancer prevention* is almost as old as that regarding carcinogenesis (i.e., occupational cancers, first reported by Percival Pott in 1775) the concept of chemoprevention emerged only recently when the possibility of reducing the incidence of experimental tumors by means of natural or synthetic chemicals was demonstrated. This new research area was rapidly developed, extended and diversified, nowadays being more correctly defined by the term of anticarcinogenesis. Neither the definition, nor its rapidly growing implications will be herein discussed. Some biochemical aspects of anticarcinogenesis are briefly reviewed in this chapter in order to support the rational development of quantitative models concerning the design of chemopreventive agents. There are actually very few attempts which could be reported in this area, most of them during the last 10 years.

The finding of effective cancer prophylactic agents is obviously linked to their screening methodology. We have to emphasize that this last aspect raises many more experimental difficulties than the screening of antitumor agents.

Actually, the strategy of chemoprevention is based mainly on a better understanding of the biochemical mechanisms governing chemical carcinogenesis. Some of these mechanisms, as well as their connections with chemoprevention are summarized in Table 1.

From the data presented here it follows that there exists a close correlation between carcinogenesis mechanisms and anticarcinogenesis strategy. Despite the growing interest for the development of this area, very few quantitative approaches for the design of chemopreventive agents are reported. Some of them will be discussed in this chapter.

II. CLASSIFICATION OF ANTICARCINOGENESIS AGENTS

In this chapter we adoped Wattenberg's[1] classification (see Table 2), which allows a rough delimitation of carcinogenesis inhibitors taking into account whether they prevent the initiation step (i.e., blocking agents, anti-initiators) or promotion step (i.e., suppressive agents, antipromoters).

In addition to these two distinct categories, the class of agents preventing the formation of (pre)carcinogens is considered. The most typical example consists in the prevention of N-nitrosoamine formation in the stomach, subsequent to nitrite ingestion.[2]

III. MECHANISMS OF ACTION FOR CARCINOGENESIS INHIBITORS

A. COMPOUNDS PREVENTING THE FORMATION OF (PRE)CARCINOGENS

This class of compounds includes derivatives able to prevent the formation of (pre)carcinogens and/or catalyze their decomposition. Such (pre)carcinogens are formed *in vivo* following the reaction between two or more reagents. A typical example of such a preventing compound is vitamin C (ascorbic acid). Empirical observations followed by epidemiological and experimental investigations have drawn attention on the correlation between the reduced incidence of some types of cancers and a certain type of diet (vegetables,

---

* The first document refering to a cancer prevention action is the *Regulation of Danish Sweepers Guild (1882)* which imposed on its members two daily baths. A lower incidence of scrotal tumors for Danish chimney sweepers relative to English sweepers resulted.

TABLE 1
Anti-Initiators Mechanisms of Action

No.	Mechanism of action	DNA protection by	Type of anticarcinogenesis inhibitors
1.	Scavenger effect	Decrease of the concentration of the carcinogenic electrophilic species	SH-group compounds, glutathione
		Decrease of (carcinogenic?) free radicals concentration	BHA, BHT
2.	Effect upon the uptake and intra- (or extra-) cellular transport of the carcinogen	Competition for specific receptors	PAH[a]
		Destruction of specific receptors (by alkylation or other chemical modifications)	Allylisopropylacetamide (AIA)
3.	Direct interaction with the enzymatic systems involved in carcinogens activation	Inhibition of activation enzymatic systems	BHA, β-NF, ethoxyquin
		Modification of their regio- and stereoselectivity by interaction with the active site of cytochromes P-450	β-NF,BHA
		Induction of a different pattern of activation (iso)enzymes	BHA
4.	Epigenetic induction of the enzymatic systems involved in carcinogens metabolism	Induction of detoxication enzymes	BHA, ethoxyquin, p-methoxyphenol, β-NF
		Increase of the amount of endogenous glutathione	BHA
		Induction of repair enzymes	AIA, isopropylvaleramide

[a] Polycyclic aromatic hydrocarbons.

TABLE 2
Classification of Chemical Carcinogenesis Inhibitors

Type	Level of interference
Inhibitors preventing ultimate carcinogens formation	Carcinogen precursors (precarcinogens)
	Carcinogenic compounds (ultimate carcinogens)
Blocking agents[a] (anti-initiators)	Reaction with critical cellular targets (cell initiation)
Suppressive agents[a] (anti-promoters)	Phenotypic effects of neoplastic type

[a] Nomenclature according to Wattenberg.[1]

fruits). It resulted that the presence of substances with carcinogenesis inhibitory properties[3] could be suspected in the respective food. N-nitrosoamine formation in the stomach was incriminated as a risk factor for tumors developing on the digestive tract. These carcinogens result following the nitrosation of ingested amines by nitrous anhydride (N_2O_3), formed from the decomposition of sodium and potassium nitrites at acidic pH, in the stomach. The yield of N-nitrosoamines thus formed is strictly dependent on several factors: pH, substrate concentration and the presence of other substances. Among the inhibitors of the nitrosation reaction one may cite: vitamin C, 1,2- and 1,4-diphenols, α-tocopherol,[5] etc. This type of action explains the prevention achieved by such agents against (fore) stomach tumors induction by piperazone, aminopyridine, ethyl- and methylurea, morpholine, etc.

Ascorbic acid is also able to inhibit *N*-ethylnitrosourea formation, as well as methylation of hepatic DNA by *N,N*-diethylnitrosoamine.

The effect of vitamin C is also exerted at the intestinal level where several carcinogenic and mutagenic substances with quite different structures are formed. In this respect, fecapentenes may be cited, which are probably involved in colorectal cancers. However, they undergo decomposition in acidic medium. This behavior is in good agreement with experimental data showing that food supplementation with vitamins C and E decreases the mutagenic capability of feces. Clinical trials also reported the decrease of colorectal cancer incidence in high risk populations (familial polyposis) following the administration of an appropriate diet consisting of vegetables and fruits (natural sources of vitamin C and fibers).

Vitamins C and E exert a protective effect even in the post-initiation step, that is when administered a long time after the carcinogen.

In C3H/10 T1/2 cells, 3-methylcholanthrene-induced transformation was prevented by treatment of cultures with vitamin C after 14 or even 23 days following the removal of the carcinogen from the medium. Vitamin E behaves similarly. However, data strongly suggest that other mechanisms of action (i.e., inhibition of the promotion step or even transformed cell reversion) could also explain the biological properties of these compounds.

B. COMPOUNDS ACTING BY SCAVENGER EFFECT

Compounds able to prevent the interaction of the direct-acting or "ultimate carcinogens" with the critical targets of the exposed cells belong to this category. In other words the scavengers decrease — by direct reaction — the concentration of the carcinogenic electrophilic species before their interaction with DNA. The scavenger agents are generally nucleophilic compounds, the most important belonging to the class of SH-group containing compounds. Because of their low toxicity they appear to be effective chemoprotective agents.[6,7]

Recently it was reported that several substances existing in edible plants (for instance, tannic acid and ellagic acid found in grapefuits, nuts, hazelnuts, raspberries)[8] inhibit BaP-induced carcinogenesis in mouse gastrointestinal tract and skin. Ellagic acid is also well tolerated by animals and humans. When administred to rats in food up to 50 mg/kg for 45 days, or to human patients intravenously at a dose of 0.2 mg/kg, no side effects were noticed.

The phenolic antioxidants are supposed to also belong to this type of compound, being known as scavengers of free radicals. However, this assumption was not confirmed because any direct interaction between these antioxidants and benzo(a)pyrene-diol-epoxide fails to be detected at physiological doses.[10] However, the possibility that phenolic antioxidants (as 2(3)*tert*-butylhydroxyanisole (BHA), 2,6-*tert*-butyl-hydroxytoluene [BHT], etc.) or ethoxyquin might also act by trapping active free radicals of oxygen could not be totally ruled out. Since the role of free radicals in initiation is still debatable, this mechanism, although not excluded, represents only a hypothesis.[11]

However, the efficiency of SH-compounds in preventing — *in vitro* — the formation of carcinogen-DNA-adducts appears reduced as compared to that of phenolic anti-initiators (acting by different mechanisms see Section III.D). Thus, in order to reduce by 50% the concentration of the adducts formed subsequent to the interaction of ^{3}H-BaP (activated *in vitro* by microsomal systems) with DNA, 10^2 fold higher anti-initiator/carcinogen ratio is required for SH-compounds as compared to BHA.[12] The compounds acting by a scavenger mechanism have to reach an effective concentration at the moment and at the place where the carcinogen is transformed to a reactive electrophilic species. However, it was shown that antioxidants are also effective if they are administered after the exposure to carcinogen. Therefore, other mechanisms of action have to also be considered for these compounds.

C. PREVENTION OF THE NUCLEAR TRANSLOCATION OF THE CARCINOGENS

The intracellular transport, particularly the nuclear tranlocation of the carcinogen itself or of its active metabolites, is not yet fully understood. A growing body of evidence[13-15] suggests the existence of a cytoplasmic proteic receptor with high affinity for BaP and probably other PAHs. This receptor seems to have the same type of functionality as the steroid hormone-receptors, but is structurally different, being without affinity for the steroidic molecules. At least three major functions in carcinogenesis initiation may be proposed for such receptors, namely:

1.	Transport of the carcinogen (or its metabolites) through cytoplasm
2.	Nuclear translocation of the intact carcinogen, this one being thus involved in the genetic modulation of the cytochrome P-450 activity and possibly of other enzymes by binding to the Ah locus in the genome
3.	Nuclear translocation of ultimate carcinogens

After its uptake in the cell, BaP binds this specific receptor, thus forming the BaP-receptor complex. The complex is translocated to the endoplasmic reticulum level, where BaP is metabolized. The same receptor may translocate the ultimate carcinogen from the metabolization place into the nucleus.* Here a promutagenic lesion is formed. Therefore by blocking these transport processes an efficient way of preventing carcinogenesis initiation could be expected. It was demonstrated that several phenols and diols resulting from activation of BaP are able to compete with BaP for this proteic receptor. Among BaP metabolites, BaP tetrols were shown to exhibit the highest affinity for the receptor. They are actually inactive hydrolyzed forms of the ultimate carcinogens (*anti-* and *syn*-BPDE). There is as yet little evidence concerning the BPDE-receptor interation. Also, the assumption that the receptor protects the ultimate carcinogen molecule against hydrolysis remains to be demonstrated, although some indirect data support such a mechanism. Nevertheless, several carcinogenesis inhibitors (i.e., BHA, ethoxyquin, BHT, β-NF and methol) also exhibit some affinity for this receptor.[16] This behavior supports a possible competition between BHA, BHT, etc. and carcinogens, for this specific receptor of carcinogens. This competition may represent an alternate mechanism of action explaining their anticarcinogenic properties. QSAR studies concerning the quantification of this substrate-receptor interaction are in progress in our laboratory, in order to determine the structural feature of BaP and inhibitor molecules responsible for this effect.

Alteration of PAH receptors might be (at least in part) responsible for the anti-initiator effect of allylisopropylacetamide and isopropylvaleramide.[17]

Disulfiram (tetraethylthiurane disulfitol) which decreases the toxicity of many alkylating agents and inhibits the tumor induction by *N*-nitroso derivatives also belongs to this category.[18,19] It was suggested that disulfiram alters the factors controlling BaP penetration through the keratine barrier.[1] Theoretically, the perturbation of intracellular transport of carcinogens appears as a specific inhibition mechanism of carcinogenesis initiation.

D. DERIVATIVES INTERACTING DIRECTLY WITH THE ENZYMATIC SYSTEMS INVOLVED IN (PRE)CARCINOGENS ACTIVATION

1. Inhibition of Carcinogens Activation

In this category are included compounds whose carcinogenesis inhibitory effect was demonstrated both *in vitro* and *in vivo*, namely: phenolic antioxidants such as BHA, BHT,[20,21] ellagic acid **1** (a phenol isolated from plants)[22] (18), clotrimazol, **2** (antifungal agent),[23] coumarin, **3**,[24] as well as α- and β-naphthoflavones, **4, 5**.

---

* Mention should be made that pro- and contra-arguments exist for this scenario.

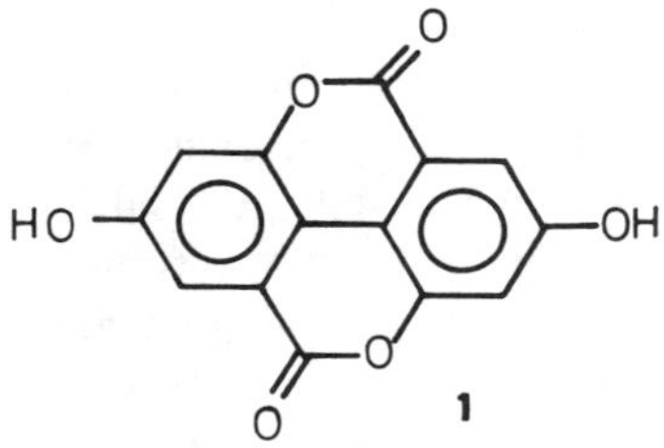

All these are inhibitors of the enzyme systems activating carcinogens and especially of the cytochrome P-450-dependent monooxygenases. The effect of BHA in the decrease of the amount of metabolized BaP was demonstrated[22] and this seems to be the principal mechanism responsible for its biological properties. These phenolic antioxidants decrease the carcinogen binding to DNA by reducing the total amount of activated carcinogens. No modifications of the usual metabolite pattern (detected by HPLC) could be established, at least for BaP.

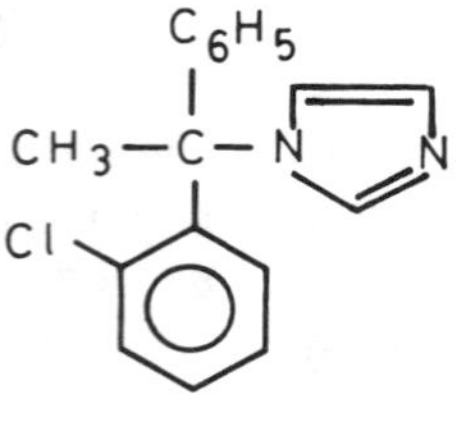

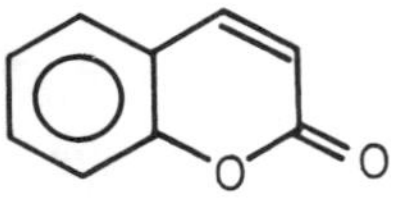

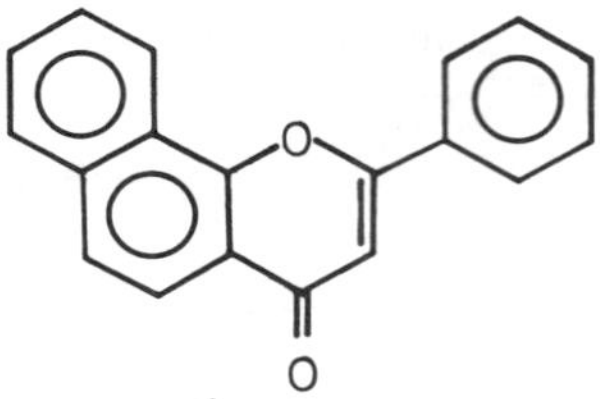

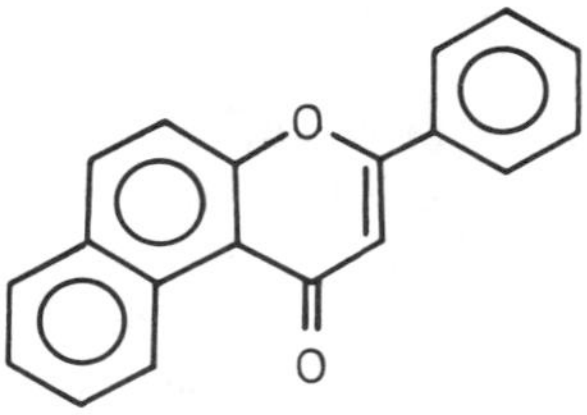

An *in vitro* prescreening test for anti-initiators acting by such a mechanism was developed in our laboratory.[12] However, the monooxygenase inhibition (by direct interaction with the enzymes) is not the sole mechanism responsible for their behavior as carcinogenesis inhibitors. Each of them exhibits a more complicated and in some way specific picture of the different ways of expressing its own biological properties. Thus, for instance, the effects of the two α- and β-naphthoflavones (α- and β-NF) (i.e., 5,6- and 7,8-benzoflavone) differ according to the experimental conditions. *In vitro* α-NF is speciospecific, inhibiting the activity of aryl hydrocarbon hydroxylase (AHH) in rat liver microsomes, but activating the same enzyme in human, rabbit and hamster liver microsomes.[26,27] An opposite effect is exerted by maackiain acetate.

The stimulation by α-NF is due in part to the influence upon the interaction between cytochrome P-450 and cytochrome P-450-reductase, which is strengthened, thus enhancing the electron transfer to cytochrome P-450.[28] This assumption is in good agreement with the fact that on using BaP as substrate for the monooxygenasic system it was demonstrated by X-ray diffraction studies that the simultaneous binding of α-NF and BaP 9,10-dihydrodiol to the catalytic site of cytochrome P-450 brings the dihydrodiol double bond closer to the activated oxygen (in comparison with the binding of the dihydrodiol alone).[29]

The inhibitory capacity of both α- and β-naphthoflavones is due to their competition with the substrate (PAH) for the catalytic site of cytochrome P-450. Both α- and β-NF possess an exocyclic oxygen atom able to interact with Fe^{2+} by a single electron pair (removing the weaker ligand). In α-NF, this oxygen atom being more exposed than in β-NF, therefore a stabler complex (enzyme $-$ α-naphthoflavone) is formed which hinders the further binding of the substrate to the enzyme catalytic site.[30] The speciospecific effect of α-NF may be explained by its requirement for a certain isoenzyme belonging to the group of cytochrome P-450 dependent monooxygenases.[31,32]

Inhibition of carcinogen activation can lead, paradoxically, to an enhanced carcinogenic effect if we agree that an increased persistence of (pre)carcinogenic species in the cell (i.e., like a retard-effect) could increase the risk of initiation. This is, however, a still debatable opinion with no clear experimental foundation. On the other hand, upon using cytochrome P-450 inhibitors for cancer prevention the organisms appear to be sensitized toward the deleterious effects of other xenobiotics detoxicated by this system. Finally, we have to consider that other enzymatic systems are also involved in the carcinogen activation (i.e., prostaglandin-synthetase, various peroxidases, etc.).[33] It would be of interest to also investigate the anticarcinogenesis effect of the specific inhibitors of these systems.

These reasons make the finding of anti-initiators which alter the regio- and stereoselectivity of enzyme-activating carcinogens more attractive.

2. Agents Affecting the Regio- and Stereoselectivity of the Activation Enzymes

A most efficient protection may be achieved by directing the metabolism of a (pre)carcinogen toward noncarcinogenic metabolites.[34,35] For instance, if the formation of 7,8-dihydrodiol during BaP metabolism might be reduced or suppressed (this diol being the direct precursor of the ultimate carcinogen, ($\pm$) *anti*-BPDE, a marked reduction of tumor incidence could be expected. In this manner one avoids all drawbacks resulting from the inhibition of the activating enzymes.

A global inhibition, but also a regioselectivity change of BaP metabolism (although not in the desired direction) was induced by the *in vitro* addition of BHA to BaP activation systems containing mouse lung microsomes. Thus at various BHA concentrations, a 50 to 70% inhibition of 9,10-diol formation was noticed, metabolization in position 4-5 is decreased by 50%, whereas the formation of 7,8-diol was inhibited by only 31%.[34] In contrast, using mouse liver microsomes stimulated by a previous administration of 3-methyl-cholanthrene, BHA inhibits 7,8-diol formation, the 4,5-diol concentration remains unchanged, whereas the production of 9,10-diol is stimulated.[36]

In vivo, oral administration of BHA followed by an analysis of BaP metabolites at short times (2 to 4 h) after administration (thus eliminating the possibility of new isoenzymes induction) showed a decrease of BaP epoxidation and a relative increase of 3-hydroxy-BaP formation (a detoxication metabolite). This fact also agrees with a possible change of the enzymatic regioselectivity to positions 1-3 of the BaP molecule.[37]

Such a mechanism could be explained if we consider that the binding of the blocking agents to the catalytic site of cytochrome P-450 produces an alteration of the binding position of the substrate, which finally leads to the modification of the epoxidated regions.[37]

E. MODULATION OF THE ENZYMATIC SYSTEMS INVOLVED IN THE ACTIVATION AND DETOXICATION OF CARCINOGENS

This class of compounds includes the carcinogenesis inhibitors acting by epigenetic mechanisms which (1) induce or suppress the (pre)carcinogen activation enzymes and (2) induce the enzymes involved in detoxication and elimination of metabolites (GST, UPD-glucuronyl-transferase, diaforase, etc.).

It is well known that the cytochrome P-450 dependent monooxygenasic system may be genetically induced by the carcinogen itself. The modulation of this system might occur by the nuclear translocation of the carcinogen-receptor complex which activates the Ah locus in the genome. Also anticarcinogenesis inhibitors which induce the transcription of the cytochrome P-450 gene could act by a similar mechanism. However, they are efficient only when combined with a very operative detoxication system.

Through a similar mechanism, the *de novo* biosynthesis of the activation enzymatic system could be hypothetically suppressed, leading to the inhibition of precarcinogen activation. It is not yet clear whether induction or suppression of activation systems represents a favorable alternative for anticarcinogenesis activity.

Activation of detoxication actually represents an alternate way of reducing the concentration of the ultimate carcinogens by eliminating more rapidly and more completely from the cell the carcinogenic metabolites or their precursors.

Hence, it is obvious that the genetic induction of enzymes involved in the detoxication process (i.e., GST, UDP-GT and even partially EH) represents a favorable event for cellular integrity.

The increase of detoxication enzyme activity (or concentration) was observed after the administration of BHA, ethoxyquin, clotrimazole, β-NF, coumarin, α-angelica-lactone and benzyl isothiocyanate to several types of animals.[38]

However, the influence of the genetic induction of the detoxication enzymes could be considered with caution because in some particular cases it could produce an opposite effect. For instance the genetic induction of epoxyhydrase (EH) which is required for diol formation from PAHs is an unfavorable event because some of the PAHs diols (i.e., 7,8-BaP-diol) are direct precursors of ultimate carcinogens. On the other hand, the same induction of the detoxication enzymes might accelerate the elimination of the antioxidant.[39]

The present discussion was based on the implicit assumption that the intact anti-initiator molecule is responsible, by a known or unknown mechanism, for the protection of DNA against the interaction with ultimate carcinogens. However, this assumption is incomplete in many cases. Recent data showed — at least for BHA — that this compound undergoes metabolization being transformed into a series of phenolic or quinonic intermediates. One of them (for instance 2-*tert*-butylhydroquinone or the corresponding quinone) is suspected to be the true carcinogenesis inhibitor. This concept may cast a different light upon the role of activation and detoxication systems in anticarcinogenesis.

This additional complication, although not changing the essence of the problem, might modify several points of view regarding the strategy of chemoprevention because the new factors contributing to the anti-initiator metabolism must also be taken into account.

Finally, compounds able to activate the natural error-free repair systems, thus decreasing the concentration of DNA-carcinogen adducts after they are formed, must also be considered.

F. COMPOUNDS INHIBITING THE PROMOTION STEP AND PRODUCING THE REVERSION OF THE EARLY STAGES OF CHEMICAL CARCINOGENESIS

These compounds were termed by Wattenberg[1] (see Table 1) as suppressor agents. They inhibit the carcinogenesis process when administered after exposure to the carcinogen, hence after the initiation or even the cellular transformation occurred. In fact, they are able to prevent, by different mechanisms, the phenotypical transformation of an initiated cell.

From the analysis of their (still unclear) mechanisms of action, it follows that the biological effects of these compounds (especially of antipromoters) are based on their interference with the regulation of (1) the differentiation and cell proliferation program; (2) the modulation of several enzyme systems; (3) the cell membrane functions; (4) the various growth factors; (5) the behavior of histonic and nonhistonic proteins; (6) the transcriptional and post-transcriptional expression; (7) the protein kinase C cascade; (8) the scavenging of oxygen free radicals often accompanying promotion (even by induction of the enzyme systems involved in this process), etc.

The most carefully investigated compounds with suppressive activity are the retinoids (vitamin A derivatives).[40] It has been known for over 50 years that retinoids are able to control both proliferation and differentiation of epithelial cells of mesenchymal origin. Old and new experimental data agree to consider that the (natural and synthetic) retinoids exert their biological effects in the cell by interfering at two main levels: cell membrane and genic expression.

Retinoids may modulate growth and differentiation by direct interaction with cyclic-AMP-dependent or calcium-dependent protein kinases associated with growth factors and their receptors. Mention should be made that protein kinase C actually represents, for phorbolic esters, a major pathway of signal transduction from cell membrane surface.

This concept might explain the multiple actions of retinoids. Moreover, it may allow the development of a unifying action system in which the trigger role of retinoids in the reversal of early stages of carcinogenesis, in some cases, would be recognized.

Another possible target for retinoids is the genome. The simplest explanation suggested by the large amount of available experimental data is that retinoids are able to modulate the expression of the genes involved in both differentiation and proliferation. The existence of specific cellular receptors (CRBP, CRABP, etc.) suggested that retinoids might modify gene expression by a mechanism very similar to that of steroidic hormones. However, in contrast with these last ones, no DNA sequence specific for retinoid receptor binding has been identified. Therefore, the way of regulating transcription is difficult to assess. However, new experimental data allowed the identification in F9 cells of a number of genes inducible by retinoids, thus confirming their possible involvement in the control mechanisms acting at the transcriptional level of several specific genes.[41]

Retinoids could also modify the oncogene transcription. Thus, *myc-c* expression is suppressed in HL-60 and ML-1 cells by retinoids being associated to the loss of proliferation ability of the cells.[42] Similarly, a decrease of the transcription of *N-myc* gene was observed in neuroblastoma cell lines treated with retinoids leading to morphological differentiation and to cell growth inhibition (both in monolayer and in semi-solid agar).

In contrast with these data, the activating effect of retinoids upon the transcriptional activity of several cellular oncogenes was reported. For instance, retinoic acid stimulates the activity and induces ODC synthesis in *ras* C_2 cells transfected with *H-ras-v* oncogene. 10 W cells, with receptors of *src-v* and *H-ras-v* oncogenes answer differently from DES-4 cells transfected with the same oncogenes. These results suggest that the pharmacological activity of retinoids might be different, depending on the cell type and/or the transforming agent.

In this respect we want to emphasize that retinoids can be very efficient suppressive agents or antipromoters for certain tissues (target tissues), and with no activity on other ones (i.e., colon, etc.). Their effects are usually reversible. Also toxic effects have to be noticed.

On this basis retinoids are considered valuable compounds in preventing several types of cancers in a high-risk population. Under certain conditions, they prove to also be able to reverse the early stage of promotion process. Vitamins C and E might also be included in this category, but their effects are significantly more restricted.[43]

IV. PREDICTION OF INHIBITORY PROPERTIES AGAINST CARCINOGENESIS BASED ON QSAR ANALYSIS

QSAR applications in the design of new biologically active compounds have been well documented,[44] especially in the area of derivatives exhibiting anticancer properties (nitrogen mustards,[45,46] triazenes,[47] platinum compounds,[48] podophylline derivatives,[49] etc.). Some progress was made in the area of carcinogenic compounds (see Chapter 5); however, little has been done to estimate the value of QSAR techniques in the field of chemical anticarcinogenesis.

However, two areas were particularly investigated in our laboratory using QSAR analysis, namely: (1) the anticarcinogenic properties of series of phenolic antioxidants (blocking agents) and (2) the carcinogenesis inhibitory properties of some synthetic retinoids.

A. QSAR ANALYSIS OF PHENOLIC ANTIOXIDANTS
Phenolic antioxidants such as: 2(3)*tert*-butyl-4-hydroxyanisole **6** (BHA),[2,50-55] 2,6-di-*tert*-butyl-hydroxytoluene **7** (BHT)[56,57] and, more recently, 4-hydroxyanisole **8** (HA)[55,58] have been recognized as powerful inhibitors of carcinogenesis against a wide range of

carcinogens (i.e., benzo(a)pyrene BaP, β-propiolactone, 7,12-dimethyl-benz(a)anthracene, etc.) in a variety of animal species and tissues (i.e., in skin, liver, lung, forestomach, etc.).[59,60]

OH   OH   OH

OCH$_3$ CH$_3$ OCH$_3$

6   **7**   **8**

Their mechanism of action is incompletely understood. However, two main hypotheses may be emphasized in this respect:

1. Current evidence suggests their ability to influence the initiation process by decreasing the concentration of the carcinogen covalently bound to DNA.[50,51,61] Three explanations are consistent with this effect: (1) a reduction or an alteration of the activation pathway[25,62-64] so that a decreased amount of ultimate carcinogen is formed; (2) a stimulation of the detoxication pathway, by increasing the activities of several enzymes involved in the detoxication of electrophilic intermediates. In fact, the activation of epoxide hydrase, UDP-glucuronyl-transferase and glutatione-S-transferase was reported:[65,66] in addition there is an increase in tissue glutathione level[67] and (3) a shift in the activation/detoxication balance, both steps being subsequently modified. If one of these mechanisms is accepted, the antioxidants would play the role of enzyme inducers or inhibitors. The possibility that antioxidants serve as nucleophiles which act as scavengers of electrophilic carcinogen intermediates remains unsupported.
2. Recently, some data claim the capacity of antioxidants to also inhibit the promotion stage,[68,69] by acting as scavengers of radicals resulting from carcinogen activation,[70] or of superoxide and other oxygen radicals involved in lipid peroxidation.[71] Both types of processes could be involved in chemical carcinogenesis, especially for those types of carcinogens for which mutagenic intermediates were not found (i.e., pesticides, etc.).[69]

A theoretical investigation of the structural and physicochemical features responsible for the biological activity of these phenolic antioxidants was undertaken in order to obtain additional information regarding their mechanism of action. The Hansch equation was used for QSAR analysis.

As biological parameters, both data obtained *in vitro* and *in vivo* regarding their carcinogenesis inhibitory properties were used, in order to obtain a deeper insight on their mechanisms of action.

The first approach[72] was undertaken considering the carcinogenic properties of 22 mono- and diphenolic antioxidants.[73] Their structures are given in Table 3.

The prevention of forestomach tumors induced with orally administered BaP (expressed as T/C, % animals with tumors) in female ICR/Ha mice was measured using equal amounts of antioxidants, given in the diet according to a uniform schedule for each case.[55] The biological activity was expressed by the formula:

$$A = \log \frac{100}{100 - T/C} \tag{1}$$

TABLE 3
Carcinogenesis Inhibitory Property and Lipophilicites of Some Phenolic Antioxidants

No.	Compound	Biological activity			Lipophilicity	
		(T/C^a)	$\log \dfrac{100}{100-T/C}$	$(\log P)$	$(\log P^b)$	$(\log P^b)$
1.	2.	3.	4.	5.	6.	7.
8.	4-Hydroxyanisole	22	0.107	0.60[c]	0.60	0.36
6.	2-*Tert*-Butyl-4-hydroxy-anisole (2BHA)	30	0.155	1.90	1.90	3.61
9.	5-Di-*tert*-butylcatechol	46	0.227	2.31	2.31	5.34
10.	2,6-Di-*tert*-butylphenol	52	0.319	3.28	3.28	10.76
11.	3-*Tert*-butyl-4-hydroxy-anisole (3BHA)	54	0.337	1.90[c]	1.90	3.61
12.	2-*Tert*-Butylhydroquinone	58	0.377	2.10[c]	2.10	4.41
13.	4-Hydroxy-3-methoxy-cinnamic acid	60	0.398	1.04[c]	−3.00	1.04
14.	2-*Tert*-Butylphenol	60	0.398	1.50	1.50	2.25
15.	3,4-Dihydrocinnamic acid	62	0.398	0.39	−3.65	0.15
16.	2-Hydroxy-cinnamic acid	66	0.420	1.26	−2.78	1.59
17.	4-Methyl-mercaptophenol	67	0.469	1.21	1.21	1.46
18.	2,3,5,6-Tetra-fluorophenol	73	0.481	0.56	0.56	0.31
19.	2,3,5,6-Tetra-methylphenol	79	0.569	2.24	2.24	5.02
20.	Di-(3,5-di-*tert*-butyl-4-hydroxyphenyl)-methane	84	0.678	6.72	6.72	45.16
21.	Fluoroglucinol	84	0.769	−0.84	−0.84	0.71
22.	4,4-Di(2,6-di-*tert*-butylphenol)	87	0.796	6.16	6.16	37.95
23.	Di-(3,5-di-*tert*-butyl-4-hydroxybenzyl)-ether	88	0.886	6.24	6.24	38.94
24.	Phenol	88	0.921	0.80[3]	0.80	0.64
25.	4,6-Di-*tert*-butylresorcinol	88	0.921	2.31	2.31	5.34
26.	Cinnamic acid	92	1.097	2.13[c]	−2.91	4.54
27.	2,4,6-Tri-*tert*-butyl-phenol	123	2.00[b]	4.71	4.71	22.18
28.	2,5-Di-*tert*-butylhydroquinone	128	2.00[b]	2.31	2.31	5.34

[a] T/C — the ratio between the number of mice with tumor in treated animals (T) with respect to the controls (C).
[b] For the T/C = 1 the expression log (100/(100 − T/C) was conventionally taken as 2.00.
[c] Experimental value.
[d] In this series $\pi_{CO^-} = -4.36$ was used for the computation of lipophilicities.

where T/C is the ratio between the number of mice with tumors in treated animals (T) and in control (C).

The following parameters were used as independent variables for the computation of the correlational equations:

1. Lipophilicity parameters — generally log P were used, calculated on the basis of the additivity properties of the π constants[59,74] when no direct experimental values were available

2.   σ-Hammett parameters — they were taken from the literature,[9] or calculated on a pK_a basis (27):

$$pK_8 = -1.298 \sum_i \sigma_i + 10.084$$

$$n = 13 \qquad s = 0.73 \qquad r = 0.965 \tag{2}$$

3.   Steric parameters — the minimal topological difference (MTD) parameter was used. For its meaning and computation see Chapter 5.D.
4.   Quantum mechanical parameters were also employed in order to substantiate a theoretical possiblity to estimate the antioxidant potency of the studied phenols. Previous studies have suggested that the antioxidant activity of substituted phenols could be related to their π-electronic structure, namely with the energy of the highest occupied orbital (see Chapter 5), which reflects the electron-donor properties of these compounds.[76,77]

Using the HMO procedure, the following parameters were calculated and used in the correlational equations: ϵ_{LEMO} — the energy of the lowest unoccupied (empty) molecular orbital; ϵ_{HOMO} — the energy of the highest occupied molecular orbital and ΔE_1 — the stabilizaion energy for a radical attack on the benzenic nucleus. This last parameter was calculated according to the formula:

$$\Delta E_1 = \sum_i^{occ} \frac{\left(\sum_r c_{i,r} \right)^2}{\lambda_i} - \sum_i^{non\ occ} \frac{\left(\sum_r c_{i,r} \right)^2}{\lambda_i} \tag{3}$$

where c_{ir} is the coefficient of the r-th atomic orbital in the ith molecular orbital, λ_i being expressed in β units; ΔE_1 is a measure of the ability of the aromatic compound to scavenge free radicals.

The correlational equations computed for these phenolic antioxidants are summarized in Table 4.

The distribution of good ($\epsilon = -1$), bad ($\epsilon = 1$) and irrelevant vertices in the hypermolecules (for its computation, see Chapter 5 and Figure 1) with only two good vertices suggest a poor steric requirement for the inhibitory activity in this class of compounds. This conclusion is also in agreement with the poor correlation obtained with MTD as sole parameter:

$$A = 0.0155 + 0.527\ (\pm 0.075)MTD$$

$$n = 20, \quad r = 0.857, \quad F = 49.60 \quad (F_{0.99} = 9.29) \tag{4}$$

Some improvement of the correlation was observed by introducing the lipophilicity parameter:

$$A = 0.029 + 0.630\ (\pm 0.068)MTD - 0.064(\pm 0.023)\pi$$

$$n = 20 \quad r = 0.892 \quad F = 20.30 \quad (F_{0.99} = 5.25) \tag{5}$$

The introduction of the quantum mechanical parameters failed to improve the correlation. Surprisingly, no correlation was found between these parameters and the *in vivo* carcinogenesis inhibitory properties of phenolic antioxidants.

In contrast, the introduction of σ-Hammett constants exerted a beneficial influence upon

TABLE 4
Correlation Parameters (r and F) of the Regression Equations Computed for the Phenolic Compounds

Independent variables used in the regression equations		Investigated samples		
		(n = 22)	(n = 20)	(n = 12[b])
MTD	r	0.750	0.857	0.919
	F	25.64	49.60	24.43
MTD, π	r	0.759	0.892	0.926
	F	12.93	32.98	15.96
MTD, HMO(3)[a]	r	0.756	0.866	—
	F	5.68	11.26	—
MTD, π,π^2	r	0.759	0.982	0.929
	F	8.17	20.73	10.47
MTD, π, HMO(3)[a]	r	0.779	0.913	—
	F	4.95	14.11	—
MTD, π, π^2, HMO(3)[a]	r	0.780	0.914	0.927
	F	3.87	11.04	3.52

[a] All three previously discussed quantum mechanical parameters (see materials and methods) were used.

[b] This series contains the Hammett parameter in all cases.

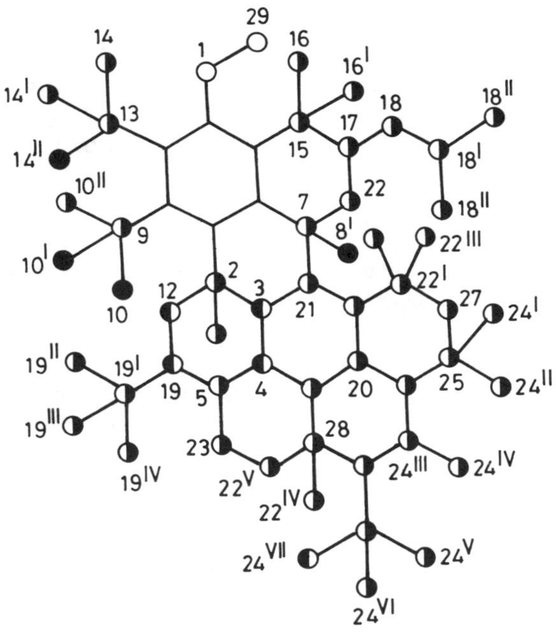

O   GOOD

◖   IRRELEVANT

●   BAD

FIGURE 1.   Hypermolecule of the investigated antioxidants.

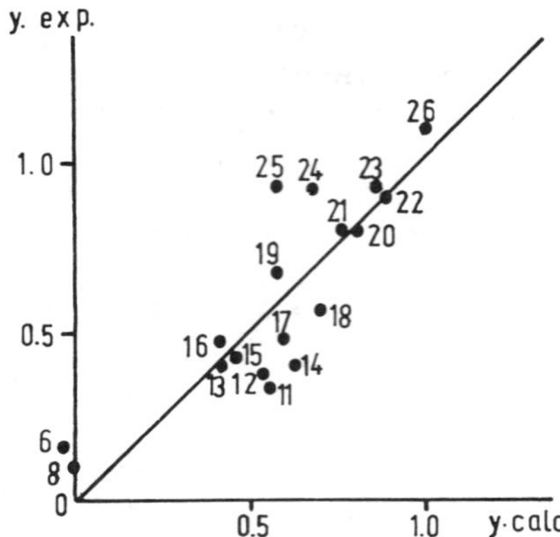

FIGURE 2.   Correlation between theoretical and experimental values of the biological parameter of the investigated phenolic antioxidants.

the correlational index (unfortunately only 12 such constants were available for our series of compounds). The following equation was obtained:

$$A = 0.0597 + 0.669(\pm 0.092)MTD - 0.087(\pm 0.071)\pi + 0.050(\pm 0.107)\sigma$$

$$n = 12 \quad r = 0.925 \quad F = 15.88 \quad (F_{0.99} = 7.59) \tag{6}$$

The correlation between the experimental and calculated data for the set of 20 antioxidant phenols (Equation 6) is given in Figure 2.

Summarizing the aforementioned aspect we want to emphasize that none of the investigated parameters has been found to be decisive for the carcinogenesis inhibitory properties of the investigated compounds. The most puzzling suggestion is that no correlation exists between the antioxidant properties of these phenols and their biological effectiveness. If we cannot rule out definitely such a possibility, we believe that this property is not involved in a rate-determining process and this assumption was submitted to further investigation.[73,79]

These data suggest that the most important mechanism of action determining the biological properties of these compounds involves their inhibitory properties against the monooxygenase-cytochrome P-450 dependent enzymatic systems. This assumption is supported by:

1.   The poor substrate selectivity of this system in good agreement with the poor correlations obtained between the biological properties and MTD parameters in this series
2.   The correlation between the monooxygenase inhibition and the experimentally found DNA-protection against MC-microsome activated BaP[80]

According to Equation 6, the addition of an extra amino group to the aromatic nucleus of the investigated phenols should afford compounds with interesting carcinogenesis inhibitory properties. In order to check the accuracy of this prediction, a series of known aminophenols was investigated, establishing whether or not they are able to protect DNA against the *in vitro* binding of (^{3}H)BaP[79] activated by MC-microsomes. The results summarized in Table 5 demonstrate that the aminophenols are also good candidates as carcinogenesis inhibitors.

However, most surprising was the observation that 4-*N*-methyl-aminophenol and 4-aminophenol solutions after being stored (for 3 to 7 days) at room temperature in the presence of air and light, exhibit much stronger inhibitory properties, so that the DNA protection

TABLE 5
Protective Effectiveness of Some Aminophenols Against Microsomal Activated G(^{3}H) BaP Binding to DNA

No.	Compound	No. of experiments	Inhibition of G(^{3}H)BaP binding, %
6.	2-*Tert*-butylhydroxyanisole (2-BHA)[a]	4	34.5 ± 0.9
7.	2,6-Di-*tert*-butyl-4-hydroxy-toluene (BHT)[a]	3	36.0 ± 1.4
8.	β-Naphthoflavone[a]	3	48.4 ± 0.1
29.	4,*N*-methylaminophenol-sulfate	3	32.0 ± 1.1
30.	4,*N*-methylaminophenol (oxidated form)	7	97.5 ± 2.2
31.	4-Aminophenol	3	31.1 ± 1.8
32.	4-Aminophenol, oxidated form	2	96.3 ± 2.4
33.	4,*N,N*-dimethylaminophenol	2	58.4 ± 6.2
34.	2-Aminophenol	2	54.7 ± 3.7
35.	3,*N,N*-dimethylaminophenol	2	43.8 ± 1.1
36.	4,*N,N*-dimethylaminoanisole	2	32.4 ± 6.3
37.	4-Aminosalicyclic acid	2	7.1 ± 2.6
38.	2-Aminoanisole	5	31.5 ± 3.5
39.	4-Aminoanisole	2	47.7 ± 6.2
40.	*N*-(4'-hydroxy-3',5'-di-*tert*-butylphenyl) 2,6-di-*tert*-butylbenziminoquinone[b]	4	79.0 ± 3.6

[a]   Antioxidants used as reference compounds.
[b]   Oxidation product of 2,6-di-*tert*-butyl-4-aminophenol.

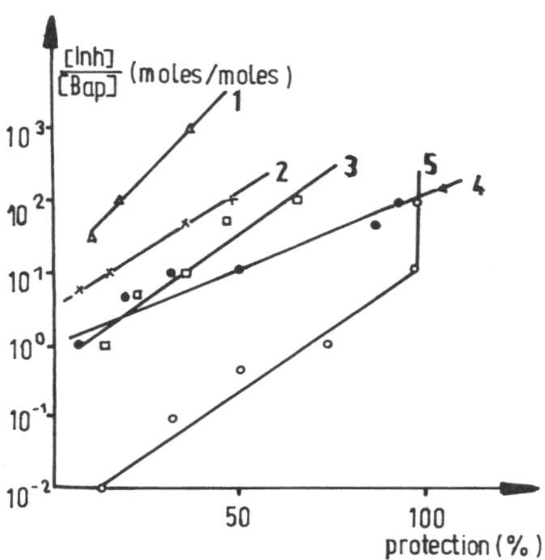

FIGURE 3.   Dose effect curves for a series of carcinogenesis inhibitors: (1) GSH; (2) 4-hydroxyanisole; (3) 2(3)-*tert*-butyl-hydroxyanisole; (4) 4-(*N*-methyl)-aminophenol; (5) 4-(*N*-methyl)-aminophenol oxidated form.

obtained using the above mentioned test (*in vitro*) exceeded 95% (see Table 5). This unusually high protection was confirmed by dose-effect curves plotted for these compounds (see Figure 3). For instance, to achieve a 50% *in vitro* protection, a BaP: anti-initiator ratio of 1:38.5 (mol/mol) is required for BHA, in contrast with 1:12.4 for *p*-aminophenol and only 1:0.27 for its oxidation products). This means a 10^2-fold increase of the protection effectiveness in the case of oxidized solutions of aminophenols.

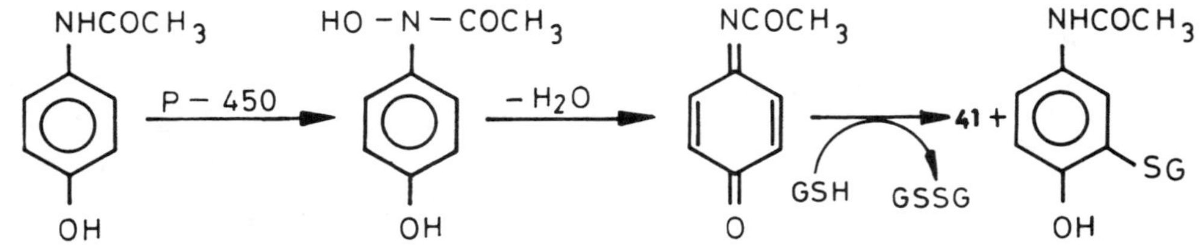

SCHEME 1.   Metabolism of acetaminophen.

Two facts have to be explained: (1) the DNA protective activity of aminophenols, and (2) why their oxidized forms are more effective than the corresponding reduced precursors.

The DNA protective activity of aminophenols measured in the previously mentioned test may be related to their ability to inhibit directly or through one of their metabolites the microsomal cytochrome P-450-dependent activation system. Some data regarding the metabolism of aminophenols are known.[81,82] For instance, it was proposed that acetaminophen **41**, a widely used analgesic, is oxidized by cytochrome P-450 to *N*-hydroxyacetaminophen **42**, which dehydrates to *N*-acetyl-p-benzoquinoneimine **43** (according to Scheme 1).

The validation of the existence *in vivo* of this latter intermediate **43** was surprisingly difficult because of its short half-life which has been reported to be no longer than 7 s in microsomal preparations.[83]

Once this quinoneimine **43** is generated it can be detoxified by covalent bonding with GSH (GSH and GSSG symbolize reduced and oxidized glutathione, respectively). The role that GSH plays in detoxication may be two-fold, according to Scheme 1. First, it may act as a nucleophile leading to 3-(glutathionyl)-acetaminophen **44**.[84] This last product was isolated recently as a biliary metabolite of acetaminophen (13). Second, GSH is a one-electron reductant in which two molecules of GSH would reduce **44** to acetaminophen and GSSG.[85]

A similar pattern of oxidation by microsomal cytochrome P-450-dependent enzymes may be suggested for the aminophenols (i.e., 4-aminophenol, 4,*N*-methylaminophenol, etc.). The corresponding quinoneimines thus formed could be potent inhibitors of the microsomal activating enzymes. However, they should be much less stable than quinoneimine **43** leading quickly to further condensation or detoxication products. It is also possible that one of these products exhibits monooxygenase inhibitory activity. Mention should also be made that the *p*-aminophenol induced cellular damage and toxicity are enhanced by autooxidation.[86] Therefore, in order to give a more complete answer to question (1), we have to assume that despite the monooxygenase inhibitory properties of aminophenols, some of the metabolite(s) formed during their oxidation by this very enzymatic system could also contribute to the observed overall DNA protection. The "pure" inhibitory effect of aminophenols upon the cytochrome P-450 monooxygenase is, for this reason, difficult to evaluate.

Despite some reports devoted to the *in vitro* oxidation of 4-aminophenol and some of its derivatives, the data concerning the structure of the products resulting from this reaction are rather confusing.[87-89] It seems that the main oxidation products are the corresponding quinoneimines which undergo further condensations to more complicated compounds. The oxidation to quinoneimines proceeds through a free-radical mechanism, involving the formation of semi-quinone radicals (i.e., radical **45** or **46**).[90] The structure of these radicals is debatable.[91]

TABLE 6
Activity of Some Phenolic Antioxidants and of Some
Aromatic Quinones

No.	Compound	No. of experiments	Inhibition of activated (^{3}H)BaP binding to DNA, %
47.	Hydroquinone	3	15.1 ± 1.0
28.	2,5-di-*tert*-butylhydroquinone	3	45.3 ± 2.7
48.	Benzoquinone	3	56.9 ± 6.3
49.	2,6-di-*tert*-butylbenzoquinone	2	93.9 ± 2.9
50.	Benzo(a)pyrene 1,6 dione	2	96.8 ± 2.9
51.	Benzo(a)pyrene 3,6 dione	2	97.4 ± 1.1
52.	Benzo(a)pyrene 6,12 dione	2	98.9 ± 0.7

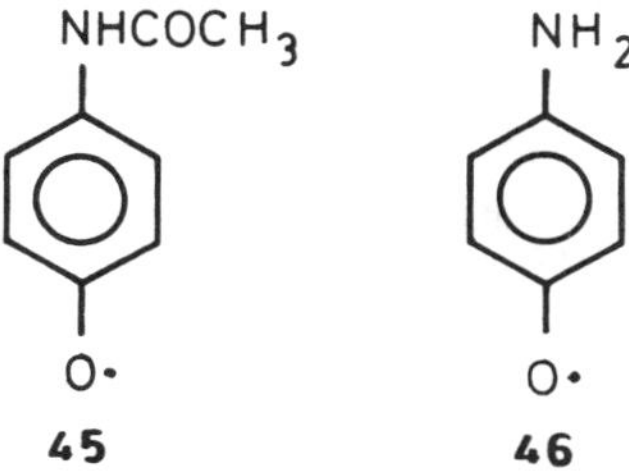

Both theoretical calculations[11] and experimental data support this oxidation pattern, as well as the intermediate formation of free radicals during oxidation.[14,24,25] These radicals and the reactive quinoneimines thus formed, or their condensation products, could be potent inhibitors of the monooxygenase cytochrome P-450-dependent system. The inhibitory species formed during the oxidation of aminophenols (by air and light) are presumably at a much higher concentration than in the microsomal preparations containing the precursor aminophenols. This fact explains why the oxidized aminophenols are more effective.

At this time we are not able to propose a tentative structure for the oxidation product(s) of 4-aminophenol or 4,*N*-methylaminophenol which possess a highly protective activity *in vitro* against the DNA binding of activated G(^{3}H)BaP. At present, we have at least four indirect arguments strongly suggesting that the quinoneimine formed during oxidation and light exposure are responsible for the inhibition of the microsomal activation enzyme.

First, as we reported previously, the procedure we use for determining the *in vitro* protecting activity of anti-initiators against DNA damaging selects the compounds which inhibit microsomal activation enzyme. Therefore, the results we discuss here show that the oxidized aminophenols are considerably more effective than their reduced precursor in inhibiting the activity of these enzymes. A similar effect was observed in the phenolic antioxidant series[78] where we demonstrated that their oxidation products (i.e., the corresponding quinones) are significantly more effective in inhibiting the microsomal activating enzymatic system than their corresponding precursors[12,78] (Table 6). Mention should be made that BaP-quinones themselves (i.e., BaP-3,6-, 3,12- and 6,12-quinones) are also potent inhibitors of these enzymes[78] (Table 6).

It was demonstrated that these BaP-diones possess significant toxicity against hamster embryo cells in culture.[93] However, this toxicity is substantially decreased or even completely abolished by the removal of molecular oxygen.[93] No direct interaction between these quinones and DNA was observed. These observations are consistent with our point of view.

Second, the 2-*tert*-butylbenzoquinone **53** which was detected during the metabolization of 2(3)-*tert*-butylhydroxyanisole could be responsible for the carcinogenesis inhibitor properties of this anti-initiator.[94]

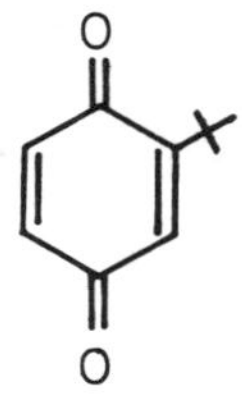

53

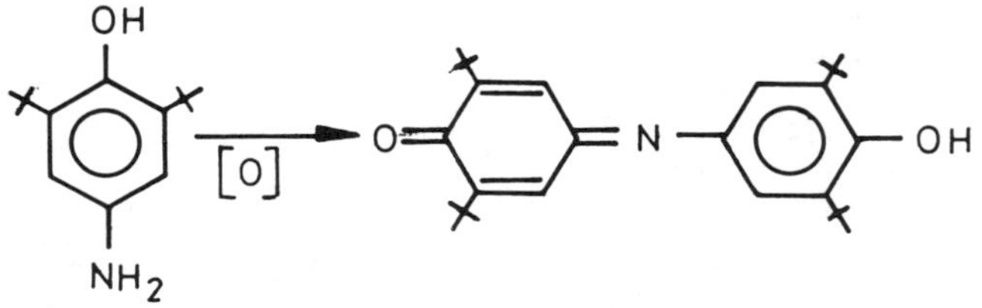

54   **55**

SCHEME 2.   Product resulted from 2,6-di-*tert*-butyl-4-aminophenol mild oxidation.

Third, as we discussed previously, the quinoneimines resulting especially from the oxidation of the *N*-unsubstituted aminophenols are very unstable compounds (with very short half-lives) leading further to condensation products, usually with unknown structures. However, for some sterically hindered aminophenols, definite condensation products with quinoneimine structures (i.e., indophenols) could be obtained in mild conditions.[95] For instance, the oxidation product of 2,6-di-*tert*-butyl-4-aminophenol **54** may be synthesized (Scheme 2).

The fact that this indophenol **55** is also more effective according to our *in vitro* text (i.e., P% = 79.0 ± 3.6%) than other aminophenols which were tested, agrees with this point of view. Finally, the fact that 4-*N,N*-dimethylaminophenol does not exhibit such an effect is also consistent with our assumption.

A final argument for this assumption is that a QSAR analysis based on an *in vitro* DNA-protection test[96] computed on a series of 27 antioxidant phenols, aminophenols and quinones (especially *t*-butyl-substituted ones) also supports this point of view.

The best correlational equation computed for this series using initiated BaP is:

$$A = -1.49(\pm 0.13)\Delta E_{\text{HO-LE}} + 2.4$$

$$n = 17 \qquad r = 0.94 \qquad F = 121.7 \tag{7}$$

where A is expressed as $\dfrac{P\%}{100 - P\%}$ and P% is the DNA protection calculated according to the relationship $P\% = (1 - \dfrac{s_o}{c_o}$; s_o is the specific activity of the sample (dpm/μg DNA) and c_o is that of control sample as determined in the absence of the anti-initiator; $\Delta E_{\text{HO-LE}} = \epsilon_{\text{HOMO}} - \epsilon_{\text{LEMO}}$, calculated by HMO.

A test series of 10 compounds randomly chosen gives the following equation:

$$A_{\text{exp}} = 1.071(\pm 0.09)A_{\text{calc}} - 0.0084$$

$$n = 10 \qquad r = 0.968 \qquad F = 119 \tag{8}$$

suggesting a good predictive potential for Equation 7.

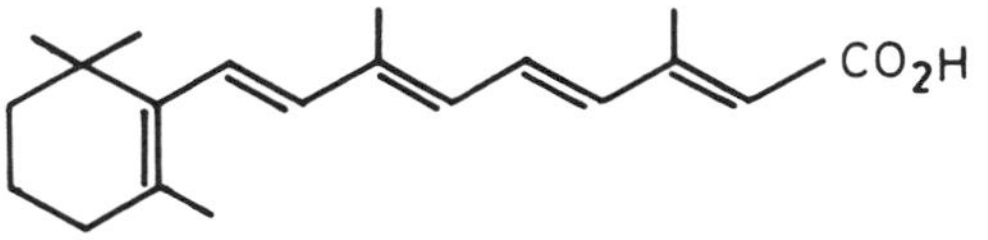

all — *trans* RA

56

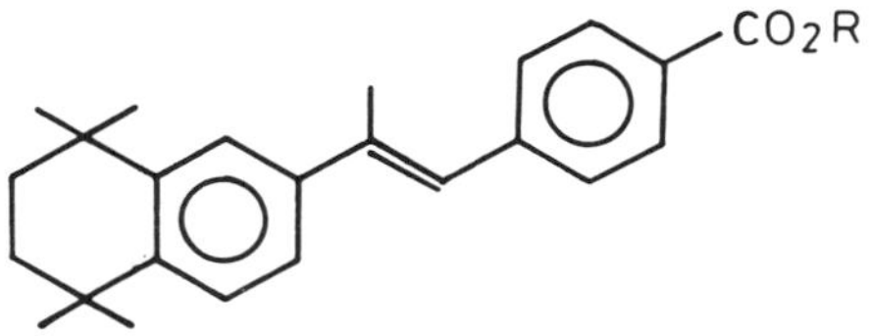

R = H   Ro 13 — 7410

R = CH_3   Ro 13 — 6289

57

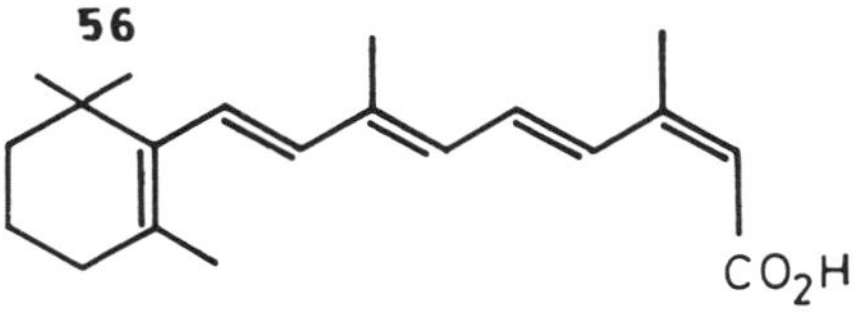

58

FIGURE 4.   Structure of retinoids.

Equation 7 reflects the very important fact that the oxidation status of the inhibitor is of prime importance in determining its biological properties. It results that the quinones and the iminoquinones are more powerful inhibitors of cytochrome P-450 dependent monooxygenases than the corresponding phenols or aminophenols.

The utility of such approaches for the design of better carcinogenesis inhibitors (belonging to the group of blocking agents) is obvious and should also be extended to other classes of compounds.

B. QSAR ANALYSIS OF SOME SYNTHETIC AND NATURAL RETINOIDS

The retinoids appear as a particularly interesting family of compounds classified as promotion step inhibitors, able to suppress the process of carcinogenesis both *in vitro* and *in vivo*[58,97] or only *in vivo*,[98,99] and also to exert an effect on certain fully transformed, invasive, neoplastic cells.[100,101] Several reviews summarized the extensive work carried out in this area.[40,99,102,103]

This class of compounds is particularly suitable to a theoretical analysis because of:

1. The great number of available structures
2. The existence of a standard biological *in vitro* test able to measure the intrinsic ability of retinoids to control epithelial cell differentiation (reversion of keratinization of hamster tracheal cells, TOC assay)
3. The particular interest presented by natural and synthetic analogs of vitamin A, for cancer prevention and perhaps also for therapy[101,104,105]

Despite these advantages, few structure-activity studies were undertaken in this area.[40,42,106]

A first QSAR-MTD analysis was performed on a sample of 68 natural and synthetic retinoids divided into an analysis series (53 compounds) and a test series (15 compounds — randomly chosen). Because of the computation difficulties the analysis series was subdivided into three groups of retinoids containing: (1) different cyclic moieties (n = 19); (2) various polyenic side chains (n = 11) and (3) endgroup modified derivatives of retinoic acid (n = 27). The main structures are presented in Figure 4.

The following parameters were used:

1. Effective dose for 50% reversion of keratinization of hamster tracheal cells (TOC assay) (mol), ED_{50}

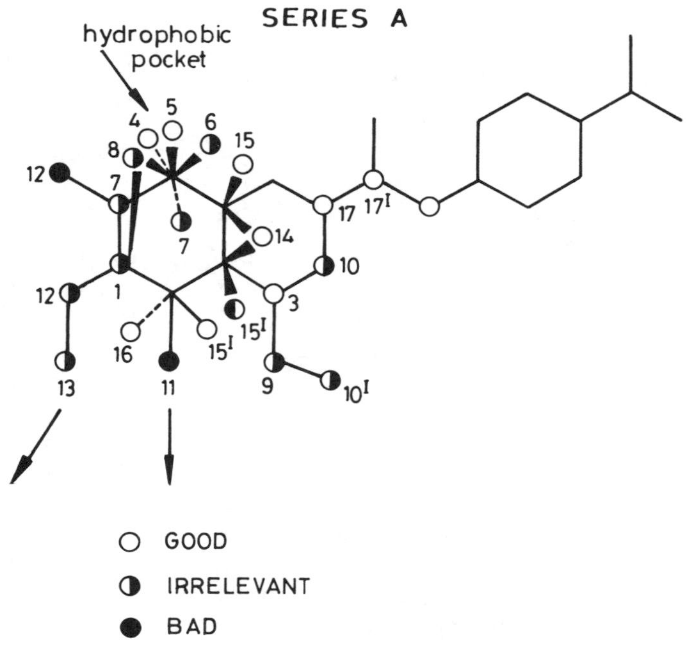

FIGURE 5. Hypermolecule for retinoic acid cyclic moiety.

2.   The lipophilicity was expressed by relative log P, a value of log P_{rel} = 0.0 being assigned to the most simple congener (all-*trans*-retinoic acid, **56**)
3.   Minimal Topological Difference MTD indices were used as steric parameters
4.   Three additional parameters (indicator variables) were employed:

- δ_1 reflecting the carboxyl group ionization (1 for ionizable carboxyl at pH 7.0 and 0 otherwise)
- δ_2 describing the degree of double bond hydrogenation (0 for noninterrupted conjugation of the polyenic chain and 1 if a double bond is hydrogenated)
- n representing the number of atoms acting as proton acceptor at the terminal functional group.

The models of all the molecules were constructed using Dreiding stereomodel; the compound with the highest activity **57** (Ro-13-7410) with a rather rigid structure was considered as a basis for the superposition procedure.

The following equations were obtained, reflecting the contribution of several parts of the retinoid molecules to the overall biological activity. The influence of the cyclic moiety (Series A):

$$\log \frac{1}{ED_{50}} = 26.11 + 0.42(\pm 0.26)\delta_1 - 104(\pm 0.11)MTD_1$$

$$n = 19 \qquad r = 0.926 \qquad F = 48.19 \tag{9}$$

If we assume that retinoids act through an effector-receptor mechanism, the distribution of the beneficial vertices in the resulted hypermolecule (see Figure 5) suggests that one or two hydrophobic pockets could be located in this region of the receptor. The influence of the polyenic chain (Series B):

$$\log \frac{1}{ED_{50}} = 30.79 - 2.40(\pm 0.42)\delta_2 - 1.31(\pm 0.17)MTD_2$$

$$n = 11 \qquad r = 0.953 \qquad F = 39.90 \tag{10}$$

One of the most important factors determining the biological activity of the investigated molecules seems to be the degree of hydrogenation of the polyenic chain. The hydrogenation of a double bond in this region of the molecule leads to less active congeners by destroying the conjugation and increasing the flexibility of the side chain. The influence of the terminal functional part of the molecule is described by the equation:

$$\log \frac{1}{ED_{50}} = 17.03 + 1.12(\pm 0.72)\delta_1 + 0.39(\pm 0.23)n_o$$

$$+ 0.53(\pm 0.19)MTD_3 + 0.04(\pm 0.15)\pi - 0.19(\pm 0.14)\pi^2$$

$$n = 27 \qquad r = 0.757 \qquad F = 5.64 \tag{11}$$

This poor correlation between the structure of the terminal part of the retinoid molecule and its activity is consistent with experimental data which have shown that molecules with very different stereochemistry of this region (i.e., all-*trans*-retinoic acid, 13-*cis*-retinoic acid **58** or Ro-13-7410, **57**, R = H) are equally effective in the considered test.

The development of a global equation (MTD = MTD$_1$ + MTD$_2$ + MTD$_3$ + const.) including all data, led to an unsatisfactory correlation although the explained variance of ED$_{50}$ remains 70%:

$$\log \frac{1}{ED_{50}} = 21.86 + 0.44(\pm 0.21)\delta_1 - 2.31(\pm 0.49)\delta_2 + 0.32(\pm 0.20)n_o$$

$$- 0.93(\pm 0.09)MTD + 0.07(\pm 0.11)\pi - 0.13(\pm 0.18)\pi^2$$

$$n = 53 \qquad r = 0.868 \qquad F = 23.11 \tag{12}$$

The small contribution of lipophilicity terms to the overall biological effects appears as somewhat unexpected. However, mention should be made that we use only relative lipophilicities (log P_{rel} = 0.0 for all-*trans*-retinoic acid). Therefore, the absolute lipophilicity is around log P = 6.60 $\pm$ 2.00. This variation means no more than 30% from the log P of RA and probably does not extensively influence the uptake and penetration across cell membranes of the considered congeners. The deletion of two aberrant points from Equation 12 gives values r = 0.918, F = 39.41 (for n = 51).

In order to check the prediction potential of this approach we calculated the ED$_{50}$ values for 15 retinoids (randomly chosen) belonging to the test series. The following equation was obtained:

$$\log \frac{1}{ED_{50,exp}} = 1.64 - 0.84 \log \frac{1}{ED_{50,calc}}$$

$$n = 15 \qquad r = 0.916 \qquad F = 60.25 \tag{13}$$

This means a satisfactory prediction capability. This QSAR analysis suggests:

1.   More effective structures could be found in this area.

2.   A passive diffusion could be expected, taking into account the high lipophilicity of the retinoids. The poor contribution of the lipophilicity terms in the developed equations is consistent with this assumption.

3.   Because of the important contribution of the MTD term in these equations, an interaction with a given receptor cavity appears to be a major event determining the biological activity of the retinoids.

4.   A cisoid conformation of the side chain as in Ro-13-7410, is necessary to obtain the best correlation indices for the computed equations.

This latter suggestion was also in agreement with a similar assumption made by Dawson et al. about the possibility that even retinoic acid (RA) assumes an active conformation in which the 9, 11, 13 E-double bond systems are planar and cisoid.[107] For this reason, a similar QSAR approach was undertaken[40] on a sample of 53 conformationally restricted retinoids synthetized by Dawson et al.[107,108,109]

Some differences were evident in this QSAR analysis compared to the previous series. Our first receptor map allowed a large variation of positions for the polyenic chain and terminal carboxyl group, without loss of biological activity. This map suggested the existence of two receptor moieties (with different cavities and a certain reciprocal mobility) as in the case of steroid receptors.[110]

For the superposition procedure, Dreiding stereomodels and computer-simulated three-dimensional structures were used.

Correlation equations were developed using MTD, δ_1, δ_3 (possibility of the endgroup being transformed into a carboxylic group, defined as 1 for esters, aldehydes, primary and secondary amines, etc., and 0 otherwise) and π term. The best equation was

$$\log \frac{1}{ED_{50}} = 16.48 + 80(\pm 0.18)\delta_1 - 0.33(\pm 0.23)\delta_3$$

$$- 1.04(\pm 0.11)MTD + 0.58(\pm 0.10)\pi$$

$$n = 29 \qquad r = 0.918 \qquad F = 32.04 \tag{14}$$

We emphasize that, as for the previous QSAR approach, a rapid *trans-cis* isomerization was postulated for retinoic acid and also for 13-*cis* congeners. This assumption significantly improved the correlation indices in this series.

Another major difference from the first approach consists in the absence of δ_2-parameter in Equation 15, which was computed for conformationally restricted retinoids especially taking into account the side chain.

$$\log \frac{1}{ED_{50}} = 13.98 + 0.77(\pm 0.22)\delta_1 - 0.73(\pm 0.08)MTD$$

$$+ 0.51(\pm 0.10)\pi - 0.10(\pm 0.06)\pi^2$$

$$n = 27 \qquad r = 0.938 \qquad F = 40.62 \tag{15}$$

This indicates that in this series the uninterrupted conjugation or a certain ridigity of the side chain is not a prerequisite condition for the activity.

This approach allowed us to point out a series of structural features that are important for the carcinogenesis inhibitory properties of these compounds. The structure of the ring moiety, as well as that of the polar terminus and the neighboring side chain (11,12- and 13,14-double bonds) are of particular importance for the biological activity of retinoids. The relative position of the carboxylic terminus (defined in polar coordinates) with respect to the ring moiety is another critical parameter for activity. The lipophilicity term has a reduced contribution in the computed equations. This fact agrees with a passive uptake of retinoids by tracheal hamster cells. Nevertheless, it appears as an important tool in describing the interaction of the cyclic moiety with the receptor cavity. These data may be of interest for the design of compounds with improved pharmacological effectiveness.

If a unified set of conformationally restricted and nonrestricted retinoids including all data is considered (n = 75), an unsatisfactory correlation resulted, not very different from that obtained for the retinoids from the first series (Equation 12):

$$\log \frac{1}{ED_{50}} = 11.99 + 0.54(\pm 0.15)\delta_1 - 2.72(\pm 0.45)\delta_2$$

$$+ 0.65(\pm 0.18)\delta_3 + 0.18(\pm 11)n_o - 0.57(\pm 0.06)MTD$$

$$+ 0.40(\pm 0.10)\pi - 0.12(\pm 0.50)\pi^2$$

$$n = 75 \qquad r = 0.847 \qquad F = 24.27 \tag{16}$$

However, it became obvious from this equation that the inclusion of the terminal group series (see Equation 11) in the overall set significantly decreased the correlation indices because of the interference between the hydrolysis process (needed for activation of the end group of modified retinoids) and the rate-determining step interaction. If this is correct, then a set containing only ring and polyenic chain modified retinoid congeners will exhibit a significantly better correlation. The following equation was obtained:

$$\log \frac{1}{ED_{50}} = 13.89 + 0.68(\pm 0.17)\delta_1 - 2.93(\pm 0.39)\delta_2 - 0.10(\pm 0.33)\delta_3$$

$$- 0.69(\pm 0.06)MTD + 0.42(\pm 0.08)\pi - 0.09(\pm 0.05)\pi^2$$

$$n = 50 \qquad r = 0.912 \qquad F = 35.58 \tag{17}$$

From the experimental data so far available and based on our contemporary concepts about cell regulation, it is most likely that two main sites are involved in the retinoid effect: the cell membrane and the nuclear chromatin.

Retinoids may modulate growth and differentiation via interaction with membrane-associated proteins, for instance by direct interaction with cyclic-AMP-dependent or calcium-dependent protein kinases associated with some growth factors and their receptors.[106,111,112] Their direct interaction with the polypeptide growth factors that control proliferation and differentiation was also suggested.[113,114] There are also arguments against this possible mode of action.[102]

Another possible target of the retinoids is the nucleus. The most simple explanation suggested by a large amount of available experimental data is that the retinods are able to modulate the expression of the genes involved in both differentiation and proliferation.[114-118] On this basis, it is logical to assume that an interaction with a receptor site at the nuclear level (by a steroid-like mechanism)[97,114-118] is responsible for the carcinogenesis inhibitory properties of the retinoids. The existence of cellular specific retinoid-binding proteins (CRBP, CRABP), etc. agrees with this mechanism of action.

Whether the transport of retinoids through the cytoplasm and their translocation to the nucleus are dependent on these binding proteins or are occurring by passive diffusion remains an open question since it has recently been demonstrated that two highly retinoid-responsive cell systems — HL60 and 10T1/2 fibroblasts — are devoid of retinoid-binding proteins.[102,119,120] The TOC assay is believed to have significant predictive value for the prevention of epithelial cancer. Some features of this assay are important, namely: (1) its high specificity and sensitivity for retinoids;[121] (2) the fairly good correlation of the activity of retinoids determined in this system with many other *in vitro* test systems such as inhibition of the growth of murine melanoma cells,[122] binding to cellular CRABP;[118] (3) the arguments that tracheal cells possess enzymes necessary to hydrolyze retinoid carboxylic acid derivatives such as esters and amides[121,123] and (4) according to Frolik et al.,[124] the ability of tracheal cells to convert retinyl acetate to retinoic acid, via retinal intermediate.

In the hamster tracheal organ culture test, the following steps could be important for the biological activity of retinoids; (1) retinoid uptake and penetration across cell membranes; (2) transport through the cytoplasm and nuclear translocation, if these processes are mediated by a specific intracellular binding protein; (3) hydrolysis or metabolic conversion of the terminal group to a carboxylic group and (4) interaction with a critical target site at the nuclear level.

Our equations describe the most important (rate-determining) process of the previously mentioned steps. Also, they are developed on the implicit assumption that all the considered retinoids act in the TOC assay by the same mechanism. This seems to be a reasonable hypothesis despite the suggestion that a retinoid may act by different mechanisms in different cell systems.[102] Because of the important contribution of MTD terms in the equations developed in this study, an interaction with a given receptor appears to be the major event determining the biological activity of the retinoids; however, which of these two types of receptors (transport or regulatory proteins) are involved in this interaction is difficult to establish. It is, therefore, interesting to speculate on theoretical models for the regulation of gene activity and also to look upon some required characteristics of the transport and regulatory proteins and the way they could be modulated by effectors.

The mechanism of RA uptake by the cells is not yet elucidated.[102] However, a passive diffusion could be expected, taking into account the high lipophilicity of retinoids. The first conclusion of our QSAR study is that lipophilicity terms make a low contribution to retinoid behavior. This conclusion agrees with the previously mentioned assumtion and also suggests that the cellular uptake of retinoid derivatives is not a rate-determining step.

A second important conclusion of our approach is the necessity of an enzymatic *trans-cis* isomerization of the side chain of RA and several other congeners in order to assume an active conformation. This result explains why compounds with the terminal carboxyl group located in very different positions by respect to that of Ro-13-7410 (the most effective retinoid) i.e., all-*trans*-RA, 13-*cis*-RA and also compounds with planar and cisoid fixed conformations, are highly active.

Measurements of the chain lengths between the C_6 atom and the terminal carbon atom of the CO_2H group, as well as the C^5-C^6-CO_2H angle using the computer-3-D-simulated retinoid molecules indicate that biological effectiveness is strongly dependent upon these two parameters and implies a relatively restricted area for the location of the carboxylic acid endgroup of the retinoid in the receptor cavity that is correlated to high biological activity.

This explanation is consistent with the activity of structurally different retinoids, for example the coordinates of the terminal moiety of RA for a planar cisoid conformation of the 11,12- and 13,14-double bonds is 10.7 Å and 107°18′, which are very close to the position of the carboxylic group of Ro-13-7410. This argument remains valid regardless of whether the retinoid receptor is a transport protein (i.e., CRABP) or a regulatory one.

A similar QSAR-MTD analysis of the results reported by Strikland et al.[113] on the ability of some aromatic retinoids to induce the differentiation of F9 teratocarcinoma and HL60 human promyelocytic leukemia cells reveals a very interesting aspect. Using the MTD parameters computed for these compounds on the basic hypermolecule previously built for the analysis of the unified set of retinoids, we obtained a reasonable correlation (r = 0.88) between their activity against F9 teratocarcinoma cells and these MTD figures. In contrast, a similar approach failed to describe the behavior of the same retinoids in the HL60 cell system. If we consider that F9 cells possess CRABP, in contrast with HL60 cells, it is possible to infer that our equations describe retinoid-CRABP interactions. However, this conclusion has to be taken with caution, because of the limited number of compounds available for this analysis (n = 9) and of the inherent limits of such an approach. More work and additional experimental systems are needed in order to elucidate this point.

Another recent approach implies the use of topological indices. Derivatives of retinoic acid wherein the carboxyl group is free ($R' = H$) or esterified with ethanol or methanol ($R' = Et$ or Me) and where the ionone group is replaced by carbocyclic or heterocyclic systems (but conserving in all cases the isoprenoid chain of four conjugated double bonds, with two methyl side groups, which joins the COOR' with the carbo/heterocyclic group R) possess a remarkable biological activity. An attempt to correlate this activity as carcinogenesis inhibitors, with the chemical structure of the group R expressed in terms of the topological index J and additional parameters gave satisfactory results. Fourteen such retinoid analogs with $-\log ED_{50}$ ranging from 6 to 9.7 were tested in terms of the JS index where the nature of heteroatoms (oxygen or nitrogen) was taken into account by means of their van der Waals radii relatively to the carbon atom (S in JS stands for steric-J). A weighting factor, $W = 0.5$, was found to optimize the correlation on multiplying the distance sum of the vertex i corresponding to the heteroatom. Thus for such a vertex the distance sum is calculated normally as for hydrocarbons (double bonds and aromatic bonds are awarded bond orders by $b = 2$, and 1.5, respectively), then it is multiplied by $W = 0.5$ and by the calculated relative van der Waals radius. The site of bonding, on the other hand, is awarded corrected distance sum $0.1\ s_i$, allowing to differentiate for instance an *n*-propyl from an isopropyl group by its J value. Finally, two other correction factors must be mentioned: (1) an indicator variable (Kronecker delta) distinguishing retinoic acids ($\delta = 1$) from their esters ($\delta = 0$) which, unlike the acids, have no hydrogen bonds and (2) the JS value is calculated only for group R, but a small correction is added for considering the R' group: 0 for acids ($R' = H$), 0.0242 for $R' = Me$, and 0.0933 for $R' = Et$; this correction results from calculating the whole molecule including groups R, R', and the isoprenoid connecting chain.

Several equations were tested; those where the structure was expressed solely by the JS value and the number v of nonhydrogen atoms in the R group gave modest correlation factors ($0.88 < r < 0.90$).

When the hydrophobicity factor π (calculated additively according to Hansch) was used in a biparametric correlation along with JS, the improvement was slight, but the indicator variable δ raised the correlation factor above 0.9. The best correlations were obtained as follows for tri- and tetra-parametric equations:

$$\log ED_{50} = 13.5321 - 1.1324\ JS + 0.3650\pi + 0.81310\delta$$

$$n = 14 \qquad r = 0.934$$

$$\log ED_{50} = 15.1263 - 1.2718\ JS - 0.095v + 0.372\pi + 0.7617\delta$$

$$n = 14 \qquad r = 0.938$$

The additional parameter v brings about an insignificant improvement of the correlation.

REFERENCES

1. **Wattenberg, L. W.**, Inhibitors of carcinogenesis, in *Carcinogens: Identification and Mechanism of Action*, Griffin C. and Shaw, Ch., Eds., Raven Press, New York, 1979, 299.
2. **Mirvish, S. S., Cordesa, A., Wellcave, L., and Shubik, P.**, Induction of mouse lung adenomas by amine or urea plus nitrite and N-nitroso compounds effects of ascorbate, gallic acid, thiocyanate and caffeine, *J. Natl. Cancer Inst.*, 55, 633, 1975.
3. **Kritchevsky, D.**, Diet and nutrition research, *Cancer*, 62, 1839, 1988.
4. **Pignatelli, B., Eriesen, M., and Walker, E. A.**, The role of phenols in catalysis of *N*-nitroso amine formation in *N-Nitroso Compounds: Analysis, Formation and Occurrence*, Walker, E. E., Griciute, L., Castegnaro, M., and Borzowsky, M., Eds., Scientific Publication No. 31, IARC, Lyon, France, 1980, 95.
5. **Scanlan, R. A.**, Formation and occurrence of nitrosoamines in food, *Cancer Res.*, (Suppl.), 2235, 1983.
6. **Voiculetz, N., Vântu, A., Stafidov, N., Niculescu-Duvăz, I., and Găldean, D.**, The protective effect of the SH-compounds upon cytotoxicity and mutagenicity of BaP and Cyclophosphamide, *Oncologia (Bucureşti)*, 1, 15, 1983.
7. **Găldean, P., Petraşincu, D., Alangiu, P., and Voiculetz, N.**, The protective effect of Thiola against the genotoxic action of benzo(a)pyrene, *Experientia (Basel)*, 42, 572, 1986.
8. **Mukhtar, H., Das, M., Khan, W. A., et al.**, Exceptional activity of tannic acid among naturally occurring plant phenols in protecting against 7,12 DMBA, BaP, 3MCh, and N-MNNU-induced skin tumorigenesis in mice, *Cancer Res.*, 48, 2361, 1988.
9. **Mukhtar, H., DelTito, B. J., Jr., Marcelo, C. L., Das, M., and Bickers, D. R.**, Ellagic acid: a potent naturally occurring inhibitor of BaP metabolism and its subsequent glucuronidation, sulfation and covalent binding to DNA in cultured BALB/c mouse keratinocytes, *Carcinogenesis*, 5(12), 1565, 1984.
10. **Stoica, G., Niculescu-Duvăz, I., and Voiculetz, N.**, Chimioprofilaxia cancerului, *Oncologia (Bucureşti)*, 81, 1987.
11. **Marnett, L. J.**, Penoxyl free radicals: potential mediators of tumor initiation and promotion, *Carcinogenesis*, 8, 1365, 1987.
12. **Safirman, C., Stoica, G., Lupu, F., Voiculetz, N., and Niculescu-Duvăz, I.**, In vitro screening of carcinogenesis inhibitors acting by inhibition of microsomal PAH activation, *Neoplasma*, 34(3), 261, 1987.
13. **Stoica, A. and Voiculetz, N.**, Rolul unor receptori în procesul de cancerizare, *Oncologia (Bucureşti)*, 3, 161, 1986.
14. **Voiculetz, N., Niculescu-Duvăz, I., Mureşan, Z., Safirman, C., and Stoica, G.**, Some molecular aspects of chemoprevention of cancer, *Oncologia (Bucureşti)*, 2, 81, 1986.
15. **Mureşan, Z., Stoica, A., Stafidov, N., and Voiculetz, N.**, Inducible high-affinity binding site for benzo(a)pyrene in cytosol from rat liver, *Neoplasma*, 34, 523, 1987.
16. **Stoica, A., Hoffman, M., and Voiculetz, N.**, High affinity binding of benzo(a)pyrene metabolites and antioxidants to the cytosolic carrier protein for benzo(a)pyrene, *Rev. Roum. Biochim.*, 25, 165, 1988.
17. **Kuszuski, Ch., Somogy, A., Nesnow, S., and Langenbach, R.**, Inhibition of BaP induced transformation of C3H/10T112 cells by Allylisopropylacetamide and Isopropylvaleramide, *Cancer Res.*, 41, 1893, 1981.
18. **Habs, H. and Habs, M.**, Effect of pretreatment with disulfiram on the toxicity and antitumor activity of 3-nitrosourea in rats, *Cancer Lett.*, 13, 63, 1981.
19. **Hacker, M. P., Erschler, W. B., Newman, R. A., and Gamelli, R. L.**, Effect of Disulfiram and Diethyldithiocarbamate on the bladder toxicity and antitumor activity of Cyclophosphamide in mice, *Cancer Res.*, 42, 4490, 1982.
20. **Anderson, M. W., Boroujerdi, M., and Wilson, A. G. E.**, Inhibition *in vivo* of the formation of adducts between metabolites of BaP and DNA by BHA, *Cancer Res.*, 41, 4309, 1981.
21. **Lam, L. K. T., Sparnins, V. L., Hochalter, J. B., and Wattenberg, L. W.**, Effects of BHA on glutathione S transferase and epoxide hydrase activities and sulphydryl levels in liver and forestomach, *Cancer Res.*, 41, 3940, 1981.
22. **DelTito, B. J., Mukhtar, H., and Bickers, D. R.**, Inhibition of epidermal metabolism and DNA binding by ellagic acid, *Biochem. Biophys. Res. Commun.*, 114, 388, 1983.
23. **Mukhtar, H., DelTito, B. J., Das, M., et al.**, Clotrimazole, an inhibitor of epidermal B(a)P metabolism and DNA binding and carcinogenicity, *Cancer Res.*, 44, 4233, 1984.
24. **Wattenberg, L. W., Lam, L. K. T., and Fladmoe, A. V.**, Inhibition of chemical-induced neoplasie by coumarins and alfa-angelica lactone, *Cancer. Res.*, 39, 1651, 1979.
25. **Dock, L., Cha, Y. N., Jernström, B., and Moldeus, P.**, Effects of BHA on BaP metabolism and DNA binding of BaP metabolites in isolated hepatocytes, *Chem. Biol. Interact.*, 41, 25, 1982.
26. **Conney, A. H.**, Induction of microsomal enzymes by foreign chemicals and carcinogens, *Cancer Res.*, 42, 4875, 1982.
27. **Huang, M. T., Johnson, E. F., Müller-Eberhardt, U., Koop, R. D., Coon, M. J., and Conney, A. H.**, Specificity of the activation and inhibition by Flavonoids of B(a)P hydroxylation by cytochrome P-450 isozymes from rabbit liver microsomes, *Br. J. Cancer*, 256, 10897, 1981.

28. **Huang, M.T., Chang, R. L., and Conney, A. H.,** Studies on the mechanisms of activation of microsomal B(a)P hydroxylation by 7,8-benzoflavone, *Fed. Proc.,* 39, 2053, 1980.
29. **Thakker, D. R., Levin, W., Bueding, M., Yagi, H., et al.,** Species specific enhancement of 7,8-benzoflavone of hepatic microsomal metabolism of BaP 9,10-dihydrodiol to bay-region diol epoxides, *Cancer Res.,* 41, 1389, 1981.
30. **Ullrich, V.,** Cytochrome P-450 and biological hydroxylation reaction, *Top. Curr. Chem.,* 83, 67, 1979.
31. **Nesuow, S.,** A preliminary structure activity of the mixed function oxidase inhibitor 7,8-benzoflavone, *J. Med. Chem.,* 22, 1244, 1979.
32. **Nesuow, S. and Bengman, H.,** Metabolism of alfa naftoflavone by rat liver microsomes, *Cancer Res.,* 41, 2621, 1981.
33. **Preuss-Schwartz, D. and Baird, W.,** Benzo(a)pyrene: DNA adduct formation in early passage Wistar rat embryo-cell cultures: evidence for multiple pathways of activation of BaP, *Cancer Res.,* 46, 545, 1986.
34. **Yang, C. S., Sydor, W., Jr., and Lewis, K. F.,** Effects of BHA on the metabolism of BaP by lung microsomes, *Cancer Res.,* 44, 134, 1984.
35. **Voiculetz, N. and Niculescu-Duvăz, I.,** Molecular basis of chemical carcinogenesis (Rom.), Scientific and Encyclopaedic Publishing House, Bucharest, Romania, in press.
36. **Wood, A. W., Levin, W., Lu A., et al.,** Metabolism of B(a)P and B(a)P derivatives to mutagenic products by highly purified hepatic microsomal enzymes, *J. Biol. Chem.,* 251, 4882, 1976.
37. **Lam, L. K., Fladmoe, A. V., Hochalter, J. B., and Wattenberg, L. W.,** Short time interval effects of BHA on the metabolism of BaP, *Cancer Res.,* 40, 2824, 1980.
38. **Wattenberg, L. W.,** Inhibition of neoplasia by minor dietary constituents, *Cancer Res.,* 43, 2448, 1983.
39. **Miller, E. C.,** Some current perspectives on chemical carcinogenesis in human and experimental animals, *Cancer Res.,* 38, 1479, 1978.
40. **Niculescu-Duvăz, I., Simon, Z., and Voiculetz, N.,** Carcinogenesis inhibitory properties of retinoids: a QSAR-MTD analysis, in *Biochemistry of Natural and Synthetic Retinoids,* Dawson, M. and Okamura, J., Eds., CRC Press, Boca Raton, FL, 1990, 546.
41. **Wang, S. Y., La Rosa, G. J., and Gudar, L. J.,** Molecular cloning of gene sequences transcriptionally regulated by retinoic acid and dibutyryl AMP in cultured mouse teratocarcinoma cells, *Der. Biol.,* 107, 75, 1985.
42. **Craic, R. W., Manc, R. J., Hromchak, A., et al.,** Decline of c-*myb* expression in human myeloblastic leukemia (ML-1) cells induced to differentiate with daunomcin, conditioned medium, or retinoic acid, *Proc. Am. Assoc. Cancer Res.,* 25, 64, 1984.
43. **Blakeslee, J. R., Yamamoto, N., and Hinuma, Y.,** Human T-cell leukemia virus I induction by 5-Iodo-2-deoxiuridine and N-methyl-N′-nitro-N-nitrosoguanidine: inhibition by retinoids, L-ascorbic acid and α-tocopherol, *Cancer Res.,* 45, 3471, 1985.
44. **Martin, V. C.,** Practitioner's perspective of the role of quantitative structure-activity analysis in medicinal chemistry, *J. Med. Chem.,* 24, 229, 1981.
45. **Leo, A., Panthananickal, A., Hansch, C., Theiss, J., Schimkin, M., and Andrews, A. W.,** A comparison of mutagenic and carcinogenic activities of aniline mustards, *J. Med. Chem.,* 24, 859, 1981.
46. **Lewis, D. P. Y.,** Molecular orbital calculations on tumor inhibitory aniline mustards: QSARs, *Xenobiotica,* 19, 243, 1989.
47. **Venger, B. H., Hansch, C., Hatheway, G., and Amrein, Y. U.,** Ames test of 1-(X-Phenyl)-3,3-dialkyltriazenes. A quantitative structure-activity study, *J. Med. Chem.,* 22, 473, 1979.
48. **Hansch, C., Venger, B. H., and Panthananikal, A.,** Mutagenicity of substituted (o-phenyldeamine)platinum dichlorides in the Ames test. A quantitative structure-activity study, *J. Med. Chem.,* 23, 459, 1980.
49. **Beard, A. R., Drew, M. G. B., Hilgard, P., Hudson, B. D., Mann, J., Neidle, S., and Wong, L. F. T.,** Podophyllotoxin analogues: synthesis and computer modelling investigation of structure-activity relationships, *Anticancer Drug Design,* 2, 247, 1987.
50. **Adrisenssens, P. I., White, C., and Anderson, M.,** Dose response relationship for binding of BaP metabolites to DNA treated mice, *Cancer Res.,* 43, 3712, 1983.
51. **Ioannou, Y. M., Wilson, A. G. E., and Anderson, M. W.,** Effect of BHA alpha-angelica lactone and beta-naphthflavone on BaP: DNA adduct formation *in vivo* in the forestomach, lung and liver of mice, *Cancer Res.,* 42, 1199, 1982.
52. **Slaga, T. J. and Bracken, W. M.,** The effects of antioxidants on skin tumor initiation and arylhydrocarbon hydroxylase, *Cancer Res.,* 37, 1631, 1977.
53. **Wattenberg, L. W., Jerina, D. M., Lam, L. K. T., et al.,** Neoplastic effects of oral administration of ± *trans* 7,8-dehydroxy-7,8-dihydrobenzo(a)pyrene and their inhibition by butylated hydroxyanisole, *J. Natl. Cancer Inst.,* 62, 1103, 1971.
54. **Wattenberg, L. W.,** Inhibition of carcinogenic and toxic effects of polycyclic hydrocarbons by phenolic antioxidants and ethoxyquin, *J. Natl. Cancer Inst.,* 48, 1425, 1972.

55. **Wattenberg, L. W., Coccia, J. B., and Lam, L. K. T.,** Inhibitory effects of phenolic compounds in benzo(a)pyrene induced neoplasia, *Cancer Res.,* 40, 2820, 1980.
56. **Maeura, Y. and Williams, G. M.,** Dose dependent reduction of N_2-fluorenyl-acetamide induced liver cancer and enhancement of bladder cancer by BHT, *Cancer Res.,* 44, 1604, 1984.
57. **Ulland, B. M., Weiberger, J. M., Yamamoto, R. S., et al.,** Antioxidants and carcinogenesis; butylated hydroxytoluene but not diphenyl-p-phenyl-endiamine, inhibits cancer induction by N-2 fluorenylacetamide and by N-hydroxy-N-2 fluorenylacetamide, *Food Cosmet. Toxicol.,* 11, 201, 1973.
58. **Wattenberg, L. W., Bouchent, P., Destafney, C., and Coccis, J. M.,** Effect of p-methoxyphenol and diet on carcinogen induced neoplasia of the mouse forestomach, *Cancer Res.,* 43, 4747, 1983.
59. **Leo, A., Hansch, C., and Elkins, P.,** The hydrophobic constants, *Chem., Rev.,* 71, 529, 1971.
60. **McCoy, P. B., King, M., Rikans, L. E., et al.,** Interactions between dietary fats and antioxidants on DMBA induced mammary carcinomas and 2 AAF-induced hyperplastic nodules and hepatomas, *J. Environ. Pathol. Toxicol.,* 3, 451, 1980.
61. **Ioannou, Y. M., Wilson, A. G. E., and Anderson, M. V.,** Effect of butylated hydroxyanisole on the *in vivo* and *in vitro* metabolism and DNA binding of benzo(a)pyrene in the A/HeJ mouse, *Carcinogenesis,* 3, 739, 1982.
62. **Batzinger, R. P., Ou, S. Y. L., and Bueding, E.,** Antimutagenic effect of 2(3) *tert*-butyl-4 hydroxyanisole and of antimocrobial agents, *Cancer Res.,* 38, 4478, 1978.
63. **Lam, L. K. and Wattenberg, L. W.,** Effect of butylated hydroxyanisole on the metabolism of benzo(a)pyrene by mouse liver microsomes, *J. Natl. Cancer, Inst.,* 58, 413, 1977.
64. **Speer, J. L. and Wattenberg, L. W.,** Alteration in microsomal metabolism of benzo(a)pyrene in mice fed by butylated hydroxyanisole, *J. Natl. Cancer Inst.,* 55, 469, 1975.
65. **Benson, A. M., Betsinger, R. P., Ou, S. Y. L., et al.,** Elevation of hepatic glutathione-S-transferase activities and protection against metabolites of benzo(a)pyrene by dietary antioxidants, *Cancer Res.,* 38, 4486, 1978.
66. **Talalay, P., Batzinger, R. P., Benson, A. M., et al.,** Biochemical studies in the mechanisms by which dietary antioxidants suppress mutagenic activity, *Adv. Enzyme Regul.,* 17, 23, 1979.
67. **Benson, A. M., Cha, Y. N., Bueding, N., et al.,** Elevation of extrahepatic glutathione-S-transferase and epoxide hydratase activities by 2(3)-*tert*-butyl-4 hydroxyanisole, *Cancer Res.,* 39, 2971, 1979.
68. **Chan, J. T. and Black, H. S.,** The mutagenic effect of dietary antioxidants and chemically induced carcinogenesis, *Experientia,* 34, 110, 1978.
69. **Kozumbo, W. J., Seed, J. L., and Kensler, T. W.,** Inhibition by BHA and other antioxidants of epidermal ornitine decarboxylase activity induced by TPA, *Cancer Res.,* 43, 2555, 1983.
70. **Trac, A. and Behna, I.,** Reactivity of free and coordinated radicals in biology and chemical carcinogenesis. II. Electron transfer from 3,4-benzopyrene to molecular oxygen and to peroxides, and interpretation of ESR signals of the intermediate radicals of oxidation, *Neoplasma,* 30, 197, 1983.
71. **Copeland, P. S.,** Free radicals in promotion. A chemical pathology study section, *Cancer Res.,* 43, 5631, 1983.
72. **Niculescu-Duvăz, I., Ionescu, A., Simon, Z., and Voiculetz, N.,** Relations quantitatives structure—oetirité dans deu classes d'inhibiteurs de la cancerogenése chimique, *Rev. Roum. Physiol.,* 22, 135, 1985.
73. **Niculescu-Duvăz, I., Simon, Z., Tiriac, S., et al.,** QSAR applications in chemical carcinogenesis, III QSAR analysis of some phenolic antioxidants, *Neoplasma,* 32, 695, 1985.
74. **Hansch, C., Leo, A., Unger, S. H., et al.,** Aromatic substituent constants for structure-activity correlations, *J. Med. Chem.,* 16, 1207, 1973.
75. **Pliev, T.,** Spectroscopic studies of the thermodynamic dissociation constants of alkyl phenols, *Dokl. A.N. SSSR,* 69, 113, 1969.
76. **Mohokuma, K., Kato, H., and Fukin, K.,** The electronic structures and antioxidizing activities of substituted phenols, *Bull. Chem., Soc. Jpn.,* 36, 541, 1963.
77. **Mracec, M.,** unpublished data.
78. **Niculescu-Duvăz, I., Safirman, C., Stoica, G., Lupu, F., Arnăutu, M., and Voiculetz, N.,** Is the antioxidant character required for chemical carcinogenesis inhibition?, *Oncologia (Bucharest),* 26, 109, 1987.
79. **Niculescu-Duvăz, I., Stoica, G., Lupu, F., Arnăutu, M., and Voiculetz, N.,** Mechanisms of carcinogenesis inhibition. II. The aminophenols and their oxidation products, *Neoplasma,* 35, 520, 1988.
80. **Niculescu-Duvăz, I. and Lupu, F.,** personal communication.
81. **Loew, G. H. and Goldblum, A.,** Metabolic activation and toxicity of acetaminophen and related analogs, *Mol. Pharmacol.,* 27, 375, 1985.
82. **Niculescu-Duvăz, I., Simon, Z., and Voiculetz, N.,** QSAR application in chemical carcinogenesis. II. QSAR analysis of a class of carcinogenesis inhibitors: retinoids, *Carcinogenesis,* 6 (4), 479, 1985.
83. **Minar, D. J. and Kissinger, P. T.,** Evidence for the involvement of N-acetyl-p-quinoneimine in acetaminophen metabolism, *Biochem. Pharmacol.,* 28, 3285, 1979.

84. **Hinson, J. A., Monks, T. J., and Hong, M.,** 3-(Glutathion-S-yl) acetaminophen. A biliary metabolite of acetaminophen, *Drug Metab. Dispos.,* 10, 47, 1982.

85. **Kosower, N. S. and Kosower, E. M.,** The glutathione status of cells, *Int. Rev. Cytol.,* 54, 109, 1978.

86. **Hayward, N. K. and Lavin, M. F.,** P-aminophenol-induced DNA damage and cytotoxicity enhanced by autooxidation, *Life Sci.,* 36, 2039, 1985.

87. **Crouk, G. and Makin, M.,** Oxidations of aromatic amines by superoxide ion, *Aust. J. Chem.,* 37, 845, 1984.

88. **Trukhin, M. F. and Trukhin, M. M.,** Free radicals of developens. 2. Free radical of *p*-aminophenols, *J. Signalaufzeichnungsmaterialen,* 6, 363, 1978.

89. **Williams, H. P. J., et al.,** Free radicals studied by Raman spectroscopy: photo-chemically generated p-substituted aniline cation radicals, *J. Raman Spectrosc.* 10, 169, 1981.

90. **Rosen, G. M., Rauckman, E. J., Ellington, S. P., et al.,** Reduction and glutathione conjugation reactions of N-acetyl-p-benzoquinoneimine and two dimethylated analogues, *Mol. Pharmacol.,* 25, 151, 1984.

91. **Tripathe, G. N. R. and Schuler, R. H.,** Resonance Raman studies of radiolytically produced p-aminophenoxyl radical, *J. Phys. Chem.,* 88, 1706, 1984.

92. **Josephy, P. D., Eling, T. E., and Mason, R. P.,** Oxidation of p-aminophenol catalysed by horseradish peroxidase and prostaglandin synthetase, *Mol. Pharmacol.,* 23, 461, 1983.

93. **Lorentzen, R. J., Leszko, S. A., McDonald, K., Ts'o, P. O. P.,** Toxicity of metabolic benzo(a)pyrene diones to cultured cells and the dependence upon molecular O_2, *Cancer Res.,* 39, 3194, 1979.

94. **Cummings, S. W., Ansani, G. A. S., Guengerich, F. P., et al.,** Metabolism of 3 tert butyl-4-hydroxyanisole by microsomal fractions and isolated rat hepatocytes, *Cancer Res.,* 45, 5617, 1985.

95. **Glebove, H. V., Vishnyebove, T. P., and Golubeva, I. A.,** Synthesis and antioxidative activity of products of the transformation of N, N bis (3,5 di-*tert*-butyl-4 hydroxyphenyl amine). I. *Neftekhimiya,* 24, 90, 1984.

96. **Niculescu-Duvăz, I. and Stoica, G.,** personal communication.

97. **Slaga, T. L., Fischer, S. M., Weeks, C. E., et al.,** Specificity and mechanism(s) of promoter inhibitors in multistage promotion, in *Carcinogenesis — A Comprehensive Survey,* Vol. 7, Hecker, E., Puseny, N., Kurz, M., and Thielman, H., Eds., Raven Press, New York, 1982, 19.

98. **Bollag, W.,** Retinoids and cancer, *Cancer Chem. Pharmacol.,* 3, 207, 1979.

99. **Sporn, M. B. and Newton, D. L.,** Chemoprevention of cancer with retinoids, *Fed. Proc.,* 38, 2538, 1979.

100. **Sporn, M. B. and Roberts, A. B.,** Role of retinoids in differentiation and carcinogenesis, *Cancer Res.,* 43, 3034, 1983.

101. **Thein, R. and Lotan, R.,** Sensitivity of human osteosarcoma and chondrosarcoma cells to retinoic acid, *Cancer Res.,* 42, 4471, 1982.

102. **Sherman, M. I.,** How do retinoids promote differentiation? in *Retinoids and Cell Differentiation,* Sherman, M. I., Ed., CRC Press, Boca Raton, FL, 1987, 161.

103. **Moon, R. C., McCormick, D. L., and Mehta, R. G.,** Inhibition of carcinogenesis by retinoids, *Cancer Res. (Suppl.),* 43, 1983, 2469.

104. **Meyskens, F., Gilmantin, E., Alberts, D. S., et al.,** Activity of Isotretinoin against squamous cell cancer and preneoplastic lesions, *Cancer Treat. Rep.,* 66, 1315, 1982.

105. **Goodman, G. E., Einsphar, J. G., Alberts, D. S., et al.,** Pharmacokinetics of 13-*cis*-retinoic in patients with advanced cancer, *Cancer Res.,* 42, 2087, 1982.

106. **Bentman, J. S.,** Structure-activity relationships among various retinoids and their ability to inhibit neoplastic transformation and increase cell adhesion in the C_3H-10 T1/2 Cl 8 cell line, *Cancer Res.,* 40, 3141, 1980.

107. **Dawson, M. I., Hobbs, P. D., Derdzinski, K., et al.,** Conformationally restricted retinoids, *J. Med. Chem.,* 27, 1516, 1984.

108. **Dawson, M. I., Hobbs, P. D., Chan, R. L., et al.,** Aromatic retinoic acid analogues, synthesis and pharmacological activity, *J. Med. Chem.,* 24, 583, 1981.

109. **Dawson, M. I., Hobbs, P. D., Chan, R. L., et al.,** Retinoic acid analogues with ring analogues with ring modification, Synthesis and pharmacological activity, *J. Med. Chem.,* 24, 1214, 1981.

110. **Mihalaş, G. I., Vlad, I., and Simon, Z.,** Trigger model for regulation of gene activity based upon interactions in the hormonal receptor protein, *J. Theor. Biol.,* 1987.

111. **Sporn, M. B., Newton, D. L., Roberts, A. B., et al.,** Retinoids suppression of the effects of polypeptide transforming factors — a new molecular approach to chemoprevention of cancer, in *Molecular Action and Targets for Cancer Chemotherapeutic Agents,* Sartorelli, A. C., Lazo, J. S., and Bertino, J. R., Eds., Academic Press, New York, 1981, 547.

112. **Jetten, A. M.,** Modulation of cells growth by retinoids and their possible mechanisms of action, *Fed. Proc.,* 43, 134, 1984.

113. **Strickland, S., Breitman, T. R., Frickel, F., Nürenbach, A., Hädiche, E., and Sporn, M. B.** Structure-activity relationships of a new series of retinoidal benzoic acid derivatives as measured by induction of differentiation of murine F 9 teratocarcinoma cells and human HL60 promyelocytic leukemia cells, *Cancer Res.,* 43, 5268, 1983.

114. **Chytil, F. and Ong, D. B.,** Cellular retinol and retinoic acid binding proteins in vitamin A action, *Fed. Proc.,* 38, 2510, 1979.
115. **Melita, R. G., Cerny, W. L., and Moon, R. C.,** Distribution of retinoic and binding proteins in normal and neoplastic tissues, *Cancer Res.,* 40, 47, 1980.
116. **Seou, B. K. and Pressman, D.,** Retinol-binding protein in the urine of cancer patients, *Cancer Res.,* 39, 4423, 1979.
117. **Omori, M. and Chytil, F.,** Mechanism of vitamin A action, *J. Biol. Chem.,* 257, 14370, 1982.
118. **Trown, P. W., Pallenoui, A. V., Bohoslawec, O., et al.,** Relationships between binding affinities to cellular retinoic acid binding protein and *in vivo* and *in vitro* properties of 18 retinoids, *Cancer Res.,* 40, 212, 1980.
119. **Dover, D. and Koeffler, H. P.,** Inhibition of the clonal growth of human myeloid leukemia cells, *J. Clin. Invest.,* 69, 277, 1982.
120. **Libby, P. R. and Bertram, J. S.,** Lack of intracellular retinoid-binding protein in a retinol sensitive cell line, *Carcinogenesis,* 3, 481, 1982.
121. **Newton, D. L., Henderson, W. R., and Sporn, M. B.,** Structure-activity relationships of retinoids in hamster tracheal organ culture, *Cancer Res.,* 40, 3413, 1980.
122. **Lotan, R., Neuman, G., and Lotan, D.,** Relationships among retinoid structure, inhibition of growth and cellular retinoic acid-binding protein in cultured S_{91} melanoma cells, *Cancer Res.,* 40, 1097, 1980.
123. **Sporn, M. B., Newton, D. L., Smith, J. M., Acton, N., Jacobson, A., and Brossi, A.,** Retinoids and cancer prevention: the importance of the terminal group of the retinoid molecule in modifying activity and toxicity, in *Carcinogens: Identification and Mechanism of Action,* Griffin, Cl. and Shaw, Ch. R., Eds., Raven Press, New York, 1979, 441.
124. **Frolik, C. A., Dant, L. L., and Sporn, M. B.,** Metabolism of all-*trans*-retinyl acetate to retinoic acid in hamster tracheal organ culture, *Biochem. Biophys. Acta,* 663, 329, 1981.

INDEX